FINDING WHAT WORKS IN HEALTH CARE

STANDARDS FOR SYSTEMATIC REVIEWS

Committee on Standards for Systematic
Reviews of Comparative Effectiveness Research

Board on Health Care Services

Jill Eden, Laura Levit, Alfred Berg, and Sally Morton, *Editors*

INSTITUTE OF MEDICINE
OF THE NATIONAL ACADEMIES

THE NATIONAL ACADEMIES PRESS
Washington, D.C.
www.nap.edu

THE NATIONAL ACADEMIES PRESS   500 Fifth Street, N.W.   Washington, DC 20001

NOTICE: The project that is the subject of this report was approved by the Governing Board of the National Research Council, whose members are drawn from the councils of the National Academy of Sciences, the National Academy of Engineering, and the Institute of Medicine. The members of the committee responsible for the report were chosen for their special competences and with regard for appropriate balance.

This study was supported by Contract No. HHSP23320042509X1 between the National Academy of Sciences and the Department of Health and Human Services. Any opinions, findings, conclusions, or recommendations expressed in this publication are those of the author(s) and do not necessarily reflect the view of the organizations or agencies that provided support for this project.

Library of Congress Cataloging-in-Publication Data

Institute of Medicine (U.S.). Committee on Standards for Systematic Reviews of Comparative Effectiveness Research.
   Finding what works in health care : standards for systematic reviews / Committee on Standards for Systematic Reviews of Comparative Effectiveness Research, Board on Health Care Services, Institute of Medicine of the National Academies ; Jill Eden ... [et al.], editors.
       p. ; cm.
   Includes bibliographical references.
   ISBN 978-0-309-16425-2 (pbk.) — ISBN 978-0-309-16426-9 (pdf) 1. Medical care—Standards—United States. 2. Medical care—United States—Quality control. I. Eden, Jill. II. Title.
   [DNLM: 1. Comparative Effectiveness Research—standards—United States. 2. Outcome and Process Assessment (Health Care)—United States. W 84.3]
   RA399.A3I565 2011
   610.28'9—dc23
                                        2011017455

Additional copies of this report are available from the National Academies Press, 500 Fifth Street, N.W., Lockbox 285, Washington, DC 20055; (800) 624-6242 or (202) 334-3313 (in the Washington metropolitan area); Internet, http://www.nap.edu.

For more information about the Institute of Medicine, visit the IOM home page at: **www.iom.edu.**

Suggested citation: IOM (Institute of Medicine). 2011. *Finding What Works in Health Care: Standards for Systematic Reviews.* Washington, DC: The National Academies Press.

"Knowing is not enough; we must apply.
Willing is not enough; we must do."
—Goethe

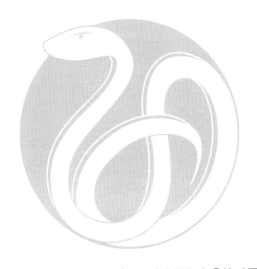

INSTITUTE OF MEDICINE
OF THE NATIONAL ACADEMIES

Advising the Nation. Improving Health.

THE NATIONAL ACADEMIES
Advisers to the Nation on Science, Engineering, and Medicine

The **National Academy of Sciences** is a private, nonprofit, self-perpetuating society of distinguished scholars engaged in scientific and engineering research, dedicated to the furtherance of science and technology and to their use for the general welfare. Upon the authority of the charter granted to it by the Congress in 1863, the Academy has a mandate that requires it to advise the federal government on scientific and technical matters. Dr. Ralph J. Cicerone is president of the National Academy of Sciences.

The **National Academy of Engineering** was established in 1964, under the charter of the National Academy of Sciences, as a parallel organization of outstanding engineers. It is autonomous in its administration and in the selection of its members, sharing with the National Academy of Sciences the responsibility for advising the federal government. The National Academy of Engineering also sponsors engineering programs aimed at meeting national needs, encourages education and research, and recognizes the superior achievements of engineers. Dr. Charles M. Vest is president of the National Academy of Engineering.

The **Institute of Medicine** was established in 1970 by the National Academy of Sciences to secure the services of eminent members of appropriate professions in the examination of policy matters pertaining to the health of the public. The Institute acts under the responsibility given to the National Academy of Sciences by its congressional charter to be an adviser to the federal government and, upon its own initiative, to identify issues of medical care, research, and education. Dr. Harvey V. Fineberg is president of the Institute of Medicine.

The **National Research Council** was organized by the National Academy of Sciences in 1916 to associate the broad community of science and technology with the Academy's purposes of furthering knowledge and advising the federal government. Functioning in accordance with general policies determined by the Academy, the Council has become the principal operating agency of both the National Academy of Sciences and the National Academy of Engineering in providing services to the government, the public, and the scientific and engineering communities. The Council is administered jointly by both Academies and the Institute of Medicine. Dr. Ralph J. Cicerone and Dr. Charles M. Vest are chair and vice chair, respectively, of the National Research Council.

www.national-academies.org

HAROLD C. SOX, Editor Emeritus, *Annals of Internal Medicine,*
American College of Physicians of Internal Medicine, Hanover, NH
PAUL WALLACE, Medical Director, The Permanente Federation, Kaiser
Permanente, Oakland, CA

Study Staff

JILL EDEN, Study Director
LAURA LEVIT, Program Officer
LEA BINDER, Research Associate (through May 2010)
MAI LE, Research Assistant (starting September 2010)
ALLISON McFALL, Senior Program Assistant (through August 2010)
JILLIAN LAFFREY, Senior Program Assistant (starting July 2010)
ROGER HERDMAN, Director, Board on Health Care Services

Consultants

JULIA KREIS, Harkness/Bosch Fellow in Health Care Policy and
Practice, Johns Hopkins Bloomberg School of Public Health,
Baltimore, MD
DAVID MOHER, Senior Scientist, Ottawa Hospital Research Institute
(OHRI), Ottawa, Ontario, Canada
ALEXANDER TSERTSVADZE, Ottawa Hospital Research Institute
(OHRI), Ottawa, Ontario, Canada
SALLY HOPEWELL, National Institute for Health Research, U.K.
Cochrane Centre, Oxford, United Kingdom
BRYAN LUCE, Senior Vice President, Science Policy, United BioSource
Corporation, Chevy Chase, MD
RACHAEL FLEURENCE, Senior Research Scientist, United BioSource
Corporation, Chevy Chase, MD

Reviewers

This report has been reviewed in draft form by individuals chosen for their diverse perspectives and technical expertise, in accordance with procedures approved by the National Research Council's Report Review Committee. The purpose of this independent review is to provide candid and critical comments that will assist the institution in making its published report as sound as possible and to ensure that the report meets institutional standards for objectivity, evidence, and responsiveness to the study charge. The review comments and draft manuscript remain confidential to protect the integrity of the deliberative process. We wish to thank the following individuals for their review of this report:

NAOMI ARONSON, Executive Director, Blue Cross and Blue Shield Association, Technology Evaluation Center

VIVIAN COATES, Vice President, Information Services and Technology Assessment, ECRI Institute

JOHN P. A. IOANNIDIS, C.F. Rehnborg Professor in Disease Prevention, Professor of Medicine, and Director, Stanford Prevention Research Center, Stanford University

ERIC B. LARSON, Executive Director, Group Health Research Institute

JOSEPH LAU, Director, Tufts Evidence-based Practice Center, Tufts Medical Center

ART LEVIN, Director, Center for Medical Consumers
ALVIN I. MUSHLIN, Professor and Chairman, Department of Public Health, Weill Medical College, Cornell University
PAUL SHEKELLE, Director, Southern California Evidence-Based Practice Center, The RAND Corporation
RICHARD N. SHIFFMAN, Associate Director, Center for Medical Informatics, Yale School of Medicine
LESLEY STEWART, Director, Centre for Reviews and Dissemination, University of York

Although the reviewers listed above have provided many constructive comments and suggestions, they were not asked to endorse the conclusions or recommendations nor did they see the final draft of the report before its release. The review of this report was overseen by **ENRIQUETA C. BOND** of the Burroughs Wellcome Fund, and **MARK R. CULLEN** of Stanford University. Appointed by the National Research Council and the Institute of Medicine, they were responsible for making certain that an independent examination of this report was carried out in accordance with institutional procedures and that all review comments were carefully considered. Responsibility for the final content of this report rests entirely with the authoring committee and the institution.

Foreword

Knowing what works in health care is of highest importance for patients, healthcare providers, and other decision makers. The most reliable way to identify benefits and harms associated with various treatment options is a systematic review of comparative effectiveness research. Increasingly recognized for their importance, systematic reviews are now being sponsored and conducted by a number of organizations across the United States. When conducted well, a systematic review identifies, appraises, and synthesizes the available body of evidence for a specific clinical question. However, not all of these reviews meet the appropriate standards of quality and methodology. At the request of the U.S. Congress, the Institute of Medicine (IOM) undertook this study to develop a set of standards for conducting systematic reviews of comparative effectiveness research.

The report will have direct implications for implementation of the *Patient Protection and Affordable Care Act of 2010*. This law established the first nonprofit, public–private Patient-Centered Outcomes Research Institute (PCORI). PCORI will be responsible for setting methodological standards for clinical effectiveness research, including systematic reviews of research findings. I hope this study will support PCORI's development of standards to ensure that systematic reviews meet a minimum level of objectivity, transparency, and scientific rigor. The IOM study should also help to inform other public sponsors of systematic reviews of comparative effectiveness research.

To conduct this study, the Institute of Medicine convened a highly qualified committee with diverse backgrounds, ably led by Alfred Berg, chair, and Sally Morton, vice chair. The committee was assisted by dedicated IOM staff led by Jill Eden. This report draws on available evidence, review of expert guidance, and careful consideration of alternative standards according to specified criteria. While this report presents an initial list of standards for improving the quality of publicly funded systematic reviews, it also calls for continued investment in methodological research to identify better practices for future reviews. A companion report establishes standards for developing clinical practice guidelines. I hope these documents will help guide a robust systematic review enterprise for health in the United States.

Harvey V. Fineberg, M.D., Ph.D.
President, Institute of Medicine
February 2011

Preface

Page through any volume of a medical journal from the 1970s and read a clinical review. The authors are likely to be recognized as experts in the field, and the introduction will often open with "we reviewed the world's medical literature," moving on to reach clinical conclusions based as much on the experience and opinions of the authors as on the published evidence. Systematic literature searches, critical appraisal, quantitative meta-analysis, and documented pathways linking the evidence to reaching clinical conclusions were virtually unknown. Today's explicit, scientifically rigorous, transparent, and publicly accountable systematic reviews (SRs) and clinical practice guidelines (CPGs) are the barely recognizable heirs to that earlier convention for giving clinical advice.

Enormous progress has been made by a large and growing international community of clinicians, methodologists, statisticians, and other stakeholders in developing SRs and CPGs, yet problems remain. There are many competing systems for evaluating and synthesizing evidence, and there are no internationally agreed-upon standards for how to conduct an SR or create a CPG. In the United States, the decades-old interest in SRs and CPGs among public and private agencies is receiving a boost from the highlighting of the importance of both in debates about healthcare reform; a specific provision in the *Medicare Improvements for Patients and Providers Act of 2008* brought two Institute of Medicine (IOM) committees into being, aimed at setting standards for SRs and CPGs. Furthermore, in the United States there is enormous interest in and high expectations for the newly created Patient-Centered Outcomes Research Institute, whose authorizing legislation specifically names SRs and CPGs as important components in developing a national program of comparative effectiveness research.

As both SR and CPG reports indicate, the term "standard" is problematic. Our two committees found a sparse evidence base that directly evaluates alternative approaches to SRs and CPGs. The SR committee thus relied on available literature, expert guidance from organizations engaged in SRs, and its own criteria and internal discussions to propose a set of standards, recognizing that any such recommendations must be considered provisional pending further development of the evidence. Collectively the standards set a high bar that will be difficult to achieve for many SRs, yet the evidence and experience are not reassuring that it is safe to cut corners if resources are limited. The standards will be especially valuable for SRs of high-stakes clinical questions with broad population impact, where the use of public funds to get the right answer justifies careful attention to the rigor with which the SR is conducted. The best practices collected in this report should be thoughtfully considered by anyone conducting an SR. In the end the most important standard is to be transparent in reporting what was done and why. Importantly, the committee concludes with recommendations that the United States invest in a program to improve both the science of SRs (with attention to both scientific rigor and feasibility/cost) and the environment that supports them, including a process to update standards as the evidence improves.

Finally, one of the most professionally satisfying benefits of leading an IOM committee is the opportunity to work with committee members with an amazing breadth and depth of experience, and IOM staff whose anticipation and completion of the next steps always appears effortless. We are deeply grateful that this committee and staff have again demonstrated the process at its best.

In conclusion, the committee believes we are at an important juncture in the development of SRs and CPGs, and that timely investment in both will produce an excellent return in improving health care and patient outcomes. We hope our recommended standards will serve as a useful milestone as the United States joins international partners to advance the science and improve the environment for SRs and CPGs.

Alfred O. Berg, *Chair*
Sally C. Morton, *Vice Chair*
Committee on Standards for Systematic
Reviews of Comparative Effectiveness Research

Acknowledgments

The committee and staff are indebted to a number of individuals and organizations for their contributions to this report. The following individuals provided testimony to the committee:

Naomi Aronson, *Executive Director, Technology Evaluation Center, Blue Cross and Blue Shield Association*

Kalipso Chalkidou, *Director, NICE International, National Institute for Health and Clinical Excellence*

Yngve Falck-Ytter, *Assistant Professor of Medicine, Case Western Reserve University; Director of Hepatology, VA Medical Center, Cleveland*

Rebekah Gee, *Assistant Professor of Clinical Medicine, Department of Obstetrics and Gynecology, Tulane University, American College of Obstetricians and Gynecologists*

Louis B. Jacques, *Director, Coverage & Analysis Group, Office of Clinical Standards & Quality, Centers for Medicare & Medicaid Services*

Sandra Zelman Lewis, *Assistant Vice President, Health & Science Policy, American College of Chest Physicians*

Virginia Moyer, *Section Head, Academic General Pediatrics, Baylor College of Medicine, American Academy of Pediatrics*

Edmund Pezalla, *National Medical Director and Chief Clinical Officer, Aetna Pharmacy Management*

Alan Rosenberg, *Vice President of Technology Assessment, Wellpoint Health Networks*
Carol Sakala, *Director of Programs, Childbirth Connection*
Gail Shearer, *Former Director, Consumer Reports Best Buy Drugs, and Former Director, Health Policy Analysis, Consumers Union*
David Shern, *President and CEO, Mental Health America*
David B. Wilson, *Crime and Justice Group Cochair, Steering Committee, The Campbell Collaboration*

We also extend special thanks to the following individuals who were essential sources of information, generously giving their time and knowledge to further the committee's efforts:

Stephanie Chang, *EPC Program Director, AHRQ*
Julian Higgins, *Senior Statistician, MRC Biostatistics Unit, Institute of Public Health, University of Cambridge*
Alison Little, *Medical Director, Drug Effectiveness Review Project*
Rose Relevo, *Research Librarian, AHRQ Scientific Resource Center*
Karen M. Schoelles, *Director, ECRI Institute Evidence-based Practice Center*
Lesley Stewart, *Director, Centre for Reviews and Dissemination*

Funding for this study was provided by the Agency for Healthcare Research and Quality (AHRQ). The committee appreciates the opportunity and support extended by AHRQ for the development of this report.
Finally, many within the Institute of Medicine were helpful to the study staff. We especially would like to thank the staff of the *Clinical Practice Guidelines We Can Trust* report for their collaborative spirit: Robin Graham, Michelle Mancher, and Dianne Wolman. Additionally, the staff would like to thank Clyde Behney, Michelle O. Crosby-Nagy, Greta Gorman, Cheryl Levey, William McLeod, Abbey Meltzer, Vilija Teel, and Lauren Tobias

Contents

APPENDIXES

Boxes, Figures, and Tables

Chapter 2

Chapter 3

Chapter 4

Chapter 5

Summary[1]

Healthcare decision makers in search of the best evidence to inform clinical decisions have come to rely on systematic reviews (SRs) of comparative effectiveness research (CER) to learn what is known and not known about the potential benefits and harms of alternative drugs, devices, and other healthcare services. An SR is a scientific investigation that focuses on a specific question and uses explicit, prespecified scientific methods to identify, select, assess, and summarize the findings of similar but separate studies. It may include a quantitative synthesis (meta-analysis), depending on the available data. Although the importance of SRs is increasingly appreciated, the quality of published SRs is variable and often poor. In many cases, the reader is unable to judge the quality of an SR because the methods are poorly documented, and even if methods are described, they may be used inappropriately, for example, in meta-analyses. Many reviews fail to assess the quality of the underlying research and also neglect to report funding sources. A plethora of conflicting approaches to evidence hierarchies and grading schemes for bodies of evidence is a further source of confusion.

In the 2008 report, *Knowing What Works in Health Care: A Roadmap for the Nation*, the Institute of Medicine (IOM) recommended that methodological standards be developed for both SRs and clini-

---

[1]This summary does not include references. Citations for the findings presected in the Summary appear in the subsequent chapters.

cal practice guidelines (CPGs). The report was followed by a congressional mandate in the *Medicare Improvements for Patients and Providers Act of 2008* for two follow-up IOM studies: one to develop standards for conducting SRs, and the other to develop standards for CPGs. This is the report of the IOM Committee on Standards for Systematic Reviews of Comparative Effectiveness Research. A companion report by the IOM Committee on Standards for Developing Trustworthy Clinical Practice Guidelines is being released in conjunction with this report.

The charge to this IOM committee was twofold: first, to assess potential methodological standards that would assure objective, transparent, and scientifically valid SRs of CER and, second, to recommend a set of methodological standards for developing and reporting such SRs (Box S-1). The boundaries of this study were defined in part by the work of the companion CPG study. The SR committee limited its focus to the development of SRs. At the same time, the CPG committee worked under the assumption that guideline developers have access to and use high-quality SRs (as defined by the standards recommended in this report).

This report presents methodological standards for SRs that are designed to inform everyday healthcare decision making, especially for patients, clinicians and other healthcare providers, and devel-

---

BOX S-1
Charge to the Committee on Standards
for Systematic Reviews of Comparative
Effectiveness Research

An ad hoc committee will conduct a study to recommend methodological standards for systematic reviews (SRs) of comparative effectiveness research (CER) on health and health care. The standards should ensure that the reviews are objective, transparent, and scientifically valid, and require a common language for characterizing the strength of the evidence. Decision makers should be able to rely on SRs of comparative effectiveness to determine what is known and not known and to describe the extent to which the evidence is applicable to clinical practice and particular patients. In this context, the committee will:

1. Assess whether, if widely adopted, any existing set of standards would assure that SRs of comparative effectiveness research are objective, transparent, and scientifically valid.
2. Recommend a set of standards for developing and reporting SRs of CER.

opers of CPGs. The focus is on the development and reporting of comprehensive, publicly funded SRs of the comparative effectiveness of therapeutic medical or surgical interventions. The recent health reform legislation underscores the imperative for establishing standards to ensure the highest quality SRs. The *Patient Protection and Affordable Care Act of 2010* (ACA) created the nation's first nonprofit, public–private Patient-Centered Outcomes Research Institute (PCORI). PCORI will be responsible for establishing and implementing a research agenda—including SRs of CER—to help patients, clinicians and other healthcare providers, purchasers, and policy makers make informed healthcare decisions. As this report was being developed, planning for PCORI was underway. An initial task of the newly appointed governing board of the institute is to establish a standing methodology committee charged with developing and improving the science and methods of CER.

The IOM committee undertook its work with the intention to inform the PCORI methodology committee's own standards development. The IOM committee also views other public sponsors of SRs of CER as key audiences for this report, including the Agency for Healthcare Research and Quality (AHRQ) Effective Health Care Program, the Centers for Medicaid and Medicare Coverage Advisory Committee, the Drug Effectiveness Research Project, the National Institutes of Health (NIH), the Centers for Disease Control and Prevention (CDC), and the U.S. Preventive Services Task Force.

PURPOSE OF SETTING STANDARDS

Organizations establish standards to set performance expectations and to promote accountability for meeting these expectations. For SRs in particular, the principal objective of setting standards is to minimize bias in identifying, selecting, and interpreting evidence. For the purposes of this report, the committee defined an SR "standard" as a process, action, or procedure that is deemed essential to producing scientifically valid, transparent, and reproducible SRs. A standard may be supported by scientific evidence, by a reasonable expectation that the standard helps achieve the anticipated level of quality in an SR, or by the broad acceptance of the practice by authors of SRs.

The evidence base for many of the steps in the SR process is sparse, especially with respect to linking characteristics of SRs to clinical outcomes, the ultimate test of quality. The committee developed its standards and elements of performance based on available research evidence and expert guidance from the AHRQ Effective

Health Care Program; the Centre for Reviews and Dissemination (CRD) (University of York, United Kingdom); the Cochrane Collaboration; the Grading of Recommendations Assessment, Development, Evaluation (GRADE) Working Group[2]; and the Preferred Reporting Items for Systematic Reviews and Meta-Analyses group (PRISMA).

The committee faced a difficult task in proposing a set of standards where in general the evidence is thin and expert guidance varies. Yet the evidence that is available does not suggest that high-quality SRs can be done quickly and cheaply. SRs conducted with methods prone to bias do indeed often miss the boat, leading to clinical advice that may in the end harm patients. All of the committee's recommended standards are based on current evidence, expert guidance, and thoughtful reasoning, and are actively used by many experts, and thus are reasonable "best practices" for reducing bias and for increasing the scientific rigor of SRs of CER. However, all of the recommended standards must be considered provisional pending better empirical evidence about their scientific validity, feasibility, efficiency, and ultimate usefulness in medical decision making.

The committee recommends 21 standards with 82 elements of performance, addressing the entire SR process, from the initial steps of formulating the topic, building a review team, and establishing a research protocol, to finding and assessing the individual studies that make up the body of evidence, to producing qualitative and quantitative syntheses of the body of evidence, and, finally, to developing the final SR report. Each standard is articulated in the same format: first, a brief statement of the step in the SR process (e.g., in Chapter 3, Standard 3.1. Conduct a comprehensive systematic search for evidence) followed by a series of elements that are essential components of the standard. These "elements" are steps that should be taken for all publicly funded SRs of CER.

Collectively the standards and elements present a daunting task. Few, if any, members of the committee have participated in an SR that fully meets all of them. Yet the evidence and experience are strong enough that it is impossible to ignore these standards or hope that one can safely cut corners. The standards will be especially valuable for SRs of high-stakes clinical questions with broad population impact, where the use of public funds to get the right answer justifies careful attention to the rigor with which the SR is conducted. Individuals involved in SRs should be thoughtful about all of the

---

[2]GRADE was a primary source for Chapter 4 only. PRISMA was a primary source for Chapter 5 only.

standards and elements, using their best judgment if resources are inadequate to implement all of them, or if some seem inappropriate for the particular task or question at hand. Transparency in reporting the methods actually used and the reasoning behind the choices are among the most important of the standards recommended by the committee.

Initiating the SR Process

The first steps in the SR process define the focus and methods of the SR and influence its ultimate utility for clinical decisions. Current practice falls far short of expert guidance; well-designed, well-executed SRs are the exception. (Note that throughout this report reference to "expert guidance" refers to the published methodological advice of the AHRQ Effective Health Care Program, CRD, and the Cochrane Collaboration.) The committee recommends eight standards for initiating the SR process, minimizing potential bias in the SR's design and execution. The standards address the creation of the SR team, user and stakeholder input, managing bias and conflict of interest (COI), topic formulation, and development of the SR protocol (Box S-2). The SR team should include individuals with appropriate expertise and perspectives. Creating a mechanism for users and stakeholders—consumers, clinicians, payers, and members of CPG panels—to provide input into the SR process at multiple levels helps to ensure that the SR is focused on real-world healthcare decisions. However, a process should be in place to reduce the risk of bias and COI from stakeholder input and in the SR team. The importance of the review questions and analytic framework in guiding the entire review process demands a rigorous approach to formulating the research questions and analytic framework. Requiring a research protocol that prespecifies the research methods at the outset of the SR process helps to prevent the effects of author bias, allows feedback at an early stage in the SR, and tells readers of the review about protocol changes that occur as the SR develops.

Finding and Assessing Individual Studies

The committee recommends six standards for identifying and assessing the individual studies that make up an SR's body of evidence, including standards addressing the search process, screening and selecting studies, extracting data, and assessing the quality of individual studies (Box S-3). The objective of the SR search is to identify all the studies (and all the relevant data from the studies) that

BOX S-2
Recommended Standards for Initiating
a Systematic Review

Standard 2.1 Establish a team with appropriate expertise and experience to conduct the systematic review
Required elements:
2.1.1 Include expertise in the pertinent clinical content areas
2.1.2 Include expertise in systematic review methods
2.1.3 Include expertise in searching for relevant evidence
2.1.4 Include expertise in quantitative methods
2.1.5 Include other expertise as appropriate

Standard 2.2 Manage bias and conflict of interest (COI) of the team conducting the systematic review
Required elements:
2.2.1 Require each team member to disclose potential COI and professional or intellectual bias
2.2.2 Exclude individuals with a clear financial conflict
2.2.3 Exclude individuals whose professional or intellectual bias would diminish the credibility of the review in the eyes of the intended users

Standard 2.3 Ensure user and stakeholder input as the review is designed and conducted
Required element:
2.3.1 Protect the independence of the review team to make the final decisions about the design, analysis, and reporting of the review

Standard 2.4 Manage bias and COI for individuals providing input into the systematic review
Required elements:
2.4.1 Require individuals to disclose potential COI and professional or intellectual bias
2.4.2 Exclude input from individuals whose COI or bias would diminish the credibility of the review in the eyes of the intended users

Standard 2.5 Formulate the topic for the systematic review
Required elements:
2.5.1 Confirm the need for a new review

may pertain to the research question and analytic framework. The search should be systematic, use prespecified search parameters, and access an array of information sources that provide both published and unpublished research reports. Screening and selecting

2.5.2 Develop an analytic framework that clearly lays out the chain of logic that links the health intervention to the outcomes of interest and defines the key clinical questions to be addressed by the systematic review

2.5.3 Use a standard format to articulate each clinical question of interest

2.5.4 State the rationale for each clinical question

2.5.5 Refine each question based on user and stakeholder input

Standard 2.6 Develop a systematic review protocol
Required elements:

2.6.1 Describe the context and rationale for the review from both a decision-making and research perspective

2.6.2 Describe the study screening and selection criteria (inclusion/exclusion criteria)

2.6.3 Describe precisely which outcome measures, time points, interventions, and comparison groups will be addressed

2.6.4 Describe the search strategy for identifying relevant evidence

2.6.5 Describe the procedures for study selection

2.6.6 Describe the data extraction strategy

2.6.7 Describe the process for identifying and resolving disagreement between researchers in study selection and data extraction decisions

2.6.8 Describe the approach to critically appraising individual studies

2.6.9 Describe the method for evaluating the body of evidence, including the quantitative and qualitative synthesis strategies

2.6.10 Describe and justify any planned analyses of differential treatment effects according to patient subgroups, how an intervention is delivered, or how an outcome is measured

2.6.11 Describe the proposed timetable for conducting the review

Standard 2.7 Submit the protocol for peer review
Required element:

2.6.9 Provide a public comment period for the protocol and publicly report on disposition of comments

Standard 2.8 Make the final protocol publicly available, and add any amendments to the protocol in a timely fashion

studies should use methods that address the pervasive problems of SR author bias, errors, and inadequate documentation of the study selection process in SRs. Study methods should be reported in sufficient detail so that searches can be replicated and appraised. Qual-

BOX S-3
Recommended Standards for Finding
and Assessing Individual Studies

Standard 3.1 Conduct a comprehensive systematic search for evidence
  Required elements:
    3.1.1 Work with a librarian or other information specialist trained in performing systematic reviews to plan the search strategy
    3.1.2 Design the search strategy to address each key research question
    3.1.3 Use an independent librarian or other information specialist to peer review the search strategy
    3.1.4 Search bibliographic databases
    3.1.5 Search citation indexes
    3.1.6 Search literature cited by eligible studies
    3.1.7 Update the search at intervals appropriate to the pace of generation of new information for the research question being addressed
    3.1.8 Search subject-specific databases if other databases are unlikely to provide all relevant evidence
    3.1.9 Search regional bibliographic databases if other databases are unlikely to provide all relevant evidence

Standard 3.2 Take action to address potentially biased reporting of research results
  Required elements:
    3.2.1 Search grey-literature databases, clinical trial registries, and other sources of unpublished information about studies
    3.2.2 Invite researchers to clarify information about study eligibility, study characteristics, and risk of bias
    3.2.3 Invite all study sponsors and researchers to submit unpublished data, including unreported outcomes, for possible inclusion in the systematic review
    3.2.4 Handsearch selected journals and conference abstracts
    3.2.5 Conduct a web search
    3.2.6 Search for studies reported in languages other than English if appropriate

Standard 3.3 Screen and select studies
  Required elements:
    3.3.1 Include or exclude studies based on the protocol's prespecified criteria
    3.3.2 Use observational studies in addition to randomized clinical trials to evaluate harms of interventions

3.3.3 Use two or more members of the review team, working independently, to screen and select studies

3.3.4 Train screeners using written documentation; test and retest screeners to improve accuracy and consistency

3.3.5 Use one of two strategies to select studies: (1) read all full-text articles identified in the search or (2) screen titles and abstracts of all articles and then read the full texts of articles identified in initial screening

3.3.6 Taking account of the risk of bias, consider using observational studies to address gaps in the evidence from randomized clinical trials on the benefits of interventions

Standard 3.4 Document the search
Required elements:

3.4.1 Provide a line-by-line description of the search strategy, including the date of every search for each database, web browser, etc.

3.4.2 Document the disposition of each report identified including reasons for their exclusion if appropriate

Standard 3.5 Manage data collection
Required elements:

3.5.1 At a minimum, use two or more researchers, working independently, to extract quantitative and other critical data from each study. For other types of data, one individual could extract the data while the second individual independently checks for accuracy and completeness. Establish a fair procedure for resolving discrepancies—do not simply give final decision-making power to the senior reviewer

3.5.2 Link publications from the same study to avoid including data from the same study more than once

3.5.3 Use standard data extraction forms developed for the specific SR

3.5.4 Pilot-test the data extraction forms and process

Standard 3.6 Critically appraise each study
Required elements:

3.6.1 Systematically assess the risk of bias, using predefined criteria

3.6.2 Assess the relevance of the study's populations, interventions, and outcome measures

3.6.3 Assess the fidelity of the implementation of interventions

ity assurance and control are essential when data are extracted from individual studies from the collected body of evidence. A thorough and thoughtful assessment of the validity and relevance of each eligible study helps ensure scientific rigor and promote transparency.

Synthesizing the Body of Evidence

The committee recommends four standards for the qualitative and quantitative synthesis and assessment of an SR's body of evidence (Box S-4). The qualitative synthesis is an often undervalued component of an SR. Many SRs lack a qualitative synthesis altogether or simply recite the facts about the studies without examining them for patterns or characterizing the strengths and weaknesses

---

BOX S-4
Recommended Standards for Synthesizing
the Body of Evidence

Standard 4.1 Use a prespecified method to evaluate the body of evidence
   Required elements:
      4.1.1 For each outcome, systematically assess the following characteristics of the body of evidence:
         • Risk of bias
         • Consistency
         • Precision
         • Directness
         • Reporting bias
      4.1.2 For bodies of evidence that include observational research, also systematically assess the following characteristics for each outcome:
         • Dose–response association
         • Plausible confounding that would change the observed effect
         • Strength of association
      4.1.3 For each outcome specified in the protocol, use consistent language to characterize the level of confidence in the estimates of the effect of an intervention

Standard 4.2 Conduct a qualitative synthesis
   Required elements:
      4.2.1 Describe the clinical and methodological characteristics of the included studies, including their size, inclusion or exclusion of important subgroups, timeliness, and other relevant factors

of the body of evidence as a whole. If the SR is to be comprehensible, it should use consistent language to describe the quality of evidence for each outcome and incorporate multiple dimensions of study quality. For readers to have a clear understanding of how the evidence applies to real-world clinical circumstances and specific patient populations, SRs should describe—in easy-to-understand language—the clinical and methodological characteristics of the individual studies, including their strengths and weaknesses and their relevance to particular populations and clinical settings. It should also describe how flaws in the design or execution of the individual studies could bias the results. The qualitative synthesis is more than a narrative description or set of tables that simply detail how many studies were assessed, the reasons for excluding other

---

4.2.2 Describe the strengths and limitations of individual studies and patterns across studies

4.2.3 Describe, in plain terms, how flaws in the design or execution of the study (or groups of studies) could bias the results, explaining the reasoning behind these judgments

4.2.4 Describe the relationships between the characteristics of the individual studies and their reported findings and patterns across studies

4.2.5 Discuss the relevance of individual studies to the populations, comparisons, cointerventions, settings, and outcomes or measures of interest

Standard 4.3 Decide if, in addition to a qualitative analysis, the systematic review will include a quantitative analysis (meta-analysis)
Required element:

4.3.1 Explain why a pooled estimate might be useful to decision makers

Standard 4.4 If conducting a meta-analysis, then do the following:
Required elements:

4.4.1 Use expert methodologists to develop, execute, and peer review the meta-analyses

4.4.2 Address the heterogeneity among study effects

4.4.3 Accompany all estimates with measures of statistical uncertainty

4.4.4 Assess the sensitivity of conclusions to changes in the protocol, assumptions, and study selection (sensitivity analysis)

NOTE: The order of the standards does not indicate the sequence in which they are carried out.

studies, the range of study sizes and treatments compared, or the quality scores of each study as measured by a risk of bias tool.

Meta-analysis is the statistical combination of results from multiple individual studies. Many published meta-analyses have combined the results of studies that differ greatly from one another. The assumption that a meta-analysis is an appropriate step in an SR should never be made. The decision to conduct a meta-analysis is neither purely analytical nor statistical in nature. It will depend on a number of factors, such as the availability of suitable data and the likelihood that the analysis could inform clinical decision making. Ultimately, authors should make this subjective judgment in consultation with the entire SR team, including both clinical and methodological perspectives. If appropriate, the meta-analysis can provide reproducible summaries of the individual study results and offer valuable insights into the patterns in the study results. A strong meta-analysis features and clearly describes its subjective components, scrutinizes the individual studies for sources of heterogeneity, and tests the sensitivity of the findings to changes in the assumptions, the set of included studies, the outcome metrics, and the statistical models.

The Final Report

Authors of all publicly sponsored SRs should produce a detailed final report. The committee recommends three standards for producing the SR final report: (1) including standards for documenting the SR process; (2) responding to input from peer reviewers, users, and stakeholders; and (3) making the final report publicly available (Box S-5). The committee's standards for documenting the SR process drew heavily on the PRISMA checklist. The committee recommends adding items to the PRISMA checklist to ensure that the report of an SR describes all of the steps and judgments required by the committee's standards (Boxes S-2, S-3, and S-4).

RECOMMENDATIONS

The evidence base supporting many elements of SRs is incomplete and, for some steps, nonexistent. Research organizations such as the AHRQ Effective Health Care Program, CRD, and the Cochrane Collaboration have published standards, but none of these are universally accepted and consistently applied during planning, conducting, reporting, and peer review of SRs. Furthermore, the SR enterprise in the United States lacks both adequate funding and coordination; many organizations conduct SRs, but do not typically work together. Thus, the committee concludes that improving the quality of SRs will require improving not only the science supporting the steps in the SR process (Boxes S-2, S-3, and S-4), but also providing a more supportive environment for the conduct of SRs. The committee proposes a framework for improving the quality of the science underpinning SRs and supporting the environment for SRs. The framework has several broad categories: strategies for involving the right people, methods for conducting reviews, methods for synthesizing and evaluating evidence, and methods for communicating and using results.

The standards and elements form the core of the committee's conclusions, but the standards themselves do not indicate how the standards should be implemented, nor do the standards address issues of improving the science for SRs or for improving the environment that supports the development and use of an SR enterprise. In consequence, the committee makes the following two recommendations:

Recommendation 1: Sponsors of SRs of CER should adopt appropriate standards for the design, conduct, and reporting of SRs and require adherence to the standards as a condition for funding.

SRs of CER in the United States are now commissioned and conducted by a vast array of private and public entities, some supported generously with adequate funding to meet the most exacting standards, others supported less generously so that the authors must make compromises at every step of the review. The committee recognizes that its standards and elements are at the "exacting" end of the continuum, some of which are within the control of the review team whereas others are contingent on the SR sponsor's compliance. However, high-quality reviews require adequate time and resources to reach reliable conclusions. The recommended standards are an appropriate starting point for publicly funded reviews in the United States (including PCORI, federal, state, and local funders) because of the heightened attention and potential clinical impact of major reviews sponsored by public agencies. The committee also recognizes that authors of SRs supported by public funds derived from nonfederal sources (e.g., state public health agencies) will see these standards as an aspirational goal rather than as a minimum requirement. SRs that significantly deviate from the standards should clearly explain and justify the use of different methods.

BOX S-5
Recommended Standards for
Reporting Systematic Reviews

Standard 5.1 Prepare final report using a structured format
Required elements:
  5.1.1 Include a report title*
  5.1.2 Include an abstract*
  5.1.3 Include an executive summary
  5.1.4 Include a summary written for the lay public
  5.1.5 Include an introduction (rationale and objectives)*
  5.1.6 Include a methods section. Describe the following:
    • Research protocol*
    • Eligibility criteria (criteria for including and excluding studies in the systematic review)*
    • Analytic framework and key questions
    • Databases and other information sources used to identify relevant studies*
    • Search strategy*
    • Study selection process*
    • Data extraction process*
    • Methods for handling missing information*
    • Information to be extracted from included studies*
    • Methods to appraise the quality of individual studies*
    • Summary measures of effect size (e.g., risk ratio, difference in means)*
    • Rationale for pooling (or not pooling) results of included studies
    • Methods of synthesizing the evidence (qualitative and meta-analysis*)
    • Additional analyses, if done, indicating which were prespecified*

Recommendation 2: The Patient-Centered Outcomes Research Institute and the Department of Health and Human Services (HHS) agencies (directed by the secretary of HHS) should collaborate to improve the science and environment for SRs of CER. Primary goals of this collaboration should include

  • Developing training programs for researchers, users, consumers, and other stakeholders to encourage more effective and inclusive contributions to SRs of CER;
  • Systematically supporting research that advances the methods for designing and conducting SRs of CER;

5.1.7 Include a results section; organize the presentation of results around key questions; describe the following (repeat for each key question):
- Study selection process*
- List of excluded studies and reasons for their exclusion*
- Appraisal of individual studies' quality*
- Qualitative synthesis
- Meta-analysis of results, if performed (explain rationale for doing one)*
- Additional analyses, if done, indicating which were prespecified*
- Tables and figures

5.1.8 Include a discussion section. Include the following:
- Summary of the evidence*
- Strengths and limitations of the systematic review*
- Conclusions for each key question*
- Gaps in evidence
- Future research needs

5.1.9 Include a section describing funding sources* and COI

Standard 5.2 Peer review the draft report
Required elements:
5.2.1 Use a third party to manage the peer review process
5.2.2 Provide a public comment period for the report and publicly report on disposition of comments

Standard 5.3 Publish the final report in a manner that ensures free public access

---

* Indicates items from the PRISMA checklist. (The committee endorses all of the PRISMA checklist items.)

- Supporting research to improve the communication and use of SRs of CER in clinical decision making;
- Developing effective coordination and collaboration between U.S. and international partners;
- Developing a process to ensure that standards for SRs of CER are regularly updated to reflect current best practice; and
- Using SRs to inform priorities and methods for primary CER.

This recommendation conveys the committee's view of how best to implement its recommendations to improve the science and support the environment for SRs of comparative effectiveness research, which is clearly in the public's interest. PCORI is specifically named because of its statutory mandate to establish and carry out a CER research agenda. As noted above, it is charged with creating a methodology committee that will work to develop and improve the science and methods of SRs of CER and to regularly update such standards. PCORI is also required to assist the Comptroller General in reviewing and reporting on compliance with its research standards, the methods used to disseminate research findings, the types of training conducted and supported in CER, and the extent to which CER research findings are used by healthcare decision makers. The HHS agencies are specifically named because AHRQ, NIH, CDC, and other sections of HHS are major funders and producers of SRs. In particular, the AHRQ EPC program has been actively engaged in coordinating high-quality SRs and in developing SR methodology. The committee assigns these groups with responsibility and accountability for coordinating and moving the agenda ahead.

The committee found compelling evidence that having high-quality SRs based on rigorous standards is a topic of international concern, and that individual colleagues, professional organizations, and publicly funded agencies in other countries make up a large proportion of the world's expertise on the topic. Nonetheless, the committee followed the U.S. law that brought this report into being, which suggests a management approach appropriate to the U.S. environment. A successful implementation of the final recommendation should result in an enterprise in the United States that participates fully and harmonizes with the international development of SRs, serving in some cases in a primary role, in others as a facilitator, and in yet others as a participant. The new enterprise should recognize that this cannot be entirely scripted and managed in advance—structures and processes must allow for innovation to arise naturally from those individuals and organizations in the United States already fully engaged in the topic.

1

Introduction

Abstract: *This chapter presents the objectives and context for this report and describes the approach that the Institute of Medicine (IOM) Committee on Standards for Systematic Reviews of Comparative Effectiveness Research used to undertake the study. The committee's charge was two-fold: first, to assess potential methodological standards that would assure objective, transparent, and scientifically valid systematic reviews (SRs) of comparative effectiveness research and, second, to recommend a set of methodological standards for developing and reporting such SRs. A companion IOM committee was charged with developing standards for trustworthy clinical practice guidelines.*

Healthcare decision makers in search of the best evidence to inform clinical decisions have come to rely on systematic reviews (SRs). Well-conducted SRs systematically identify, select, assess, and synthesize the relevant body of research, and will help make clear what is known and not known about the potential benefits and harms of alternative drugs, devices, and other healthcare services. Thus, SRs of comparative effectiveness research (CER) can be essential for clinicians who strive to integrate research findings into their daily practices, for patients to make well-informed choices about their own care, for professional medical societies and other organizations that develop CPGs, and for payers and policy makers.[1] A brief overview of the current producers and users of SRs is provided at the end of the chapter. SRs can also inform medical coverage decisions and be used to set agendas and funding for primary research by highlighting gaps in evidence. Although the importance of SRs is gaining appreciation, the quality of published SRs is variable and often poor (Glasziou et al., 2008; Hopewell et al., 2008b; Liberati et al., 2009; Moher et al., 2007). In many cases, the reader cannot judge the quality of an SR because the methods are poorly documented (Glenton et al., 2006). If methods are described, they may be used inappropriately, such as in meta-analyses (Glenny et al., 2005; Laopaiboon, 2003). One cannot assume that SRs, even when published in well-regarded journals, use recommended methods to minimize bias (Bassler et al., 2007; Colliver et al., 2008; Roundtree et al., 2008; Song et al., 2009; Steinberg and Luce, 2005; Turner et al., 2008). Many SRs fail to assess the quality of the included research (Delaney et al., 2007; Mallen et al., 2006; Tricco et al., 2008) and neglect to report funding sources (Lundh et al., 2009; Roundtree et al., 2008). A plethora of conflicting approaches to evidence hierarchies and grading schemes for bodies of evidence is a further source of confusion (Glasziou et al., 2004; Lohr, 2004; Schünemann et al., 2003).

In its 2008 report, *Knowing What Works in Health Care: A Roadmap for the Nation*, the Institute of Medicine (IOM) recommended that methodological standards be developed for SRs that focus on research on the effectiveness of healthcare interventions and for CPGs (IOM, 2008). The report concluded that decision makers would be helped significantly by development of standards for both SRs and CPGs, especially with respect to transparency, minimizing bias and conflict of interest, and clarity of reporting. The IOM report was soon followed by a congressional mandate in the *Medicare Improvements for Patients and Providers Act of 2008*[2] for two follow-up IOM studies: one, to develop standards for conducting SRs, and the other to develop standards for CPGs. The legislation directs the IOM to recommend methodological standards to ensure that SRs and CPGs "are objective, scientifically valid, and consistent."

In response to this congressional directive, the IOM entered into a contract with the Agency for Healthcare Research and Quality (AHRQ) in July 2009 to produce both studies at the same time.

---

[1] The IOM Committee on Standards for Developing Trustworthy Clinical Practice Guidelines defines CPGs as "statements that include recommendations intended to optimize patient care that are informed by an SR of evidence and an assessment of the benefits and harms of alternative care options."

[2] Public Law 110-275, Section 304.

The IOM appointed two independent committees to undertake the projects. The 16-member[3] Committee on Standards for Systematic Reviews of Comparative Effectiveness Research included experts in biostatistics and epidemiology, CER, CPG development, clinical trials, conflict of interest, clinical care and delivery of healthcare services, consumer perspectives, health insurance, implementation science, racial and ethnic disparities, SR methods, and standards of evidence. Brief biographies of the SR committee members are presented in Appendix I. This report presents the findings and recommendations of the SR committee. A companion report, *Clinical Practice Guidelines We Can Trust*, presents the findings and recommendations of the Committee on Standards for Developing Trustworthy Clinical Practice Guidelines.

COMMITTEE CHARGE

The charge to the SR committee was two-fold: first, to assess potential methodological standards that would assure objective, transparent, and scientifically valid SRs of CER, and second, to recommend a set of methodological standards for developing and reporting such SRs (Box 1-1).

WHAT IS COMPARATIVE EFFECTIVENESS RESEARCH?

In recent years, various terms such as evidence-based medicine, health technology assessment, clinical effectiveness research, and comparative effectiveness research have been used to describe healthcare research that focuses on generating or synthesizing evidence to inform real-world clinical decisions (Luce et al., 2010). While the legislation that mandated this study used the term *clinical* effectiveness research, the committee could not trace the ancestry of the phrase and was uncertain about its meaning separate from the phrase *comparative* effectiveness research in general use by clinicians, researchers, and policy makers. Thus, this report adopts the more commonly used terminology—*comparative effectiveness research* and defines CER as proposed in the IOM report, *Initial National Priorities for Comparative Effectiveness Research* (IOM, 2009, p. 42):

> CER is the generation and synthesis of evidence that compares the benefits and harms of alternative methods to prevent, diagnose, treat, and monitor a clinical condition or

---

[3] One member stepped down from the committee in July 2010.

BOX 1-1
Charge to the Committee on Standards for Systematic
Reviews of Comparative Effectiveness Research

An ad hoc committee will conduct a study to recommend methodological standards for systematic reviews (SRs) of comparative effectiveness research on health and health care. The standards should ensure that the reviews are objective, transparent, and scientifically valid, and require a common language for characterizing the strength of the evidence. Decision makers should be able to rely on SRs of comparative effectiveness to know what is known and not known and to describe the extent to which the evidence is applicable to clinical practice and particular patients. In this context, the committee will:

1. Assess whether, if widely adopted, any existing set of standards would assure that SRs of comparative effectiveness research are objective, transparent, and scientifically valid.
2. Recommend a set of standards for developing and reporting SRs of comparative effectiveness research.

---

to improve the delivery of care. The purpose of CER is to assist consumers, clinicians, purchasers, and policy makers to make informed decisions that will improve health care at both the individual and population levels.

Research that is compatible with the aims of CER has six defining characteristics (IOM, 2009):

1. The objective is to inform a specific clinical decision.
2. It compares at least two alternative interventions, each with the potential to be "best practice."
3. It addresses and describes patient outcomes at both a population and a subgroup level.
4. It measures outcomes that are important to patients, including harms as well as benefits.
5. It uses research methods and data sources that are appropriate for the decision of interest.
6. It is conducted in settings as close as possible to the settings in which the intervention will be used.

Body of Evidence for Systematic Reviews of Comparative Effectiveness Research

The body of evidence for an SR of CER includes randomized controlled trials (RCTs) and observational studies such as cohort studies, cross-sectional studies, case-control studies, registries, and SRs themselves (Box 1-2). RCTs have an ideal design to answer questions about the comparative effects of different interventions across a wide variety of clinical circumstances. However, to be applicable to real-world clinical decision making, SRs should assess well-

---

BOX 1-2
Types of Comparative Effectiveness Research Studies

Experimental study: A study in which the investigators actively intervene to test a hypothesis.
- **Controlled trials** are experimental studies in which a group receives the intervention of interest while one or more comparison groups receive an active comparator, a placebo, no intervention, or the standard of care, and the outcomes are compared. In head-to-head trials, two active treatments are compared.
- In a **randomized controlled trial (RCT),** participants are randomly allocated to the experimental group or the comparison group. Cluster randomized trials are RCTs in which participants are randomly assigned to the intervention or comparison in groups (clusters) defined by a common feature, such as the same physician or health plan.

Observational study: A study in which investigators simply observe the course of events.
- In **cohort studies,** groups with certain characteristics or receiving certain interventions (e.g., premenopausal woman receiving chemotherapy for breast cancer) are monitored over time to observe an outcome of interest (e.g., loss of fertility).
- In **case-control studies,** groups with and without an event or outcome are examined to see whether a past exposure or characteristic is more prevalent in one group than in the other.
- In **cross-sectional studies,** the prevalence of an exposure of interest is associated with a condition (e.g., prevalence of hysterectomy in African American versus white women) and is measured at a specific time or time period.

Systematic review (SR): A scientific investigation that focuses on a specific question and that uses explicit, planned scientific methods to identify, select, assess, and summarize the findings of similar but separate studies. It may or may not include a quantitative synthesis (meta-analysis) of the results from separate studies.
- A **meta-analysis** is an SR that uses statistical methods to combine quantitatively the results of similar studies in an attempt to allow inferences to be made from the sample of studies and be applied to the population of interest.

SOURCE: Adapted from Last (1995).

designed research on the comparative effectiveness of alternative treatments that includes a broad range of participants, describes results at both the population and subgroup levels, and measures outcomes (both benefits and harms) that are important to patients, and reflects results in settings similar to those in which the intervention is used in practice. Many RCTs lack these features (IOM, 2009). As a result, in certain situations and for certain questions, decision makers find it limiting to use SRs that are confined to RCTs.

Observational research is particularly useful for identifying an intervention's potential for unexpected effects or harms because many adverse events are too rare to be observed during typical RCTs or do not occur until after the trial ends (Chou et al., 2010; Reeves

---

BOX 1-3
Four Examples of the Use of Observational Studies in Systematic Reviews of Comparative Effectiveness Research

Important outcomes are not captured in randomized controlled trials (RCTs)
More than 50 RCTs of triptans focused on the speed and degree of migraine pain relief related to a few isolated episodes of headache. These trials provided no evidence about two outcomes important to patients: the reliability of migraine relief from episode to episode over a long period of time, and the overall effect of use of the triptan on work productivity. The best evidence for these outcomes came from a time-series study based on employment records merged with prescription records comparing work days lost before and after a triptan became available. Although the study did not compare one triptan with another, the study provided data that a particular triptan improved work productivity—information that was not available in RCTs.

Available trials of antipsychotic medications for schizophrenia included a narrow spectrum of participants and only evaluated short-term outcomes

In a systematic review (SR) of antipsychotic medications, 17 short-term efficacy trials evaluated a relatively narrow spectrum of patients with schizophrenia, raising a number of questions: Is the effect size observed in the RCTs similar to that observed in practice? Do groups of patients excluded from the trials respond as frequently and as well as those included in the trials? Are long-term outcomes similar to short-term outcomes? For a broad spectrum of patients with schizophrenia who are initiating treatment with an atypical antipsychotic medication, which drugs have better persistency and sustained effectiveness for longer term follow-up (e.g., 6 months to 2 years)? Given the many questions not addressed by RCTs, these review authors determined that they would examine and include observational studies. Meta-analyses of RCTs were conducted where appropriate, but most of the data were summarized qualitatively.

et al., 2008). Moreover, observational studies may provide evidence about the performance of an intervention in everyday practice or about outcomes that were not evaluated in available RCTs (Box 1-3). Despite their potential advantages, however, observational studies are at greater risk of bias compared to randomized studies for determining intervention effectiveness.

STUDY SCOPE

This report presents methodological standards for SRs that are designed to inform everyday healthcare decision making, especially for patients, clinicians and other healthcare providers, and develop-

---

Participants in trials comparing percutaneous coronary intervention (PCI) versus coronary artery bypass graft (CABG) differed from patients seen in community practices

An SR of PCI versus CABG for coronary disease identified 23 relevant RCTs. At the outset, cardiothoracic surgical experts raised concerns that the trials enrolled patients with a relatively narrow spectrum of disease (generally single- or two-vessel disease) relative to patients receiving the procedures in current practice. Thus, the review included 96 articles reporting findings from 10 large cardiovascular registries. The registry data confirmed that the choice between the two procedures in the community varied substantially with extent of coronary disease. For patients similar to those enrolled in the trials, mortality results in the registries reinforced the findings from trials (i.e., no difference in mortality between PCI and CABG). At the same time, the registries reported that the relative mortality benefits of PCI versus CABG varied markedly with extent of disease, raising caution about extending trial conclusions to patients with greater or lesser disease than those in the trial population.

Paucity of trial data on using a commonly prescribed drug for a specific indication, that is, heparin for burn injury

In an SR on heparin to treat burn injury, the review team determined very early in its process that observational data should be included. Based on preliminary, cursory reviews of the literature and input from experts, the authors determined that there were few (if any) RCTs on the use of heparin for this indication. Therefore, they decided to include all types of studies that included a comparison group before running the main literature searches.

SOURCES: Adapted from Norris et al. (2010), including Bravata et al. (2007); Helfand and Peterson (2003); McDonagh et al. (2008); and Oremus et al. (2006).

ers of CPGs. The focus is on the development and reporting of comprehensive, publicly funded SRs of the comparative effectiveness of therapeutic medical or surgical interventions.

The recent health reform legislation underscores the imperative for establishing SR standards, calling for a new research institute similar to the national program envisioned in *Knowing What Works*. *The Patient Protection and Affordable Care Act* of 2010[4] created the nation's first nonprofit, public–private Patient-Centered Outcomes Research Institute (PCORI). It will be responsible for establishing and implementing a research agenda—including SRs of CER—to help patients, clinicians, policy makers, and purchasers in making informed healthcare decisions. As this report was being developed, the plans for PCORI were underway. An initial task of the newly appointed PCORI governing board is to establish a standing methodology committee charged with developing and improving the science and methods of CER. The IOM committee undertook its work with the intention to inform the PCORI methodology committee's own standards development. The IOM committee also views other public sponsors of SRs of CER as key audiences for this report, including the AHRQ Effective Health Care Program, Medicare Evidence Development & Coverage Advisory Committee (MEDCAC), Drug Effectiveness Research Project (DERP), National Institutes of Health, Centers for Disease Control and Prevention, and U.S. Preventive Services Task Force. See Table 1-1 for a brief overview of the statutory requirements for PCORI.

Outside the Scope of the Study

As noted earlier, this report focuses on methods for producing comprehensive, publicly funded SRs of the comparative effectiveness of therapeutic interventions. The report's recommended standards are not intended for SRs initiated and conducted for purely academic purposes. Nor does the report address SR methods for synthesizing research on diagnostic tests, disease etiology or prognosis, systems improvement, or patient safety practices. The evidence base and expert guidance for SRs on these topics is considerably less advanced. For example, while the Cochrane Collaboration issued its fifth edition of its handbook for SRs of interventions in 2008 (Higgins and Green, 2008), a Cochrane diagnostics handbook is still under development (Cochrane Collaboration Diagnostic Test

---

[4]Public Law 111-148.

TABLE 1-1 Statutory Requirements for the Patient-Centered Outcomes Research Institute

Topic	Provisions

Purpose	• To assist patients, clinicians, policy makers, and purchasers in making informed health decisions by identifying and analyzing:
	  o National research priorities
	  o New clinical evidence and evidentiary gaps
	  o Relevance of evidence and economic effects

Organization	• Nonprofit corporation • Not an agency or establishment of the U.S. government
Funding	• Fiscal years (FYs) 2010–2012: Direct appropriations of $10 million, $50 million, and $150 million per year, respectively • FYs 2013–2019: Trust fund with annual inflow of $150 million in appropriations plus annual per-capita charges per enrollee from Medicare, health insurance, and self-insured health plans • After FY 2019: No funds available from trust fund
Oversight	• Public–private board of governors; 19 members include Agency for Healthcare Research and Quality (AHRQ) and National Institutes of Health (NIH) designees • Methodology committee to develop and update science-based methodological standards; include AHRQ and NIH
Research	• Will award contracts for peer-reviewed research • Authorized to enter into contracts with outside entities to manage funding and conduct research; preference given to AHRQ and NIH if research is authorized by their governing statutes
Dissemination and transparency	• Make research findings available within 90 days • AHRQ, in consultation with NIH, will broadly disseminate research findings • Provide public comment periods for major actions • Establish publicly available resource database

SOURCE: Clancy and Collins (2010).

Accuracy Working Group, 2011). AHRQ methods guidance for SRs of diagnostics and prognosis is also underway.

Finally, the utility of an SR is only as good as the body of individual studies available. A considerable literature documents the shortcomings of reports of individual clinical trials and observational research (Altman et al., 2001; Glasziou et al., 2008; Hopewell et al., 2008b; Ioannidis et al., 2004; Plint et al., 2006; von Elm et al., 2007). This report will emphasize that the quality of individual studies must be scrutinized during the course of an SR. However, it is beyond the scope of this report to examine the many quality-scoring systems that have been developed to measure the quality of individual research studies (Brand, 2009; Hopewell et al., 2008a; Moher et al., 2010).

Relationship with the Committee on Standards for Developing Trustworthy Clinical Practice Guidelines

The boundaries of this study were defined in part by the work of the companion CPG study (Box 1-4). A coordinating group[5] for the two committees met regularly to consider the interdependence of SRs and CPGs and to minimize duplication of effort. The coordinating group agreed early on that SRs are critical inputs to the guideline development process. It also decided that the SR committee would limit its focus to the development of SRs, starting with the formulation of the research question and ending with the completion of a final report—while paying special attention to the role of SRs in supporting CPGs. At the same time, the CPG committee would work under the assumption that guideline developers have access to high- quality SRs (as defined by the SR committee's recommended standards) that address their specific research questions, and would discuss what steps in an SR are particularly important for a CPG. In Chapter 2 of this report, the SR committee addresses how the SR and CPG teams may interact when an SR is being conducted to inform a specific CPG.

CONCEPTUAL FRAMEWORK

Fundamentals of Systematic Reviews

Experts agree on many of the key attributes of a high-quality SR (CRD, 2009; Higgins and Green, 2008; Owens et al., 2010). The objective of an SR is to answer a specific research question by using an explicit, preplanned protocol to identify, select, assess, and summarize the findings of similar but separate studies. SRs often include—but do not require—a quantitative synthesis (meta-analysis). The SR process can be summarized in six steps:

Step 1: Initiate the process, organize the review team, develop a process for gathering user and stakeholder input, formulate the research question, and implement procedures for minimiz-

---

[5] The six-member coordinating group included the chair, vice chair, and one other individual from each committee.

BOX 1-4
Charge to the Committee on Standards for Developing
Trustworthy Clinical Practice Guidelines

An ad hoc committee will conduct a study to recommend standards for developing clinical practice guidelines and recommendations. The standards should ensure that clinical practice guidelines are unbiased, scientifically valid, and trustworthy and also incorporate separate grading systems for characterizing quality of available evidence and strength of clinical recommendations. In this context, the committee should:

1. Assess whether, if widely adopted, any existing set of standards would assure the development of unbiased, scientifically valid, and trustworthy clinical practice guidelines.
2. Endorse an existing set of standards for developing clinical practice guidelines. If the committee judges current standards to be inadequate, it will develop a new set of standards.
3. Determine best practices for promoting voluntary adoption of the standards.

---

ing the impact of bias and conflict of interests (see standards in Chapter 2).

Step 2: Develop the review protocol, including the context and rationale for the review and the specific procedures for the search strategy, data collection and extraction, qualitative synthesis and quantitative data synthesis (if a meta-analysis is done), reporting, and peer review (see standards in Chapter 2).

Step 3: Systematically locate, screen, and select the studies for review (see standards in Chapter 3).

Step 4: Appraise the risk of bias in the individual studies and extract the data for analysis (see standards in Chapter 3).

Step 5: Synthesize the findings and assess the overall quality of the body of evidence (see standards in Chapter 4).

Step 6: Prepare a final report and have the report undergo peer review (see standards in Chapter 5).

SRs of CER can be narrow in scope and consist of simple comparisons, such as drug X versus drug Y. They can also address broader topics including comparisons of the effectiveness of drugs versus surgery for a condition, or "watchful waiting" when it is a reasonable strategy in a clinical context (IOM, 2009). These more complex reviews often include multiple clinical questions that will each need a separate review of the literature, analysis, and synthesis. The committee's standards apply to both narrow and broad SRs of CER.

The Purpose of Setting Standards

Most disciplines establish standards to articulate their agreed-on performance expectations and to promote accountability for meeting these expectations. Users of SRs and the public have the right to expect that SRs meet minimum standards for objectivity, transparency, and scientific rigor (as the legislative mandate for this study required). For the purposes of this report, the committee defined an SR "standard" as meaning:

> A process, action, or procedure for performing SRs that is deemed essential to producing scientifically valid, transparent, and reproducible results. A standard may be supported by scientific evidence, by a reasonable expectation that the standard helps achieve the anticipated level of quality in an SR, or by the broad acceptance of the practice in SRs.

The principal objectives of applying standards to SR methods are: (1) to improve the usefulness of SRs for patients, clinicians, and guideline developers; (2) to increase the impact of SRs on clinical outcomes; (3) to encourage stakeholder "buy-in" and trust in SRs; and (4) to minimize the risks of error and bias. The fourth objective is an essential precursor to the first three. An SR must minimize bias in identifying, selecting, and interpreting evidence to be credible.

METHODS OF THE STUDY

The committee deliberated during four in-person meetings and numerous conference calls between October 2009 and October 2010. During its second meeting, the committee convened a public workshop to learn how various stakeholders use and develop SRs. Panels of SR experts, professional specialty societies, payers, and consumer advocates provided testimony in response to a series of questions posed by the committee in advance of the event. Appendix C provides the workshop agenda and questions. Other experts from selected organizations were also interviewed by committee staff.[6]

---

[6] The organizations included the Aetna Health plan; the American Academy of Neurology; the American College of Cardiology; the American College of Chest Physicians; the American College of Obstetrics and Gynecology; Blue Cross and Blue

Developing the SR Standards

The committee faced a difficult task in proposing a set of standards where in general the evidence is thin especially with respect to linking characteristics of SRs to clinical outcomes, the ultimate test of quality. There have been important advances in SR methods in recent years. However, the field remains a relatively young one and the evidence that is available does not suggest that high-quality SRs can be done quickly and cheaply. For example, literature searching and data extraction, two fundamental steps in the SR process, are very resource intensive but there is little research to suggest how to make the processes more efficient. Similarly, as noted earlier, observational data can alert researchers to an intervention's potential for harm but there is little methodological research on ways to identify, assess, or incorporate high-quality observational data in an SR. Moreover, whereas this report concerns the production of comprehensive SR final reports, most research on SR methods focuses on the abridged, page-limited versions of SRs that appear in peer-reviewed journals.

Thus, the committee employed a multistep process to identify, assess, and select potential SR standards. It began by developing a set of assessment criteria, described below, to guide its selection of SR standards (Table 1-2). The next steps were to document expert guidance and to collect the available empirical research on SR methods. In addition, the committee commissioned two reports: one on the role of consumers in developing SRs in the United States and another that helped identify the evidence base for the steps in the SR process.[7]

Criteria for Assessing Potential Standards

The overarching goals of the criteria are to increase the usefulness of SRs for patient and clinician decisions while minimizing

Shield Technical Evaluation Center; the ECRI Institute; Geisinger health care system; Institute for Clinical Systems Improvement; Kaiser Permanente (Southern California); Medicare Evidence Development & Coverage Advisory Committee; National Comprehensive Cancer Network; National Heart, Lung, and Blood Institute; and the Veteran's Health Administration.

[7]Julia Kreis, Harkness/Bosch Fellow in Health Care Policy and Practice, Johns Hopkins Bloomberg School of Public Health, Johns Hopkins Bloomberg School of Public Health, contributed a paper on the role of U.S. consumers in systematic reviews. David Moher, Ph.D., and Alexander Tsertsvadze, M.D., of the Ottawa Health Research Institute and Sally Hopewell, Ph.D., of the U.K. Cochrane Centre helped identify methodological research on the conduct of SRs.

TABLE 1-2 Committee Criteria for Assessing Potential Standards and Elements for Systematic Reviews

Acceptability or credibility	Cultivates stakeholder understanding and acceptance of findings
Applicability or generalizability	Is consistent with the aim of comparative effectiveness research (CER): to assist consumers, clinicians, purchasers, and policy makers to make informed decisions that will improve health care at both the individual and population levels
Efficiency of conducting the review	Avoids unnecessary burden and cost of the process of conducting the review, and allows completion of the review in a timely manner
Patient-centeredness	Shows respect for and responsiveness to individual patient preferences, needs, and values; helps ensure that patient values and circumstances guide clinical decisions
Scientific rigor	Improves objectivity, minimizes bias, provides reproducible results, and fosters more complete reporting
Timeliness	Ensures currency of the review
Transparency	Ensures that methods are explicitly defined, consistently applied, and available for public review so that observers can readily link judgments, decisions, or actions to the data on which they are based; allows users to assess the strengths and weaknesses of the systematic review or clinical practice guideline

the risks of error and bias. The following describes the committee's rationale for each criterion:

- **Acceptability (credibility):** If clinicians, guideline developers, or patients are unlikely to accept the findings of SRs, the costs of conducting the SRs could be for naught. Some SR standards are necessary to enhance the review's overall credibility. For example, a standard requiring that the review team solicit consumer input as it formulates the review questions enhances credibility.
- **Applicability (generalizability):** Healthcare interventions found to be effective in one patient population may not be effective in other patient populations. SRs should address the relevance of the available evidence to actual patients. Evidence on how outcomes vary among different types of patients is essential to developing usable CPGs and oth-

er types of clinical advice (Boyd et al., 2005; Tinetti et al., 2004; Vogeli et al., 2007). Patients seen in everyday clinical practice are more diverse than participants in clinical trials, particularly with respect to age, gender, race and ethnicity, health status, comorbidities, and other clinically relevant factors (Pham et al., 2007; Slone Survey, 2006; Vogeli et al., 2007).

- **Efficiency:** Despite the potential benefit of standardizing some aspects of SRs, the decision to impose a standard must consider the cost implications, both in time and economic resources. Some standards, such as requiring two reviewers to screen individual studies, may require additional cost, but be necessary because empirical evidence shows that the standard would meaningfully improve the reliability of the SR (Edwards et al., 2002). Or, the evidence may suggest that the additional expense is not always warranted. For example, for some topics, collecting and translating non-English literature may ensure a comprehensive collection of research, but it may not be worth the cost if the research question is confined to an English-language only region (e.g., school lunches) (Moher et al., 2000, 2003; Morrison et al., 2009).

- **Patient-centeredness:** Patients want to know what health-care services work best for them as individuals. Focusing on the patient is integral to improving the quality of health care (IOM, 2001, 2008). SRs of research on comparative effectiveness should focus on informing the decisions about the care patients receive by addressing the questions of consumers, practicing clinicians, and developers of CPGs. For example, a standard that requires the review team to solicit feedback from patients about which clinical outcomes to address in review would enhance patient-centeredness.

- **Scientific rigor:** Potential standards should be considered if evidence shows that they increase the scientific rigor of the review. SRs are most likely to benefit patient care if the underlying methods are objective and fully reported, minimize risk of bias, and yield reproducible results. For example, a standard that requires use of appropriate statistical techniques to synthesize data from the body of research enhances scientific rigor.

- **Timeliness:** If an SR is out of date, it may not analyze important new clinical information of the benefits or harms of an intervention. Decision makers require up-to-date information. When new discoveries reveal serious risk of harm

or introduce a new and superior alternative treatment, updating the review or commissioning a new one is critical.
For example, a standard that requires a review to consider
relevant research within a recent timeframe would enhance
timeliness.

- **Transparency:** Without transparency, the integrity of an SR
  remains in question. Transparency requires that methods
  be reported in detail and be available to the public. This
  enables readers to judge the quality of the review and to
  interpret any decisions based on the review's conclusions.
  For example, standards that require thorough reporting of
  review methods, funding sources, and conflicts of interest
  would facilitate transparency.

Expert Guidance

The committee's next step was to consult with and review the
published methods manuals of leading SR experts—at AHRQ, Centre for Reviews and Dissemination (CRD) (University of York, UK),
and the Cochrane Collaboration—to document state-of-the-art guidance on best practices. Experts at other organizations were also consulted to finalize the committee's detailed list of essential steps and
considerations in the SR process. These organizations were DERP,
the ECRI Institute, National Institute for Health and Clinical Excellence (UK), and several Evidence-based Practice Centers (EPCs)
(with assistance from AHRQ staff).

With this information, the committee's assessment criteria,
and the research of commissioned authors and staff, the committee
evaluated and revised the list of steps and best practices in the SR
process through several iterations. The committee took a cautious
approach to developing standards. All of the committee's recommended standards are based on current evidence, expert guidance
(and are actively used by many experts), and thoughtful reasoning,
Thus, the proposed standards are reasonable "best practices" for
reducing bias and for increasing the scientific rigor of SRs of CER.

In its use of the term "standard," the committee recognizes that
its recommendations will not be the final word. Standards must
always be considered provisional, pending additional evidence and
experience. The committee supports future research that would
identify better methods that meet both the goals of scientific rigor
and efficiency in producing SRs.

The committee's proposed standards are presented in Chapters
2–5. Each standard is articulated in the same format: first, a brief state-

ment of the step in the SR process (e.g., in Chapter 3, Standard 3.1. Conduct a comprehensive systematic search for evidence) followed by a series of elements of performance. These elements are essential components of the standard that should be taken for all publicly funded SRs of CER. Thus, Standard 3.1, for example, includes several elements that are integral to conducting a comprehensive search (e.g., "design a search strategy to address each key research question," "search bibliographic databases"). Box 1-5 describes the committee's numbering system for the recommended standards.

Collectively the standards and elements present a daunting task. Few, if any, members of the committee have participated in an SR that fully meets all of them. Yet the evidence and experience are strong enough that it is impossible to ignore these standards or hope that one can safely cut corners. The standards will be especially valuable for SRs of high-stakes clinical questions with broad population impact, where the use of public funds to get the right answer justifies careful attention to the rigor with which the SR is conducted. Individuals involved in SRs should be thoughtful about all of the standards and elements, using their best judgment if resources are

---

BOX 1-5
Numbering System for the Committee's
Recommended Systematic Review Standards

The recommended systematic review (SR) standards are presented in Chapters 2–5. For easy reference within the report, the recommended standards and related elements of performance are numbered according to chapter number and sequence within chapters using the convention "x.y.z." The first number (x) refers to the chapter number; the second number (y) refers to the standard; and the third number (z) refers to the essential element of the standard, where applicable.

For example, the first standard in Chapter 3 is:

Standard 3.1 Conduct a comprehensive systematic search for evidence
Required elements:
  3.1.1 Work with a librarian or other information specialist training in performing SRs to plan the search strategy
  3.1.2 Design the search strategy to address each key research question
  3.1.3 Use an independent librarian or information specialist to peer review the search strategies

etc.

inadequate to implement all of them, or if some seem inappropriate for the particular task or question at hand. Transparency in reporting the methods actually used and the reasoning behind the choices are among the most important of the standards recommended by the committee.

CURRENT LANDSCAPE

This section provides a brief overview of the major producers, users, and other stakeholders involved in SRs.

Producers of Systematic SRs

A number of public- and private-sector organizations produce SRs. As noted earlier, the committee focused much of its review on the methods of AHRQ, the Cochrane Collaboration, and CRD. However, many other organizations play a key role in sponsoring, conducting, and disseminating SRs. Some of the key U.S. and international organizations are described below.

U.S. Organizations

In the United States, the federal government funds a number of SRs, primarily through the AHRQ EPCs (Table 1-3). Private organizations also conduct SRs of CER, including the Blue Cross and Blue Shield Association's Technology Evaluation Center, the ECRI Institute, and Hayes, Inc. (Table 1-4).

International Organizations

The U.S. SR enterprise is part of a larger international effort focused on SRs. Many international organizations have advanced and highly sophisticated SR programs that not only produce SRs, but also focus on how best to conduct SRs. Table 1-5 describes several leading international SR organizations.

Users and Stakeholders

This report uses the terms "users" and "stakeholders" to refer to individuals and organizations that are likely to consult a specific SR to guide decision making or who have a particular interest in the outcome of an SR. Table 1-6 lists examples of user and stakeholder organizations that use SRs to inform decision making. The

TABLE 1-3 Examples of U.S. Governmental Organizations That Produce Systematic Reviews

Organization	Description
Agency for Healthcare Research and Quality (AHRQ) Effective Health Care Program	In 1997, AHRQ established 12 Evidence-based Practice Centers (EPCs) to promote evidence-based practice in everyday care. AHRQ awards 5-year contracts to EPCs to develop evidence reports and technology assessments. Currently, there are 14 EPCs in university and private settings. The U.S. Department of Veterans Affairs, the U.S. Preventive Services Task Force, and the Centers for Medicare & Medicaid Services use EPC reviews.
Centers for Disease Control and Prevention (CDC)	The CDC supports two programs for systematic reviews, the *Guide to Community Preventive Services,* initiated in 1996 and focusing on synthesizing evidence related to public health interventions, and the *HIV/AIDS Prevention Research Synthesis,* established in 1996 to review and summarize HIV behavioral prevention research literature.
Substance Abuse and Mental Health Services Administration (SAMHSA)	Since 1997 SAMHSA has provided information about the scientific basis and practicality of interventions that prevent or treat mental health and substance abuse disorders through the National Registry of Evidence-based Programs and Practices.

SOURCES: Adapted from GAO (2009), IOM (2008).

report focuses on four major categories of users and stakeholders: (1) consumers, including patients, families, and informal (or unpaid) caregivers; (2) clinicians, including physicians, nurses, and other healthcare professionals; (3) payers; and (4) policy makers, including guideline developers and other SR sponsors.

ORGANIZATION OF THE REPORT

Chapter Objectives

This introductory chapter has described the background, charge to the committee, study scope, conceptual framework, current landscape, and methods for this report. Chapter 2 through Chapter 5 present the committee's review of and recommended standards for the basic steps in an SR. Chapter 6 provides a summary of the committee's conclusions and recommendations.

TABLE 1-4 Examples of Private U.S. Organizations That Produce Systematic Reviews

Organization	Description
Blue Cross and Blue Shield Association (BCBSA), Technology Evaluation Center (TEC)	BCBSA founded TEC in 1985 to provide decision makers with objective assessments of comparative effectiveness. TEC serves a wide range of clients in both the private and public sectors, including Kaiser Permanente and the Centers for Medicare & Medicaid Services. TEC is a designated Evidence-based Practice Center (EPC), and its products are publicly available.
ECRI Institute	The ECRI Institute is a nonprofit organization that provides technology assessments and cost-effectiveness analyses to ECRI Institute members and clients, including hospitals; health systems; public and private payers; U.S. federal and state government agencies; and ministries of health, voluntary-sector organizations, associations, and accrediting agencies. Its products and methods are generally not available to the public. The ECRI Institute is a designated EPC and is also a Collaborating Center for the World Health Organization.
Hayes, Inc.	Hayes, Inc., is a for-profit organization, established in 1989, to develop health technology assessments for health organizations, including health plans, managed-care companies, hospitals, and health networks. Hayes, Inc., produces several professional products, including the *Hayes Briefs*, the *Hayes Directory*, and the *Hayes Outlook*. Its products and methods are generally not available to the public.

SOURCE: Adapted from IOM (2008).

Chapter 2, Standards for Initiating a Systematic Review, focuses on the early steps in an SR that define the objectives of the review and influence its ultimate relevance to clinical decisions: establishing the review team, ensuring user and stakeholder input, managing bias and conflict of interest, and formulating the research topic and review protocol.

Chapter 3, Standards for Finding and Assessing Individual Studies, focuses on a central step in the SR process: the identification, collection, screening, and appraisal of the individual studies that make up an SR's body of evidence.

Chapter 4, Standards for Synthesizing the Body of Evidence, focuses on considerations in the synthesis and assessment of the body of evidence that are key to ensuring objectivity, transparency, and scientific rigor.

TABLE 1-5 Examples of International Organizations That Produce Systematic Reviews

Organization	Description
Cochrane Collaboration	Founded in 1993, the Cochrane Collaboration is an independent, nonprofit multinational organization that produces systematic reviews (SRs) of healthcare interventions. Cochrane SRs are prepared by researchers who work with one or more of 52 Cochrane Review Groups that are overseen by an elected Steering Committee. Editorial teams oversee the preparation and maintenance of the SRs and the application of quality standards. Cochrane's global contributors and centers are funded by government agencies and private sources; its central infrastructure is supported by subscriptions to *The Cochrane Library*. Commercial funding of review groups is not allowed. Cochrane review abstracts and plain-language summaries are free; complete SRs are available via subscription. The *Cochrane Database of SRs* includes more than 6,000 protocols and SRs.
Centre for Reviews and Dissemination (CRD)	CRD is part of the National Institute for Health Research (NIHR) and a department of the University of York in the UK. Founded in 1994, CRD produces SRs of health interventions, SR methods research, and guidance for conducting SRs. CRD also produces the *Database of Abstracts of Reviews of Effects* (DARE), the *National Health Service Economic Evaluation Database*, and the *Health Technology Assessment Database*, which are used internationally by health professionals, policy makers, and researchers. An international prospective registry of SRs utilizing existing database infrastructure is also under development. The DARE includes over 19,000 records of SRs of health care interventions, including more than 10,000 critical abstracts, which summarize the methods and findings of published reviews—highlighting their strengths and weaknesses. Approximately 1,200 new critical abstracts are added to DARE annually. CRD is funded primarily through NIHR with some funding from other government agencies. To avoid conflict of interest, CRD has a policy not to undertake research for or receive funds from the pharmaceutical or medical devices industries.
Campbell Collaboration	The Campbell Collaboration is an international research network that produces SRs of the effects of social interventions. It was established in 2000 and has five Coordinating Groups: Social Welfare, Crime and Justice, Education, Methods, and Users. The Coordinating Groups oversee the production, scientific merit, and relevance of the SRs. Final SRs are published in the peer-reviewed monograph series, *Campbell Systematic Reviews*. The International Secretariat is hosted by the Norwegian Centre for the Health Services.

continued

TABLE 1-5 Continued

Organization	Description
National Institute for Health and Clinical Excellence (NICE)	NICE was established in 1999 as part of the U.K.'s National Health Service (NHS). It provides guidance to NHS, sets quality standards, and manages a national database to improve health and prevent and treat ill health. NICE commissions SRs on new and existing technologies from independent academic centers. NICE then uses the SRs to make recommendations to NHS on how a technology should be used in NHS.

SOURCES: Information on the Cochrane Collaboration was adapted from IOM (2008). Information on CRD and the Campbell Collaboration: The Campbell Collaboration (2010); CRD (2010); NICE (2010).

TABLE 1-6 Examples of Organizations That Use Systematic Reviews

Organization	Description
Drug Effectiveness Review Project (DERP)	DERP is a collaboration of public and private organizations, including 13 state programs, which develops reports assessing the comparative effectiveness and safety of drugs within particular drug classes. Evidence-based Practice Centers (EPCs) conduct evidence reviews for DERP. State Medicaid programs have used this information to develop their drug formularies.
Medicare Evidence Development & Coverage Advisory Committee (MedCAC)	The Centers for Medicare & Medicaid (CMS) established the Medicare Coverage Advisory Committee (now the Medicare Evidence Development & Coverage Advisory Committee [MedCAC]) in 1998 to provide independent expert advice to CMS on specific clinical topics. MedCAC reviews and evaluates the medical literature and technology assessments on medical items and services that are under evaluation at CMS, including systematic reviews (SRs) produced by the EPCs and other producers of SRs. MedCAC can be an integral part of the national coverage determination process. MedCAC is advisory in nature; CMS is responsible for all final decisions.
NIH Consensus Development Program (CDP)	CDP produces consensus statements on the effects of healthcare interventions. CDP convenes independent panels of researchers, health professionals, and public representatives who consider the literature reviews conducted by EPCs, as well as expert testimony. Topics are chosen based on their public health importance, prevalence, controversy, potential to reduce gaps between knowledge and practice, availability of scientific information, and potential impact on healthcare costs.

TABLE 1-6 Continued

Organization	Description
Performance measurement organizations	Performance measurement organizations track and evaluate provider performance by measuring providers' actual clinical practices against the recommended practices. To conduct this work, these organizations typically establish standards of care based on SRs, against which the performance of providers can be assessed. Examples of performance measurement organizations include the AQA Alliance and the National Quality Forum.
Professional medical societies	Many professional medical societies have instituted processes and directed resources to developing clinical practice guidelines on the basis of systematic reviews. Examples of societies with well-established guideline development procedures include the American College of Cardiology/American Heart Association, American College of Chest Physicians, American Academy of Neurology, and American Academy of Pediatrics.
U.S. Preventive Services Task Force (USPSTF)	The USPSTF consists of a panel of private-sector experts that makes recommendations about which preventive services should be incorporated routinely into primary medical care. Its evidence-based recommendations are regarded as the "gold standard" for clinical preventive services. USPSTF is supported by an EPC, which conducts systematic reviews on relevant clinical prevention topics.

SOURCE: Adapted from IOM (2008).

Chapter 5, Standards for Reporting Systematic Reviews, focuses on the components of an SR final report that are fundamental to its eventual utility for patients, clinicians, and others.

Chapter 6, Improving the Quality of Systematic Reviews: Discussion, Conclusions, and Recommendations, presents the committee's conclusions and recommendations for advancing the science underlying SR methods and for providing a more supportive environment for the conduct of SRs.

REFERENCES

Altman, D. G., K. F. Schulz, D. Moher, M. Egger, F. Davidoff, D. Elbourne, P. C. Gøtzsche, and T. Lang. 2001. The revised CONSORT statement for reporting randomized trials: Explanation and elaboration. *Annals of Internal Medicine* 134(8):663–694.

Bassler, D., I. Ferreira-Gonzalez, M. Briel, D. J. Cook, P. J. Devereaux, D. Heels-Ansdell, H. Kirpalani, M. O. Meade, V. M. Montori, A. Rozenberg, H. J. Schünemann, and G. H. Guyatt. 2007. Systematic reviewers neglect bias that results from trials stopped early for benefit. *Journal of Clinical Epidemiology* 60(9):869–873.

Boyd, C. M., J. Darer, C. Boult, L. P. Fried, L. Boult, and A. W. Wu. 2005. Clinical practice guidelines and quality of care for older patients with multiple comorbid diseases: Implications for pay for performance. *JAMA* 294(6):716–724.

Brand, R. A. 2009. Standards of reporting: The CONSORT, QUORUM, and STROBE guidelines. *Clinical Orthopaedics and Related Research* 467(6):1393–1394.

Bravata, D. M., K. M. McDonald, A. L. Gienger, V. Sundaram, M. V. Perez, R. Varghese, J. R. Kapoor, R. Ardehali, M. C. McKinnon, C. D. Stave, D. K. Owens, and M. Hlatky. 2007. *Comparative effectiveness of percutaneous coronary interventions and coronary artery bypass grafting for coronary artery disease.* Rockville, MD: AHRQ.

The Campbell Collaboration. 2010. *About us.* http://www.campbellcollaboration.org/about_us/index.php (accessed September 22, 2010).

Chou, R., N. Aronson, D. Atkins, A. S. Ismaila, P. Santaguida, D. H. Smith, E. Whitlock, T. J. Wilt, and D. Moher. 2010. Assessing harms when comparing medical interventions: AHRQ and the Effective Health-Care Program. *Journal of Clinical Epidemiology* 63(5):502–512.

Clancy, C., and F. S. Collins. 2010. Patient-Centered Outcomes Research Institute: The intersection of science and health care. *Science Translational Medicine* 2(37): 37cm18.

Cochrane Collaboration Diagnostic Test Accuracy Working Group. 2011. Handbook for DTA reviews. http://srdta.cochrane.org/handbook-dta-reviews (accessed March 15, 2011).

Colliver, J. A., K. Kucera, and S. J. Verhulst. 2008. Meta-analysis of quasi-experimental research: Are systematic narrative reviews indicated? *Medical Education* 42(9):858–865.

CRD (Centre for Reviews and Dissemination). 2009. *Systematic reviews: CRD's guidance for undertaking reviews in health care.* York, U.K.: York Publishing Services, Ltd.

CRD. 2010. *About CRD.* http://www.york.ac.uk/inst/crd/about_us.htm (accessed September 22, 2010).

Delaney, A., S. M. Bagshaw, A. Ferland, K. Laupland, B. Manns, and C. Doig. 2007. The quality of reports of critical care meta-analyses in the Cochrane Database of Systematic Reviews: An independent appraisal. *Critical Care Medicine* 35(2):589–594.

Edwards, P., M. Clarke, C. DiGuiseppi, S. Pratap, I. Roberts, and R. Wentz. 2002. Identification of randomized controlled trials in systematic reviews: Accuracy and reliability of screening records. *Statistics in Medicine* 21:1635–1640.

GAO (Government Accountability Office). 2009. *Program evaluation: A variety of rigorous methods can help identify effective interventions.* Vol. GAO-10-30. Washington, DC: GAO.

Glasziou, P., J. Vandenbroucke, and I. Chalmers. 2004. Assessing the quality of research. *BMJ* 328(7430):39–41.

Glasziou, P., E. Meats, C. Heneghan, and S. Shepperd. 2008. What is missing from descriptions of treatment in trials and reviews? *BMJ* 336(7659):1472–1474.

Glenny, A. M., D. G. Altman, F. Song, C. Sakarovitch, J. J. Deeks, R. D'Amico, M. Bradburn, and A. J. Eastwood. 2005. Indirect comparisons of competing interventions. *Health Technology Assessment* 9(26):1–134.

Glenton, C., V. Underland, M. Kho, V. Pennick, and A. D. Oxman. 2006. Summaries of findings, descriptions of interventions, and information about adverse effects would make reviews more informative. *Journal of Clinical Epidemiology* 59(8):770–778.

Helfand, M., and K. Peterson. 2003. *Drug class review on the triptans: Drug Effectiveness Review Project.* Portland, OR: Oregon Evidence-based Practice Center.

Higgins, J. P. T., and S. Green, eds. 2008. *Cochrane handbook for systematic reviews of interventions.* Chichester, UK: John Wiley & Sons.

Hopewell, S., M. Clarke, D. Moher, E. Wager, P. Middleton, D. G. Altman, and K. F. Schulz. 2008a. CONSORT for reporting randomized controlled trials in journal and conference abstracts: Explanation and elaboration. *PLoS Medicine* 5(1):e20.

Hopewell, S., L. Wolfenden, and M. Clarke. 2008b. Reporting of adverse events in systematic reviews can be improved: Survey results. *Journal of Clinical Epidemiology* 61(6):597–602.

Ioannidis, J. P., J. W. Evans, P. C. Gøtzsche, R. T. O'Neill, D. Altman, K. Schulz, and D. Moher. 2004. Better reporting of harms in randomized trials: An extension of the CONSORT Statement. *Ann Intern Med* 141:781–788.

IOM (Institute of Medicine). 2001. *Crossing the quality chasm: A new health system for the 21st century.* Washington, DC: National Academy Press.

IOM. 2008. *Knowing what works in health care: A roadmap for the nation.* Edited by J. Eden, B. Wheatley, B. J. McNeil, and H. Sox. Washington, DC: The National Academies Press.

IOM. 2009. *Initial national priorities for comparative effectiveness research.* Washington, DC: The National Academies Press.

Laopaiboon, M. 2003. Meta-analyses involving cluster randomization trials: A review of published literature in health care. *Statistical Methods in Medical Research* 12(6):515–530.

Last, J. M., ed. 1995. *A dictionary of epidemiology*, 3rd ed. New York: Oxford University Press.

Liberati, A., D. G. Altman, J. Tetzlaff, C. Mulrow, P. C. Gøtzsche, J. P. A. Ioannidis, M. Clarke, P. J. Devereaux, J. Kleijnen, and D. Moher. 2009. The PRISMA statement for reporting systematic reviews and meta-analyses of studies that evaluate health care interventions: Explanation and elaboration. *Annals of Internal Medicine* 151(4):W1–W30.

Lohr, K. N. 2004. Rating the strength of scientific evidence: Relevance for quality improvement programs. *International Journal for Quality in Health Care* 16(1):9–18.

Luce, B. R., M. Drummond, B. Jönsson, P. J. Neumann, J. S. Schwartz, U. Siebert, and S. D. Sullivan. 2010. EBM, HTA, and CER: Clearing the confusion. *Milbank Quarterly* 88(2):256–276.

Lundh, A., S. L. Knijnenburg, A. W. Jorgensen, E. C. van Dalen, and L. C. M. Kremer. 2009. Quality of systematic reviews in pediatric oncology—A systematic review. *Cancer Treatment Reviews* 35(8):645–652.

Mallen, C., G. Peat, and P. Croft. 2006. Quality assessment of observational studies is not commonplace in systematic reviews. *Journal of Clinical Epidemiology* 59(8):765–769.

McDonagh, M., K. Peterson, S. Carson, R. Fu, and S. Thakurta. 2008. *Drug class review: Atypical antipsychotic drugs. Update 3.* Portland, OR: Oregon Evidence-based Practice Center.

Moher, D., B. Pham, T. P. Klassen, K. F. Schulz, J. A. Berlin, A. R. Jadad, and A. Liberati. 2000. What contributions do languages other than English make on the results of meta-analyses? *Journal of Clinical Epidemiology* 53 (9):964–972.

Moher, D., B. Pham, M. L. Lawson, and Klassen T. P. 2003. The inclusion of reports of randomised trials published in languages other than English in systematic reviews. *Health Technology Assessment* 7 (41):1–90.

Moher, D., J. Tetzlaff, A. C. Tricco, M. Sampson, and D. G. Altman. 2007. Epidemiology and reporting characteristics of systematic reviews. *PLoS Medicine* 4(3):447–455.

Moher, D., K. F. Schulz, I. Simera, and D. G. Altman. 2010. Guidance for developers of health research reporting guidelines. *PLoS Med* 7(2):e1000217.

Morrison, A., K. Moulton, M. Clark, J. Polisena, M. Fiander, M. Mierzwinski-Urban, S. Mensinkai, T. Clifford, and B. Hutton. 2009. *English-language restriction when conducting systematic review-based meta-analyses: Systematic review of published studies*. Ottawa, CA: Canadian Agency for Drugs and Technologies in Health.

NICE (National Institute for Health and Clinical Excellence). 2010. *About NICE*. http://www.nice.org.uk/aboutnice/about_nice.jsp (accessed October 27, 2010).

Norris, S., D. Atkins, W. Bruening, S. Fox, E. Johnson, R. Kane, S. C. Morton, M. Oremus, M. Ospina, G. Randhawa, K. Schoelles, P. Shekelle, and M. Viswanathan. 2010. Selecting observational studies for comparing medical interventions. In *Methods guide for comparative effectiveness reviews*. http://effectivehealthcare.ahrq.gov/ehc/products/196/454/MethodsGuideNorris_06042010.pdf (accessed November 8, 2010).

Oremus, M., M. Hanson, R. Whitlock, E. Young, A. Gupta, A. Dal Cin, C. Archer, and P. Raina. 2006. *The uses of heparin to treat burn injury*. Evidence Report/Technology Assessment No. 148. AHRQ Publication No. 07-E004. Rockville, MD: AHRQ.

Owens, D. K., K. N. Lohr, D. Atkins, J. R. Treadwell, J. T. Reston, E. B. Bass, S. Chang, and M. Helfand. 2010. AHRQ Series Paper 5: Grading the strength of a body of evidence when comparing medical interventions: AHRQ and the Effective Health-Care Program. *Journal of Clinical Epidemiology* 63 (5):513–523.

Pham, H. H., D. Schrag, A. S. O'Malley, B. Wu, and P. B. Bach. 2007. Care patterns in Medicare and their implications for pay for performance. *New England Journal of Medicine* 356(11):1130–1139.

Plint, A. C., D. Moher, A. Morrison, K. Schulz, D. G. Altman, C. Hill, and I. Gaboury. 2006. Does the CONSORT checklist improve the quality of reports of randomised controlled trials? A systematic review. *Medical Journal of Australia* 185(5):263–267.

Reeves, B. C., J. J. Deeks, J. Higgins, and G. A. Wells. 2008. Chapter 13: Including non-randomized studies. In *Cochrane handbook for systematic reviews of interventions*, edited by J. P. T. Higgins and G. S. West. Chichester, UK: John Wiley & Sons.

Roundtree, A. K., M. A. Kallen, M. A. Lopez-Olivo, B. Kimmel, B. Skidmore, Z. Ortiz, V. Cox, and M. E. Suarez-Almazor. 2008. Poor reporting of search strategy and conflict of interest in over 250 narrative and systematic reviews of two biologic agents in arthritis: A systematic review. *Journal of Clinical Epidemiology* 62(2):128–137.

Schünemann, H., D. Best, G. Vist, and A. D. Oxman. 2003. Letters, numbers, symbols and words: How to communicate grades of evidence and recommendations. *Canadian Medical Association Journal* 169(7):677–680.

Slone Survey. 2006. *Patterns of medication use in the United States*. Boston, MA: Slone Epidemiology Center.

Song, F., Y. K. Loke, T. Walsh, A. M. Glenny, A. J. Eastwood, and D. G. Altman. 2009. Methodological problems in the use of indirect comparisons for evaluating healthcare interventions: Survey of published systematic reviews. *BMJ* 338:b1147.

Steinberg, E. P., and B. R. Luce. 2005. Evidence based? Caveat emptor! [editorial]. *Health Affairs (Millwood)* 24(1):80–92.

Tinetti, M. E., S. T. Bogardus, Jr., and J. V. Agostini. 2004. Potential pitfalls of disease-specific guidelines for patients with multiple conditions. *New England Journal of Medicine* 351(27):2870–2874.

Tricco, A. C., J. Tetzlaff, M. Sampson, D. Fergusson, E. Cogo, T. Horsley, and D. Moher. 2008. Few systematic reviews exist documenting the extent of bias: A systematic review. *Journal of Clinical Epidemiology* 61(5):422–434.

Turner, E. H., A. M. Matthews, E. Linardatos, R. A. Tell, and R. Rosenthal. 2008. Selective publication of antidepressant trials and its influence on apparent efficacy. *New England Journal of Medicine* 358(3):252–260.

Vogeli, C., A. Shields, T. Lee, T. Gibson, W. Marder, K. Weiss, and D. Blumenthal. 2007. Multiple chronic conditions: Prevalence, health consequences, and implications for quality, care management, and costs. *Journal of General Internal Medicine* 22(Suppl. 3):391–395.

von Elm, E., D. G. Altman, M. Egger, S. J. Pocock, P. C. Gotzsche, and J. P. Vandenbroucke. 2007. The strengthening the reporting of observational studies in epidemiology (STROBE) statement: Guidelines for reporting observational studies. *Annals of Internal Medicine* 147(8):573–577.

2

Standards for Initiating a Systematic Review

Abstract: *This chapter describes the initial steps in the systematic review (SR) process. The committee recommends eight standards for ensuring a focus on clinical and patient decision making and designing SRs that minimize bias: (1) establishing the review team; (2) ensuring user and stakeholder input; (3) managing bias and conflict of interest (COI) for both the research team and (4) the users and stakeholders participating in the review; (5) formulating the research topic; (6) writing the review protocol; (7) providing for peer review of the protocol; and (8) making the protocol publicly available. The team that will conduct the review should include individuals with appropriate expertise and perspectives. Creating a mechanism for users and stakeholders—consumers, clinicians, payers, and members of clinical practice guideline panels—to provide input into the SR process at multiple levels helps to ensure that the SR is focused on real-world healthcare decisions. However, a process should be in place to reduce the risk of bias and COI from user and stakeholder input and in the SR team. The importance of the review questions and analytic framework in guiding the entire review process demands a rigorous approach to formulating the research questions and analytic framework. Requiring a research protocol that prespecifies the research methods at the outset of the SR process helps prevent the effects of bias.*

The initial steps in the systematic review (SR) process define the focus of the complete review and influence its ultimate use in making clinical decisions. Because SRs are conducted under varying circumstances, the initial steps are expected to vary across different reviews, although in all cases a review team should be established, user and stakeholder input gathered, the topic refined, and the review protocol formulated. Current practice falls far short of recommended guidance[1]; well-designed, well-executed SRs are the exception. At a workshop organized by the committee, representatives from professional specialty societies, consumers, and payers testified that existing SRs often fail to address questions that are important for real-world healthcare decisions.[2] In addition, many SRs fail to develop comprehensive plans and protocols at the outset of the project, which may bias the reviews (Liberati et al., 2009; Moher et al., 2007). As a consequence, the value of many SRs to healthcare decisions makers is limited.

The committee recommends eight standards for ensuring a focus on clinical and patient decision making and designing SRs that minimize bias. The standards pertain to: establishing the review team, ensuring user and stakeholder input, managing bias and conflict of interest (COI) for both the research team and users and stakeholders, formulating the research topic, writing the review protocol, providing for peer review of the protocol, and making the protocol publicly available. Each standard includes a set of requirements composed of elements of performance (Box 2-1). A *standard* is a process, action, or procedure for performing SRs that is deemed essential to producing scientifically valid, transparent, and reproducible results. A standard may be supported by scientific evidence; by a reasonable expectation that the standard helps to achieve the anticipated level of quality in an SR; or by the broad acceptance of the practice in SRs. Each standard includes elements of performance that the committee deems essential.

---

[1] Unless otherwise noted, expert guidance refers to the published methods of the Evidence-based Practice Centers in the Agency for Healthcare and Research Quality Effective Health Care Program, the Centre for Reviews and Dissemination (University of York, UK), and the Cochrane Collaboration. The committee also consulted experts at other organizations, including the Drug Effectiveness Review Project, the ECRI Institute, the National Institute for Health and Clinical Excellence (UK), and several Evidence-Based Practice Centers (with assistance from staff from the Agency for Healthcare Research and Quality). See Appendix D for guidance.

[2] On January 14, 2010, the committee held a workshop that included four panels with representatives of organizations engaged in using and/or developing systematic reviews, including SR experts, professional specialty societies, payers, and consumer groups. See Appendix C for the complete workshop agenda.

ESTABLISHING THE REVIEW TEAM

The review team is composed of the individuals who will manage and conduct the review. The objective of organizing the review team is to pull together a group of researchers as well as key users and stakeholders who have the necessary skills and clinical content knowledge to produce a high-quality SR. Many tasks in the SR process should be performed by multiple individuals with a range of expertise (e.g., searching for studies, understanding primary study methods and SR methods, synthesizing findings, performing meta-analysis). Perceptions of the review team's trustworthiness and knowledge of real-world decision making are also important for the final product to be used confidently by patients and clinicians in healthcare decisions. The challenge is in identifying all of the required areas of expertise and selecting individuals with these skills who are neither conflicted nor biased and who are perceived as trustworthy by the public.

This section of the chapter presents the committee's recommended standards for organizing the review team. It begins with background on issues that are most salient to setting standards for establishing the review team: the importance of a multidisciplinary review team, the role of the team leader, and bias and COI. The rationale for the recommended standards follows. Subsequent sections address standards for involving various users and stakeholders in the SR process, formulating the topic of the SR, and developing the SR protocol. The evidence base for these initial steps in the SR process is sparse. The committee developed the standards by reviewing existing expert guidance and weighing the alternatives according to the committee's agreed-on criteria, especially the importance of improving the acceptability and patient-centeredness of publicly funded SRs (see Chapter 1 for a full discussion of the criteria).

A Multidisciplinary Review Team

The review team should be capable of defining the clinical question and performing the technical aspects of the review. It should be multidisciplinary, with experts in SR methodology, including risk of bias, study design, and data analysis; librarians or information specialists trained in searching bibliographic databases for SRs; and clinical content experts. Other relevant users and stakeholders should be included as feasible (CRD, 2009; Higgins and Green, 2008; Slutsky et al., 2010). A single member of the review team can have multiple areas of expertise (e.g., SR methodology and quantitative analysis). The size of the team will depend on the number and com-

---

BOX 2-1
Recommended Standards for Initiating
a Systematic Review

Standard 2.1 Establish a team with appropriate expertise and experience to conduct the systematic review
Required elements:
  2.1.1   Include expertise in the pertinent clinical content areas
  2.1.2   Include expertise in systematic review methods
  2.1.3   Include expertise in searching for relevant evidence
  2.1.4   Include expertise in quantitative methods
  2.1.5   Include other expertise as appropriate

Standard 2.2 Manage bias and conflict of interest (COI) of the team conducting the systematic review
Required elements:
  2.2.1   Require each team member to disclose potential COI and professional or intellectual bias
  2.2.2   Exclude individuals with a clear financial conflict
  2.2.3   Exclude individuals whose professional or intellectual bias would diminish the credibility of the review in the eyes of the intended users

Standard 2.3 Ensure user and stakeholder input as the review is designed and conducted
Required element:
  2.3.1   Protect the independence of the review team to make the final decisions about the design, analysis, and reporting of the review

Standard 2.4 Manage bias and COI for individuals providing input into the systematic review
Required elements:
  2.4.1   Require individuals to disclose potential COI and professional or intellectual bias
  2.4.2   Exclude input from individuals whose COI or bias would diminish the credibility of the review in the eyes of the intended users

Standard 2.5 Formulate the topic for the systematic review
Required elements:
  2.5.1   Confirm the need for a new review

---

plexity of the question(s) being addressed. The number of individuals with a particular expertise needs to be carefully balanced so that one group of experts is not overly influential. For example, review teams that are too dominated by clinical content experts are more likely to hold preconceived opinions related to the topic of the SR,

2.5.2 Develop an analytic framework that clearly lays out the chain of logic that links the health intervention to the outcomes of interest and defines the key clinical questions to be addressed by the systematic review

2.5.3 Use a standard format to articulate each clinical question of interest

2.5.4 State the rationale for each clinical question

2.5.5 Refine each question based on user and stakeholder input

Standard 2.6 Develop a systematic review protocol
Required elements:

2.6.1 Describe the context and rationale for the review from both a decision-making and research perspective

2.6.2 Describe the study screening and selection criteria (inclusion/exclusion criteria)

2.6.3 Describe precisely which outcome measures, time points, interventions, and comparison groups will be addressed

2.6.4 Describe the search strategy for identifying relevant evidence

2.6.5 Describe the procedures for study selection

2.6.6 Describe the data extraction strategy

2.6.7 Describe the process for identifying and resolving disagreement between researchers in study selection and data extraction decisions

2.6.8 Describe the approach to critically appraising individual studies

2.6.9 Describe the method for evaluating the body of evidence, including the quantitative and qualitative synthesis strategies

2.6.10 Describe and justify any planned analyses of differential treatment effects according to patient subgroups, how an intervention is delivered, or how an outcome is measured

2.6.11 Describe the proposed timetable for conducting the review

Standard 2.7 Submit the protocol for peer review
Required element:

2.7.1 Provide a public comment period for the protocol and publicly report on disposition of comments

Standard 2.8 Make the final protocol publicly available, and add any amendments to the protocol in a timely fashion

spend less time conducting the review, and produce lower quality SRs (Oxman and Guyatt, 1993).

Research examining dynamics in clinical practice guideline (CPG) groups suggests that the use of multidisciplinary groups is likely to lead to more objective decision making (Fretheim et al.,

2006a; Hutchings and Raine, 2006; Murphy et al., 1998; Shrier et al., 2008). These studies are relevant to SR teams because both the guideline development and the SR processes involve group dynamics and subjective judgments (Shrier et al., 2008). Murphy and colleagues (1998), for example, conducted an SR that compared judgments made by multi- versus single-disciplinary clinical guideline groups. They found that decision-making teams with diverse members consider a wider variety of alternatives and allow for more creative decision making compared with single disciplinary groups. In a 2006 update, Hutchings and Raine identified 22 studies examining the impact of group members' specialty or profession on group decision making and found similar results (Hutchings and Raine, 2006). Guideline groups dominated by medical specialists were more likely to recommend techniques that involve their specialty than groups with more diverse expertise. Fretheim and colleagues (2006a) identified six additional studies that also indicated medical specialists have a lower threshold for recommending techniques that involve their specialty. Based on this research, a guideline team considering interventions to prevent hip fracture in the elderly, for example, should include family physicians, internists, orthopedists, social workers, and others likely to work with the patient population at risk.

The Team Leader

Minimal research and guidance have been done on the leadership of SR teams. The team leader's most important qualifications are knowledge and experience in proper implementation of an SR protocol, and open-mindedness about the topics to be addressed in the review. The leader should also have a detailed understanding of the scope of work and be skilled at overseeing team discussions and meetings. SR teams rely on the team leader to act as the facilitator of group decision making (Fretheim et al., 2006b).

The SR team leader needs to be skilled at eliciting meaningful involvement of all team members in the SR process. A well-balanced and effective multidisciplinary SR team is one where every team member contributes (Fretheim et al., 2006b). The Institute of Medicine (IOM) directs individuals serving on its committees to be open to new ideas and willing to learn from one another (IOM, 2005). The role of the leader as facilitator is particularly important because SR team members vary in professional roles and depth of knowledge (Murphy et al., 1998). Pagliari and Grimshaw (2002) observed a multidisciplinary committee and found that the chair made the largest contributions to group discussion and was pivotal in ensuring inclusion of the views of all parties. Team members with less specialization, such as primary care physicians and nurses, tended to be less active in the group discussion compared with medical specialists.

Bias and Conflicts of Interest

Minimizing bias and COI in the review team is important to ensure the acceptability, credibility, and scientific rigor of the SR.[3] A recent IOM report, *Conflict of Interest in Medical Research, Education, and Practice*, defined COI as "a set of circumstances that creates a risk that professional judgment or actions regarding a primary interest will be unduly influenced by a secondary interest" (IOM, 2009a, p. 46). Disclosure of individual financial, business, and professional interests is the established method of dealing with researchers' COI (IOM, 2009a). A recent survey of high-impact medical journals found that 89 percent required authors to disclose COIs (Blum et al., 2009). The International Committee of Medical Journal Editors (ICMJE) recently created a universal disclosure form for all journals that are members of ICMJE to facilitate the disclosure process (Box 2-2) (Drazen et al., 2009, 2010; ICMJE, 2010). Leading guidance from producers of SRs also requires disclosure of competing interest (CRD, 2009; Higgins and Green, 2008; Whitlock et al., 2010). The premise of disclosure policies is that reporting transparency allows readers to judge whether these conflicts may have influenced the results of the research. However, many authors fail to fully disclose their COI despite these disclosure policies (Chimonas et al., 2011; McPartland, 2009; Roundtree et al., 2008). Many journals only require disclosure of financial conflicts, and do not require researchers to disclose intellectual and professional biases that may be similarly influential (Blum et al., 2009).

Because of the importance of preventing bias from undermining the integrity of biomedical research, a move has been made to strengthen COI policies. The National Institutes of Health (NIH), for example, recently announced it is revising its policy for managing financial COI in biomedical research to improve compliance, strengthen oversight, and expand transparency in this area (Rockey and Collins, 2010). There is also a push toward defining COI to include potential biases beyond financial conflicts. The new ICMJE policy requires that authors disclose "any other relationships or

---

[3] Elsewhere in this report, the term "bias" is used to refer to bias in reporting and publication (see Chapter 3).

BOX 2-2
International Committee of Medical Journal Editors
Types of Conflict-of-Interest Disclosures

- Associations with commercial entities that provided support for the work reported in the submitted manuscript. Should include both resources received directly and indirectly (via your institution) that enabled the author to complete the work.
- Associations with commercial entities that could be viewed as having an interest in the general area of the submitted manuscript.
- Other relationships or activities that readers could perceive to have influenced, or that give the appearance of potentially influencing, what the author wrote in the submitted work.

SOURCE: ICMJE (2010).

---

activities that readers could perceive to influence, or that give the appearance of potentially influencing" the research, such as personal, professional, political, institutional, religious, or other associations (Drazen et al., 2009, 2010, p. 268). The Cochrane Collaboration also requires members of the review team to disclose "competing interests that they judge relevant" (The Cochrane Collaboration, 2006). Similarly, the Patient-Centered Outcomes Research Institute (PCORI), created by the 2010 *Patient Protection and Affordable Care Act*, will require individuals serving on the Board of Governors, the methodology committee, and expert advisory panels to disclose both financial and personal associations.[4]

Secondary interests, such as the pursuit of professional advancement, future funding opportunities, and recognition, and the desire to do favors for friends and colleagues, are also important potential conflicts (IOM, 2009a). Moreover, mere disclosure of a conflict does not resolve or eliminate it. Review teams should also evaluate and act on the disclosed information. Eliminating the relationship, further disclosure, or restricting the participation of a researcher with COI may be necessary. Bias and COI may also be minimized by creating review teams that are balanced across relevant expertise and perspectives as well as competing interests (IOM, 2009a). The Cochrane Collaboration, for example, requires that if a member of

---

[4] *The Patient Protection and Affordable Care Act,* Public Law 111-148, 111th Cong., Subtitle D, § 6301 (March 23, 2010).

the review team is an author of a study that is potentially eligible for the SR, there must be other members of the review team who were not involved in that study. In addition, if an SR is conducted by individuals employed by a pharmaceutical or device company that relates to the products of that company, the review team must be multidisciplinary, with the majority of the members not employed by the relevant company. Individuals with a direct financial interest in an intervention may not be a member of the review team conducting an SR of that intervention (The Cochrane Collaboration, 2006). Efforts to prevent COI in health research should focus on not only whether COI actually biased an individual, but also whether COI has the potential for bias or appearance of bias (IOM, 2009a).

RECOMMENDED STANDARDS FOR ORGANIZING THE REVIEW TEAM

The committee recommends two standards for organizing the review team:

Standard 2.1—Establish a team with appropriate expertise and experience to conduct the systematic review

Required elements:

2.1.1 Include expertise in pertinent clinical content areas
2.1.2 Include expertise in systematic review methods
2.1.3 Include expertise in searching for relevant evidence
2.1.4 Include expertise in quantitative methods
2.1.5 Include other expertise as appropriate

Standard 2.2—Manage bias and conflict of interest (COI) of the team conducting the systematic review

Required elements:

2.2.1 Require each team member to disclose potential COI and professional or intellectual bias
2.2.2 Exclude individuals with a clear financial conflict
2.2.3 Exclude individuals whose professional or intellectual bias would diminish the credibility of the review in the eyes of the intended users

Rationale

The team conducting the SR should include individuals skilled in group facilitation who can work effectively with a multidisciplinary review team, an information specialist, and individuals skilled in project management, writing, and editing (Fretheim et al., 2006a). In addition, at least one methodologist with formal training and experience in conducting SRs should be on the team. Performance of SRs, like any form of biomedical research, requires education and training, including hands-on training (IOM, 2008). Each of the steps in conducting an SR should be, as much as possible, evidence based. Methodologists (e.g., epidemiologists, biostatisticians, health services researchers) perform much of the research on the conduct of SRs and are likely to stay up-to-date with the literature on methods. Their expertise includes decisions about study design and potential for bias and influence on findings, methods to minimize bias in the SR, qualitative synthesis, quantitative methods, and issues related to data collection and data management.

For SRs of comparative effectiveness research (CER), the team should include people with expertise in patient care and clinical decision making. In addition, as discussed in the following section, the team should have a clear and transparent process in place for obtaining input from consumers and other users and stakeholders to ensure that the review is relevant to patient concerns and useful for healthcare decisions. Single individuals might provide more than one area of required expertise. The exact composition of the review team should be determined by the clinical questions and context of the SR. The committee's standard is consistent with guidance from the Agency for Healthcare Research and Quality (AHRQ) Evidence-based Practice Center (EPC), the United Kingdom's Centre for Reviews and Dissemination (CRD), and the Cochrane Collaboration (CRD, 2009; Higgins and Green, 2008; Slutsky et al., 2010). It is also integral to the committee's criteria of scientific rigor by ensuring the review team has the skills necessary to conduct a high-quality SR.

The committee believes that minimizing COI and bias is critical to credibility and scientific rigor. Disclosure alone is insufficient. Individuals should be excluded from the review team if their participation would diminish public perception of the independence and integrity of the review. Individuals should be excluded for financial conflicts as well as for professional or intellectual bias. This is not to say that knowledgeable experts cannot participate. For example, it may be possible to include individual orthopedists in reviews of the efficacy of back surgery depending on the individual's specific employment, sources of income, publications, and public image. Other orthopedists may have to be excluded if they may benefit from the conclusions of the SR or may undermine the credibility of the SR. This is consistent with the recent IOM recommendations (IOM, 2009a). However, this standard is stricter than all of the major organizations' guidance on this topic, which emphasize disclosure of professional or intellectual bias, rather than requiring the exclusion of individuals with this type of competing interest (CRD, 2009; Higgins and Green, 2008; Slutsky et al., 2010). In addition, because SRs may take a year or more to produce, the SR team members should update their financial COI and personal biases at regular intervals.

ENSURING USER AND STAKEHOLDER INPUT

The target audience for SRs of CER include consumers, patients, and their caregivers; clinicians; payers; policy makers; private industry; organizations that develop quality indicators; SR sponsors; guideline developers; and others involved in "deciding what medical therapies and practice are approved, marketed, promoted, reimbursed, rewarded, or chosen by patients" (Atkins, 2007, p. S16). The purpose of CER, including SRs of CER, is to "assist consumers, clinicians, purchasers, and policy makers to make informed decisions that will improve health care at both the individual and populations levels" (IOM, 2009b, p. 41). Creating a clear and explicit mechanism for users and stakeholders to provide input into the SR process at multiple levels, beginning with formulating the research questions and analytic framework, is essential to achieving this purpose. A broad range of views should be considered in deciding on the scope of the SR. Often the organization(s) that nominate or sponsor an SR may be interested in specific populations, interventions, comparisons, and outcomes. Other users and stakeholders may bring a different perspective on the appropriate scope for a review. Research suggests that involving decision makers directly increases the relevance of SRs to decision making (Lavis et al., 2005; Schünemann et al., 2006).

Some SR teams convene formal advisory panels with representation from relevant user and stakeholder groups to obtain their input. Other SR teams include users and stakeholders on the review team, or use focus groups or conduct structured interviews with individuals to elicit input. Whichever model is used, the review team must include a skilled facilitator who can work effectively with consumers and other users and stakeholders to develop the questions and scope for the review. Users and stakeholders may have conflicting interests or very different ideas about what outcomes are relevant, as may other members of the review team, to the point that reconciling all of the different perspectives might be very challenging.

AHRQ has announced it will spend $10 million on establishing a Community Forum for CER to engage users and stakeholders formally, and to expand and standardize public involvement in the entire Effective Health Care Program (AHRQ, 2010). Funds will be used to conduct methodological research on the involvement of users and stakeholders in study design, interpretation of results, development of products, and research dissemination. Funds also will be used to develop a formal process for user and stakeholder input, to convene community panels, and to establish a workgroup on CER to provide formal advice and guidance to AHRQ (AHRQ, 2010).

This section of the chapter presents the committee's recommended standards for gathering user and stakeholder input in the review process. It begins with a discussion of some issues relevant to involving specific groups of users and stakeholders in the SR process: consumers, clinicians, payers, representatives of clinical practice guideline teams, and sponsors of reviews. There is little evidence available to support user and stakeholder involvement in SRs. However, the committee believes that user and stakeholder participation is essential to ensuring that SRs are patient centered and credible, and focus on real-world clinical questions.

Consumer Involvement

Consumer involvement is increasingly recognized as essential in CER. The IOM Committee on Comparative Effectiveness Research Prioritization recommended that "the CER program should fully involve consumers, patients, and caregivers in key aspects of CER, including strategic planning, priority setting, research proposal development, peer review, and dissemination" (IOM, 2009b, p. 143). It also urged that strategies be developed to engage and prepare consumers effectively for these activities (IOM, 2009b).

Despite the increasing emphasis on the importance of involving consumers in CER, little empiric evidence shows how to do this most effectively. To inform the development of standards for SRs, the IOM committee commissioned a paper to investigate what is known about consumer involvement in SRs in the United States and key international organizations.[5] The study sampled 17 organizations and groups ("organizations") that commission or conduct SRs (see Box 2-3 for a list of the organizations). Information about these organizations was retrieved from their websites and through semi-structured interviews with one or more key sources from each

---

[5] This section was excerpted and adapted from the paper commissioned by the IOM Committee: Kreis, Julia, a Harkness/Bosch Fellow in Health Care Policy and Practice at Johns Hopkins Bloomberg School of Public Health (2010). Consumer Involvement in Systematic Reviews.

BOX 2-3
Organizations and Groups Included in the
Commissioned Paper on Consumer Involvement in
Systematic Reviews

Agency for Healthcare Research and Quality*
American Academy of Pediatrics
American College of Chest Physicians
Blue Cross and Blue Shield Association, Technology Evaluation Center
Campbell Collaboration*
Centers for Medicare & Medicaid Services
Cochrane Collaboration (Steering Group)*
Cochrane Musculoskeletal Group*
Cochrane Pregnancy and Childbirth Group*
ECRI Institute
Hayes, Inc.
Johns Hopkins Evidence-based Practice Center*
Kaiser Permanente
Mayo Clinic, Knowledge and Encounter Research Unit
Office of Medical Applications of Research, National Institutes of Health
Oregon Evidence-based Practice Center*
U.S. Department of Veterans Affairs

---

* Organizations reporting that they usually involve consumers.

---

organization. Key sources for 7 of the 17 organizations (AHRQ, Oregon Evidence-based Practice Center, Johns Hopkins EPC, Campbell Collaboration, Cochrane Collaboration, Cochrane Musculoskeletal Group, and Cochrane Pregnancy and Childbirth Group) reported that their organization has a process in place to involve consumers on a regular basis. The other 10 organizations reported that their organizations do not usually involve consumers in the SR process, although some of them do so occasionally or they involve consumers regularly in other parts of their processes (e.g., when making coverage decisions).

The organizations that do involve consumers indicated a range of justifications for their procedures. For example, consumer involvement aims at ensuring that the research questions and outcomes included in the SR protocol reflect the perspectives and needs of the people who will receive the care and require this information to make real-world and optimally informed decisions. Several key sources noted that research questions and outcomes identified by consumers with a personal experience with the condition or treatment being studied are often different from the questions and outcomes identified by researchers and clinicians.

Consumers have been involved in all stages of the SR process. Some key sources reported that consumers should be involved early in the SR process, such as in topic formulation and refinement and in identification of the research questions and outcomes. Others involve consumers in reviewing the draft protocol. However, some noted, by the time the draft protocol is ready for review, accommodating consumer comments may be difficult because so much has already been decided. Some organizations also involve consumers in reviewing the final report (see Chapter 5). A few organizations reported instances in which consumers have participated in the more technical and scientific steps of an SR process, or even authored an SR. However, these instances are rare, and some key sources indicated they believed involving consumers is not necessary in these aspects of the review.

The term "consumer" has no generally accepted definition. Organizations that involve consumers have included patients with a direct personal experience of the condition of interest, and spouses and other family members (including unpaid family caregivers) who have direct knowledge about the patient's condition, treatment, and care. Involving family members and caregivers may be necessary in SRs studying patients who are unable to participate themselves because of cognitive impairment or for other reasons. However, family members and caregivers may also have different perspectives than patients about research questions and outcomes for an SR. Key sources reported that they have involved representatives from patient organizations as well as individual patients. The most important qualifications for the consumers to be involved in SRs—as pointed out by key sources—included a general interest, willingness to engage, and ability to participate.

The extent to which consumers are compensated for the time spent on SR activities depended on the organization and on the type of input the consumer provided. For example, in SRs commissioned by AHRQ, consumers who act as peer reviewers or who are involved in the process of translating the review results into consumer-friendly language are financially compensated for their time, generally at a fairly modest level. Other organizations do not provide any financial compensation. The form of involvement also differed across organizations, with, for example, consumers contributing as part of a user and stakeholder group, as part of an advisory group to a specific review or group of reviews, and as individuals.

A few organizations provide some initial orientation toward the review process or more advanced training in SR methodology for consumers, and one is currently developing training for researchers about how to involve or work with consumers and other stakeholders in the SR process.

Expert guidance on SRs generally recommends that consumers be involved in the SR process. The EPCs involve consumers in SRs for CER at various stages in the SR process, including in topic formulation and dissemination (Whitlock et al., 2010). Likewise, the Cochrane Collaboration encourages consumer involvement, either as part of the review team or in the editorial process (Higgins and Green, 2008). Both organizations acknowledge, however, that many questions about the most effective ways of involving consumers in the SR process remain unresolved (Higgins and Green, 2008; Whitlock et al., 2010).

Various concerns have been raised about involving consumers in the health research process (Entwistle et al., 1998). For example, some have argued that one consumer, or even a few consumers, cannot represent the full range of perspectives of all potential consumers of a given intervention (Bastian, 2005; Boote et al., 2002). Some consumers may not understand the complexities and rigor of research, and may require training and mentoring to be fully involved in the research process (Andejeski et al., 2002; Boote et al., 2002). Consumers may also have unrealistic expectations about the research process and what one individual research project can achieve. In addition, obtaining input from a large number of consumers may add considerably to the cost and amount of time required for a research project (Boote et al., 2002).

Based on this review of current practice, the committee concluded that although there are a variety of ways to involve consumers in the SR process, there are no clear standards for this involvement. However, gathering input from consumers, through *some* mechanism, is essential to CER. Teams conducting publicly funded SRs of CER should develop a process for gathering meaningful input from consumers and other users and stakeholders. The Cochrane Collaboration has conducted a review of its Consumer Network, which included process issues, and its newly hired consumer coordinator may undertake a close review of processes and impacts. The AHRQ Community Forum may also help establish more uniform standards in this area based on the results of methodological research addressing the most effective methods of involving consumers (AHRQ, 2010). In Chapter 6, the committee highlights the need for a formal evaluation of the effectiveness of the various methods of consumer involvement currently in practice, and of the impact of consumer involvement on the quality of SRs.

Clinician Involvement

Clinicians (e.g., physicians, nurses, and others who examine, diagnose, and treat patients) rely on SRs to answer clinical questions and to understand the limitations of evidence for the outcomes of an intervention. Although there is little empirical evidence, common sense suggests that their participation in the SR process can increase the relevance of research questions to clinical practice, and help identify real-world healthcare questions. Clinicians have unique insights because of their experiences in treating and diagnosing illness and through interacting with patients, family members, and their caregivers. In addition, getting input from clinicians often elucidates assumptions underlying support for a particular intervention. Eliciting these assumptions and developing questions that address them are critical elements of scoping an SR.

If the review team seeks clinician input, the team should hear from individuals representing multiple disciplines and types of practices. Several studies suggest that clinical specialists tend to favor and advocate for procedures and interventions that they provide (Fretheim et al., 2006b; Hutchings and Raine, 2006). Evidence also suggests that primary care physicians are less inclined than specialists to rate medical procedures and interventions as appropriate care (Ayanian et al., 1998; Kahan et al., 1996). In addition, clinicians from tertiary care institutions may have perspectives that are very different from clinicians from community-based institutions (Srivastava et al., 2005).

Payer Involvement

The committee heard from representatives of several payers at its workshop[6] and during a series of informal interviews with representatives from Aetna, Kaiser Permanente, Geisinger, Blue Cross and Blue Shield's Technology Evaluation Center, Centers for Medicare & Medicaid Services, and the Veterans Health Administration. Many of these organizations rely on publicly available SRs for decision making. They use SRs to make evidence-based coverage determinations and medical benefit policy and to provide clinician and patient

---

[6] See Appendix C.

decision support. For example, if there is better evidence for the efficacy of a procedure in one clinical setting over another, then the coverage policy is likely to reflect this evidence. Similarly, payers use SRs to determine pharmaceutical reimbursement levels and to manage medical expenditures (e.g., by step therapy or requiring prior authorization). Obtaining input from individuals that represents the purchaser perspective is likely to improve the relevance of an SR's questions and concerns.

Involvement of the Clinical Practice Guidelines Team

If an SR is a prerequisite to developing a CPG, it is important that the SR team be responsive to the questions of the CPG panel. There are various models of interaction between the CPG and SR teams in current practice, ranging from no overlap between the two groups (e.g., the NIH Consensus Development Conferences), to the SR and CPG teams interacting extensively during the evidence review and guideline writing stages (e.g., National Kidney Foundation [NKF], Kidney Disease: Improving Global Outcomes), to numerous variations in between (e.g., American College of Chest Physicians [ACCP]) (Box 2-4). Table 2-1 describes three general models of interaction: more complete isolation, moderate, and unified. Each model has benefits and drawbacks. Although the models have not been formally evaluated, the committee believes that a moderate level of interaction is optimal because it establishes a mechanism for communication between the CPG panel and the SR team, while also protecting against inappropriate influence on the SR methods.

Separation of the SR and the CPG teams, such as the approach used by NIH Consensus Development Conferences to develop evidence-based consensus statements, may guard against the CPG panel interfering in the SR methods and interpretation, but at the risk of producing an SR that is unresponsive to the guidelines team's questions. By shutting out the CPG panel from the SR process, particularly in the analysis of the evidence and preparation of the final report, this approach reduces the likelihood that the primary audience for the SR will understand the nuances of the existing evidence. The extreme alternative, unrestricted interaction between the review team and the guidelines team, or when the same individuals conduct the SR and write the CPG, risks biasing the SR and the review team is more likely to arrive at the answers the guideline team wants.

Some interaction, what the committee refers to as "moderate," allows the SR team and the CPG team to maintain separate identities and to collaborate at various stages in the SR and guideline

BOX 2-4
Examples of Interaction Between Systematic Review (SR)
and Clinical Practice Guideline (CPG) Teams

More Isolation: The National Institutes of Health (NIH) Consensus Development Conferences
- An initial panel of experts appointed by the NIH works with the review team to formulate research questions.
- An Agency for Healthcare Research and Quality's (AHRQ's) Evidence-based Practice Center (EPC) conducts the SRs based on the research questions. The NIH panel chair sits on the EPC to provide a communication bridge between the two groups.
- An independent panel of experts evaluates the SRs, gets input from expert presentations at a consensus development conference, and develops the evidence-based consensus statements.

Moderate: American College of Chest Physicians (ACCP)
- An ACCP panel of experts defines CPG chapter topics and assigns each chapter to an SR methodologist and clinical content editors (the CPG chapter leaders).
- The CPG chapter leaders work with an AHRQ EPC to formulate key questions. The AHRQ EPC searches the literature, selects and extracts data from relevant studies, and summarizes the findings in evidence tables.
- The evidence tables are delivered to the CPG chapter leaders:
  o The clinical content editors provide input into preparing, summarizing, and interpreting the evidence.
  o The SR methodologists are responsible for the final presentation of evidence and rating the quality of evidence.
- During the deliberations that ultimately determine the direction and strength of the CPG recommendations:
  o The clinical content editors are excluded if they have any relevant biases and conflicts of interest.
  o The SR methodologists are present, and are responsible for ensuring that the CPG panel is exposed to presentations and interpretations of the evidence that are free of bias. They do not make recommendations.

Unified: National Kidney Foundation, Kidney Disease: Improving Global Outcomes
- SR methodologists are on the CPG team. They conduct the SR and grade the evidence.
- There is no firewall to guarantee that the SR methodologists are responsible for the final presentation of the evidence.

SOURCES: Guyatt et al. (2010); KDIGO (2010); NIH (2010).

TABLE 2-1 Models of Interaction Between Systematic Review (SR) and Clinical Practice Guideline (CPG) Teams

	General Models of Interaction Between Developers of SRs and CPGs		
	More Isolatation	Moderate	Unified
Level of interaction	• SR and CPG teams confer about key questions; firewall between SR and CPG until a draft SR report is produced	• CPG and SR teams collaborate at various stages; a firewall is created by giving the methodologists final say on interpreting the evidence	• CPG team members may conduct the SR; no firewall
Potential benefits	• Deters inappropriate CPG influence over the collection and interpretation of evidence	• Helps ensure that SR research protocol responds to questions and information needs of the CPG team • SR team assures that prespecified research protocol is followed (protecting against bias)	• Ensures that the SR research protocol responds to questions and information needs of the CPG team • CPG team may better understand the limitations of the evidence
Potential drawbacks	• SR may not be fully responsive to all CPG concerns • CPG team will have only limited understanding of the body of evidence	• SR may not be fully responsive to all CPG concerns	• Fewer protections against bias in the SR • CPG developers may lack the skills and resources needed to produce SRs as well as CPGs

development process. Moderate interaction can occur in numerous ways, including, for example, having one or more CPG liaison(s) regularly communicate with the SR team, holding joint meetings of the SR and CPG team, or including a CPG representative on the SR team. At this level of interaction, the CPG team has input into the SR topic formulation, inclusion/exclusion criteria, and organization of the review, but it does not have control over the methods and conclusions of the final SR report (see Chapter 5). The SR team can be available to answer the CPG team's questions regarding the evidence during the drafting of the guideline. An additional example of moderate interaction is including members of the SR team on the CPG team. Some professional societies, such as the ACCP (see Box 2-4), allow both SR methodologists and clinical content experts from the CPG team to have input into preparing the SR report. Bias and COI is prevented because the SR methodologists, not the clinical content experts, have final responsibility for the interpretation and presentation of the evidence (Guyatt et al., 2010).

Sponsors of SRs

As discussed above, professional specialty societies and other private healthcare organizations, such as ACCP and NKF, often sponsor SRs to inform the development of CPGs. AHRQ and other government agencies also sponsor many SRs, as will PCORI, that are intended to inform patient and clinician decisions, but not specifically for a CPG. While an SR should respond to the sponsor's questions, the sponsor should not overly influence the SR process. The relationship between the sponsor and the SR review team needs to be carefully managed to balance the competing goals of maintaining the scientific independence of the SR team and the need for oversight to ensure the quality and timeliness of their work.

To protect the scientific integrity of the SR process from sponsor interference, the types of interactions permitted between the sponsor and SR team should be negotiated and refined before the finalization of the protocol and the undertaking of the review. The sponsor should require adherence to SR standards, but should not impose requirements that may bias the review. Examples of appropriate mechanisms for managing the relationship include oversight by qualified project officers, an independent peer review process, and the use of grants as well as contracts for funding SRs. Qualified project officers at the sponsoring organization should have knowledge and experience about how to conduct an SR and a high internal standard of respect for science, and not interfere in the conduct of the SR. An independent peer review process allows a neutral party to determine whether an SR follows appropriate scientific standards and is responsive to the needs of the sponsor. All feedback to the SR team should be firsthand via peer review. The use of grants and other mechanism to fund SRs allows the SR team to have more scientific independence in conducting the review than traditional contracts.

Sponsors should not be allowed to delay or prevent publication of an SR in a peer-reviewed journal and should not interfere with the journal's peer review process. This promotes the committee's criteria of transparency by making SR results widely available. The ICMJE publication requirements for industry-sponsored clinical trials should be extended to publicly funded SRs (ICMJE, 2007). Except where prohibited by a journal's policies, it is reasonable for the authors to provide the sponsor with a copy of the proposed journal submission, perhaps with the possibility of the sponsor offering nonbinding comments. If a paper is accepted by a journal after delivery of the final report, discrepancies between the journal article and the report may legitimately result from the journal's peer review process. The agreement between the sponsor and the SR team should give the SR team complete freedom to publish despite any resulting discrepancies.

RECOMMENDED STANDARDS FOR ENSURING USER AND STAKEHOLDER INPUT

The committee recommends two standards for ensuring user and stakeholder input in the SR process:

Standard 2.3—Ensure user and stakeholder input as the review is designed and conducted
  Required element:
      2.3.1. Protect the independence of the review team to make the final decisions about the design, analysis, and reporting of the review

Standard 2.4—Manage bias and COI for individuals providing input into the systematic review
  Required elements:
      2.4.1. Require individuals to disclose potential COI and professional or intellectual bias
      2.4.2. Exclude input from individuals whose COI or bias would diminish the credibility of the review in the eyes of the intended users

Rationale

All SR processes should include a method for collecting feedback on research questions, topic formulation, inclusion/exclusion criteria, and the organization of the SR from individuals with relevant perspectives and expertise. Users and stakeholders need not be consulted in interpreting the science, in drawing conclusions, or in conducting the technical aspects of the SR. User and stakeholder feedback can be collected through various techniques, such as a formal advisory group, the use of focus groups or structured interviews, the inclusion of users and stakeholders on the review team, or peer review. Various users and stakeholders bring different perspectives and priorities to the review, and these views should help shape the research question and outcomes to be evaluated so that they are more focused on clinical and patient-centered decision making. The EPCs, CRD, and Cochrane Collaboration experts recognize that engaging a range of users and stakeholders—such as consumers, clinicians, payers, and policy makers—is likely to make reviews of higher quality and more relevant to end users (CRD, 2009; Higgins and Green, 2008; Whitlock et al., 2010). User and stakeholder involvement is also likely to improve the credibility of the review. The type of users and stakeholders important to consult, and the decision on whether to create a formal or informal advisory group, depend on the topic and circumstances of the SR.

Getting input from relevant CPG teams (as appropriate) and SR sponsors helps to ensure that SRs are responsive to these groups' questions and needs. However, the independence of the review team needs to be protected to ensure that this feedback does not interfere with the scientific integrity of the review. This is consistent with guidance from the Cochrane Collaboration, which prohibits sponsorship by any commercial sources with financial interests in the conclusions of Cochrane reviews. It also states that sponsors should not be allowed to delay or prevent publication of a review, or interfere with the independence of the authors of reviews (The Cochrane Collaboration, 2006; Higgins and Green, 2008).

Avoiding bias and COI is as important for the users and stakeholders providing input into SR process as it is for those actually conducting the review. Individuals providing input should publicly acknowledge their potential biases and COI, and should be excluded from the review process if their participation would diminish the credibility of the review in the eyes of the intended user. In some cases, it may be possible to balance feedback from individuals with strong biases or COI across competing interests if their viewpoints are important for the review team to consider. For example, users and stakeholders with strong financial and personal connections with industry should not participate in reviews. This is consistent with the EPC guidance, which requires that participants, consultants, subcontractors, and other technical experts disclose in writing any financial and professional interests that are related to the subject matter of the review (Slutsky et al., 2010). The next edition of the CRD guidance will also make explicit that users and stakeholders should declare all biases, and steps should be taken to ensure that these do not impact the review.[7] In addition, as mentioned above, managing bias and COI is critical to transparency, credibility, and scientific rigor.

FORMULATING THE TOPIC

Informative and relevant SRs of CER require user and other stakeholder input as the review's research questions are being developed and designed. CER questions should address diverse populations of study participants, examine interventions that are feasible to implement in a variety of healthcare settings, and measure a broad range of health outcomes (IOM, 2009b). Well-formulated questions are particularly important because the questions determine many other components of the review, including the search for studies, data extraction, synthesis, and presentation of findings (Counsell, 1997; Higgins and Green, 2008; IOM, 2008; Liberati et al., 2009).

Topic formulation, however, is a challenging process that often takes more time than expected. The research question should be precise so that the review team can structure the other components of the SR. To inform decision making, research questions should focus on the uncertainties that underlie disagreement in practice, and the outcomes and interventions that are of interest to patients and clinicians. Also important is ensuring that the research questions are addressing novel issues, and not duplicating existing SRs or other ongoing reviews (CRD, 2009; Whitlock et al., 2010).

Structured Questions

Well-formulated SR questions use a structured format to improve the scientific rigor of an SR, such as the PICO(TS) mnemonic: population, intervention, comparator, outcomes, timing, and

---

[7] Personal communication with Lesley Stewart, Director, CRD (March 15, 2010).

TABLE 2-2 PICO Format for Formulating an Evidence Question

PICO Component	Tips for Building Question	Example
Patient population or problem	"How would I describe this group of patients?" Balance precision with brevity	"In patients with heart failure from dilated cardiomyopathy who are in sinus rhythm . . . "
Intervention (a cause, prognostic factor, treatment, etc.)	"Which main intervention is of interest?" Be specific	" . . . would adding anti-coagulation with warfarin to standard heart failure therapy . . . "
Comparison intervention (if necessary)	"What is the main alternative to be compared with the intervention?" Be specific	" . . . when compared with standard therapy alone . . . "
Outcomes	"What do I hope the intervention will accomplish?" "What could this exposure really affect?" Be specific	" . . . lead to lower mortality or morbidity from thromboembolism? Is this enough to be worth the increased risk of bleeding?"

SOURCE: Adapted from the *Evidence-based Practice Center Partner's Guide* (AHRQ, 2009).

setting (Counsell, 1997; IOM, 2008; Richardson et al., 1995; Whitlock et al., 2010).[8] Table 2-2 provides an example.

Identifying the population requires selecting the disease or condition of interest as well as specifying whether the review will focus on a specific subpopulation of individuals (e.g., by age, disease severity, existence of comorbidities). If there is good reason to believe a treatment may work differently in diverse subpopulations, the review protocol should structure the review so that these populations are examined separately. Focusing SRs on subgroups, such as individuals with comorbidities, can help to identify patients who are likely to benefit from an intervention in real-world clinical situations. SRs may address conditions and diseases that have the greatest impact on the health of the U.S. population, or on conditions and diseases that disproportionately and seriously affect subgroups and underserved members of the populations (IOM, 2009b).

---

[8] Some producers of SR have expanded PICO to PICOS or PICOTS, with "T" standing for timing and "S" standing for either "study design" or "setting."

For an SR to meet the definition of CER, it should compare at least two alternative interventions, treatments, or systems of care (IOM, 2009b). The interventions and comparators should enable patients and clinicians to balance the benefits and harms of potential treatment options. Cherkin and colleagues, for example, compared three treatment alternatives of interest to patients with lower back pain: physical therapy, chiropractic care, and self-care (Cherkin et al., 1998). The study found minimal differences between the treatments in terms of numbers of days of reduced activity or missed work, or in recurrences of back pain.

The SR should seek to address all outcomes that are important to patients and clinicians, including benefits, possible adverse effects, quality of life, symptom severity, satisfaction, and economic outcomes (IOM, 2009b; Schünemann et al., 2006; Tunis et al., 2003). Patients faced with choosing among alternative prostate cancer treatments, for example, may want to know not only prognosis, but also potential adverse effects such as urinary incontinence and impotence. The SR team should obtain a wide range of views about what outcomes are important to patients (Whitlock et al., 2010). Whether or not every outcome important to patients can actually be addressed in the review depends on whether those outcomes have been included in the primary studies.

If the research question includes timing of the outcome assessment and setting, this helps set the context for the SR. It also narrows the question, however, and the evidence examined is limited as a result. The timing should indicate the time of the intervention and of the follow-up, and the setting should indicate primary or specialty care, inpatient or outpatient treatment, and any cointerventions (Whitlock et al., 2010).

Analytic Framework

An analytic framework (also called "logic framework") is helpful to developing and refining the SR topic, especially when more than one question is being asked. It should clearly define the relevant patient and contextual factors that might influence the outcomes or treatment effects and lay out the chain of logic underlying the mechanism by which each intervention may improve health outcomes (Harris et al., 2001; IOM, 2008; Mulrow et al., 1997; Sawaya et al., 2007; Whitlock et al., 2002; Woolf et al., 1996). This visual representation of the question clarifies the researchers' assumptions about the relationships among the intervention, the intermediate outcomes (e.g., changes in levels of blood pressure or bone density),

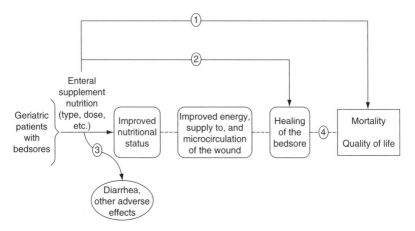

FIGURE 2-1 Analytic framework for a new enteral supplement to heal bedsores.
SOURCE: Helfand and Balshem (2010).

and health outcomes (e.g., myocardial infarction and strokes). It can also help clarify the researchers' implicit beliefs about the benefits of a healthcare intervention, such as quality of life, morbidity, and mortality (Helfand and Balshem, 2010). It increases the likelihood that all contributing elements in the causal chain will be examined and evaluated. However, the analytic framework diagram may need to evolve to accurately represent SRs of CER that compare alternative treatments and interventions.

Figure 2-1 shows an analytic framework for evaluating studies of a new enteral supplement to heal bedsores (Helfand and Balshem, 2010). On the left side of the analytic framework is the population of interest: geriatric patients with bedsores. Moving from left to right across the framework is the intervention (enteral supplement nutrition), intermediate outcomes (improved nutritional status, improved energy/blood supply to the wound, and healing of the bedsore), and final health outcomes of interest (reduction in mortality, quality of life). The lines with arrows represent the researchers' questions that the evidence must answer at each phase of the review. The dotted lines indicate that the association between the intermediate outcomes and final health outcomes are unproven, and need to be linked by evaluating several bodies of evidence. The squiggly line denotes the question that addresses the harms of the intervention (e.g., diarrhea or other adverse effects). In this example, the lines and arrows represent the following key research questions:

Line 1   Does enteral supplementation improve mortality and quality of life?

Line 2   Does enteral supplementation improve wound healing?

Line 3   How frequent and severe are side effects such as diarrhea?

Line 4   Is wound healing associated with improved survival and quality of life?

Evidence that directly links the intervention to the final health outcome is the most influential (Arrow 1). Arrows 2 and 4 link the treatments to the final outcomes *in*directly: from treatment to an intermediate outcome, and then, separately, from the intermediate outcome to the final health outcomes. The nutritional status and improved energy/blood supply to the wound are only important outcomes if they are in the causal pathway to improved healing, reduced mortality, and a better quality of life. The analytic framework does not have corresponding arrows to these intermediate outcomes because studies measuring these outcomes would only be included in the SR if they linked the intermediate outcome to healing, mortality, or quality of life.

RECOMMENDED STANDARDS FOR FORMULATING THE TOPIC

The importance of the research questions and analytic framework in determining the entire review process demands a rigorous approach to topic formulation. The committee recommends the following standard:

Standard 2.5—Formulate the topic for the systematic review
   Required elements:
   2.5.1   Confirm the need for a new review
   2.5.2   Develop an analytic framework that clearly lays out the chain of logic that links the health intervention to the outcomes of interest and defines the key clinical questions to be addressed by the systematic review
   2.5.3   Use a standard format to articulate each clinical question of interest
   2.5.4   State the rationale for each clinical question
   2.5.5   Refine each question based on user and stakeholder input

Rationale

SRs of CER should focus on specific research questions using a structured format (e.g., PICO[TS]), an analytic framework, and a clear rationale for the research question. Expert guidance recommends using the PICO(TS) acronym to articulate research questions (CRD, 2009; Higgins and Green, 2008; Whitlock et al., 2010). Developing an analytic framework is required by the EPCs to illustrate the chain of logic underlying the research questions (AHRQ, 2007; Helfand and Balshem, 2010; IOM, 2008). Using a structured approach and analytic framework also improves the scientific rigor and transparency of the review by requiring the review team to clearly articulate the clinical questions and basic assumptions in the SR.

The AHRQ EPC program, CRD, and the Cochrane Collaboration all have mechanisms for ensuring that new reviews cover novel and important topics. AHRQ, for example, specifically requires that topics have strong potential for improving health outcomes (Whitlock et al., 2010). CRD recommends that researchers undertaking reviews first search for existing or ongoing reviews and evaluate the quality of any reviews on similar topics (CRD, 2009). The Cochrane Collaboration review groups require approval by the "coordinating editor" (editor in chief) of the relevant review group for new SRs (Higgins and Green, 2008). Confirming the need for a new review is consistent with the committee's criterion of efficiency because it prevents the burden and cost of conducting an unnecessary, duplicative SR (unless the "duplication" is considered necessary to improve on earlier efforts). If the SR registries now in development become fully operational, this requirement will become much easier for the review team to achieve in the near future (CRD, 2010; HHS, 2010; Joanna Briggs Institute, 2010; NPAF, 2011; PIPC, 2011).

DEVELOPING THE SYSTEMATIC REVIEW PROTOCOL

The SR protocol is a detailed description of the objectives and methods of the review (CRD, 2009; Higgins and Green, 2008; Liberati et al., 2009). The protocol should include information regarding the context and rationale for the review, primary outcomes of interest, search strategy, inclusion/exclusion criteria, data synthesis strategy, and other aspects of the research plan. The major challenge to writing a comprehensive research protocol is accurately specifying the research questions and methods before the study begins. Developing the protocol is an iterative process that requires communication with users and stakeholders, input from the general public, and a preliminary review of the literature before all of the components of the protocol are finalized (CRD, 2009). Researchers' decisions to undertake an SR may be influenced by prior knowledge of results of available studies. The inclusion of multiple perspectives on the review team and gathering user and stakeholder input helps prevent choices in the protocol that are based on such prior knowledge.

The use of protocols in SRs is increasing, but is still not standard practice. A survey of SRs indexed in MEDLINE in November, 2004 found that 46 percent of the reviews reported using a protocol (Moher et al., 2007), a significant rise from only 7 percent of reviews in an earlier survey (Sacks et al., 1987).

Publication of the Protocol

A protocol should be made publicly available at the start of an SR in order to prevent the effects of author bias, allow feedback at an early stage in the SR, and tell readers of the review about protocol changes that occur as the SR develops. It also gives the public the chance to examine how well the SR team has used input from consumers, clinicians, and other experts to develop the questions and PICO(TS) the review will address. In addition, a publicly available protocol has the benefit that other researchers can identify ongoing reviews, and thus avoids unnecessary duplication and encourages collaboration. This transparency may provide an opportunity for methodological and other research (see Chapter 6) (CRD, 2010).

One of the most efficient ways to publish protocols is through an SR protocol electronic registration. However, more than 80 percent of SRs are conducted by organizations that do not have existing registries (CRD, 2010). The Cochrane Collaboration and AHRQ have created their own infrastructure for publishing protocols (Higgins and Green, 2008; Slutsky et al., 2010). Review teams conducting SRs funded through PCORI[9] will also be required to post research protocols on a government website at the outset of the SR process.

Several electronic registries under development intend to publish all SR protocols, regardless of the funding source (CRD, 2010; Joanna Briggs Institute, 2010). CRD is developing an international registry of ongoing health-related SRs that will be open to all prospective registrations and will offer free public access for electronic searching. Each research protocol will be assigned a unique identifi-

---

[9] *The Patient Protection and Affordable Care Act*, Public Law 111-148, 111th Cong., Subtitle D, § 6301 (March 23, 2010).

cation number, and an audit trail of amendments will be part of each protocol's record. The protocol records will also link to the resulting publication. The Preferred Reporting Items for Systematic Reviews and Meta-Analyses (PRISMA) Statement reflects the growing recognition of the importance of prospective registration of protocols, and requires that published SRs indicate whether a review protocol exists and if and where it can accessed (e.g., web address), and the registration information and number (Liberati et al., 2009).

Amendments to the Protocol

Often the review team needs to make amendments to a protocol after the start of the review that result from the researchers' improved understanding of the research questions or the availability of pertinent evidence (CRD, 2009; Higgins and Green, 2008; Liberati et al., 2009). Common amendments include extending the period of the search to include older or newer studies, broadening eligibility criteria, and adding new analyses suggested by the primary analysis (Liberati et al., 2009). Researchers should document such amendments with an explanation for the change in the protocol and completed review (CRD, 2009; Higgins and Green, 2008; Liberati et al., 2009).

In general, researchers should not modify the protocol based on knowledge of the results of analyses. This has the potential to bias the SR, for example, if the SR omits a prespecified comparison when the data indicate that an intervention is more or less effective than the retained comparisons. Similar problems occur when researchers modify the protocol by adding or deleting certain study designs or outcome measures, or change the search strategy based on prior knowledge of the data. Researchers may be motivated to delete an outcome when its results do not match the results of the other outcome measures (Silagy et al., 2002), or to add an outcome that had not been prespecified. Publishing the protocol and amendments allows readers to track the changes and judge whether an amendment has biased the review. The final SR report should also identify those analyses that were prespecified and those that were not, and any analyses requested by peer reviewers (see Chapter 5).

RECOMMENDED STANDARDS FOR DEVELOPING THE SYSTEMATIC REVIEW PROTOCOL

The committee recommends three standards related to the SR protocol:

Standard 2.6—Develop a systematic review protocol
Required elements:
- 2.6.1 Describe the context and rationale for the review from both a decision-making and research perspective
- 2.6.2 Describe the study screening and selection criteria (inclusion/exclusion criteria)
- 2.6.3 Describe precisely which outcome measures, time points, interventions, and comparison groups will be addressed
- 2.6.4 Describe the search strategy for identifying relevant evidence
- 2.6.5 Describe the procedures for study selection
- 2.6.6 Describe the data extraction strategy
- 2.6.7 Describe the process for identifying and resolving disagreement between researchers in study selection and data extraction decisions
- 2.6.8 Describe the approach to critically appraising individual studies
- 2.6.9 Describe the method for evaluating the body of evidence, including the quantitative and qualitative synthesis strategy
- 2.6.10 Describe and justify any planned analyses of differential treatment effects according to patient subgroups, how an intervention is delivered, or how an outcome is measured
- 2.6.11 Describe the proposed timetable for conducting the review

Standard 2.7—Submit the protocol for peer review
Required element:
- 2.7.1 Provide a public comment period for the protocol and publicly report on disposition of comments

Standard 2.8—Make the final protocol publicly available, and add any amendments to the protocol in a timely fashion

Rationale

The majority of these required elements are consistent with leading guidance, and ensure that the protocol provides a detailed description of the objectives and methods of the review (AHRQ,

2009; CRD, 2009; Higgins and Green, 2008).[10] The committee added the requirement to identify and justify planned subgroup analyses to examine whether treatment effects vary according to patient group, the method of providing the intervention, or the approach to measuring an outcome, because evidence on variability in treatment effects across subpopulations is key to directing interventions to the most appropriate populations. The legislation establishing PCORI requires that "research shall be designed, as appropriate, to take into account the potential for differences in the effectiveness of health-care treatments, services, and items as used with various subpopulations, such as racial and ethnic minorities, women, age, and groups of individuals with different comorbidities, genetic and molecular subtypes, or quality of life preferences."[11] The protocol should state a hypothesis that justifies the planned subgroup analyses, including the direction of the suspected subgroup effects, to reduce the possibility of identifying false subgroup effects. The subgroup analyses should also be limited to a small number of hypothesized effects (Sun et al., 2010). The committee also added the requirement that the protocol include the proposed timetable for conducting the review because this improves the transparency, efficiency, and timeliness of publicly funded SRs.

The draft protocol should be reviewed by clinical and methodological experts as well as relevant users and stakeholders identified by the review team and sponsor. For publicly funded reviews, the public should also have the opportunity to comment on the protocol to improve the acceptability and transparency of the SR process. The review team should be responsive to peer reviewers and public comments and publicly report on the disposition of the comments. The review team need not provide a public response to every question; it can group questions into general topic areas for response. The period for peer review and public comment should be specified so that the review process does not delay the entire SR process.

Cochrane requires peer review of protocols (Higgins and Green, 2008). The EPC program requires that the SR research questions and protocol be available for public comment (Whitlock et al., 2010).[12] All of the leading guidance requires that the final protocol be pub-

---

[10] The elements are all discussed in more detail in Chapters 3 through 5.

[11] *The Patient Protection and Affordable Care Act*, Public Law 111-148, 111th Cong., Subtitle D, § 6301(d)(2)(D) (March 23, 2010).

[12] Information on making the protocol public comes from Mark Helfand, Director, Oregon Evidence-Based Practice Center, Professor of Medicine and Medical Informatics and Clinical Epidemiology, Oregon Health and Science University, Portland, Oregon.

licly available (CRD, 2009; Higgins and Green, 2008; Whitlock et al., 2010).

REFERENCES

AHRQ (Agency for Healthcare Research and Quality). 2007. *Methods reference guide for effectiveness and comparative effectiveness reviews, Version 1.0.* Rockville, MD: AHRQ.

AHRQ. 2009. *AHRQ Evidence-based Practice Centers partner's guide.* Rockville, MD: AHRQ.

AHRQ. 2010. *Reinvestment Act investments in comparative effectiveness research for a citizen forum.* Rockville, MD: AHRQ. http://ftp.ahrq.gov/fund/cerfactsheets/cerfsforum.htm (accessed August 30, 2010).

Andejeski, Y., E. S. Breslau, E. Hart, N. Lythcott, L. Alexander, I. Rich, I. Bisceglio, H. S. Smith, and F. M. Visco. 2002. Benefits and drawbacks of including consumer reviewers in the scientific merit review of breast cancer research. *Journal of Women's Health & Gender-Based Medicine* 11(2):119–136.

Atkins, D. 2007. Creating and synthesizing evidence with decision makers in mind: Integrating evidence from clinical trials and other study designs. *Medical Care* 45(10 Suppl 2):S16–S22.

Ayanian, J. Z., M. B. Landrum, S. T. Normand, E. Guadagnoli, and B. J. McNeil. 1998. Rating the appropriateness of coronary angiography—Do practicing physicians agree with an expert panel and with each other? *New England Journal of Medicine* 338(26):1896–1904.

Bastian, H. 2005. Consumer and researcher collaboration in trials: Filling the gaps. *Clinical Trials* 2(1):3–4.

Blum, J. A., K. Freeman, R. C. Dart, and R. J. Cooper. 2009. Requirements and definitions in conflict of interest policies of medical journals. *JAMA* 302(20):2230–2234.

Boote, J., R. Telford, and C. Cooper. 2002. Consumer involvement in health research: A review and research agenda. *Health Policy* 61(2):213–236.

Cherkin, D. C., R. A. Deyo, M. Battié, J. Street, and W. Barlow. 1998. A comparison of physical therapy, chiropractic manipulation, and provision of an educational booklet for the treatment of patients with low back pain. *New England Journal of Medicine* 339(15):1021–1029.

Chimonas, S., Z. Frosch, and D. J. Rothman. 2011. From disclosure to transparency: The use of company payment data. *Archives of Internal Medicine* 171(1):81–86.

The Cochrane Collaboration. 2006. *Commercial sponsorship and The Cochrane Collaboration.* http://www.cochrane.org/about-us/commercial-sponsorship (accessed January 11, 2011).

Counsell, C. 1997. Formulating questions and locating primary studies for inclusion in systematic reviews. *Annals of Internal Medicine* 127(5):380–387.

CRD (Centre for Reviews and Dissemination). 2009. *Systematic reviews: CRD's guidance for undertaking reviews in health care.* York, UK: York Publishing Services, Ltd.

CRD. 2010. *Register of ongoing systematic reviews.* http://www.york.ac.uk/inst/crd/projects/register.htm (accessed June 17, 2010).

Drazen, J., M. B. Van Der Weyden, P. Sahni, J. Rosenberg, A. Marusic, C. Laine, S. Kotzin, R. Horton, P. C. Hebert, C. Haug, F. Godlee, F. A. Frozelle, P. W. Leeuw, and C. D. DeAngelis. 2009. Uniform format for disclosure of competing interests in ICMJE journals. *New England Journal of Medicine* 361(19):1896–1897.

Drazen, J. M., P. W. de Leeuw, C. Laine, C. D. Mulrow, C. D. DeAngelis, F. A. Frizelle, F. Godlee, C. Haug, P. C. Hébert, A. James, S. Kotzin, A. Marusic, H. Reyes, J. Rosenberg, P. Sahni, M. B. Van Der Weyden, and G. Zhaori. 2010. Toward more uniform conflict disclosures: The updated ICMJE conflict of interest reporting form. *Annals of Internal Medicine* 153(4):268–269.

Entwistle, V. A., M. J. Renfrew, S. Yearley, J. Forrester, and T. Lamont. 1998. Lay perspectives: Advantages for health research. *BMJ* 316(7129):463–466.

Fretheim, A., H. J. Schünemann, and A. D. Oxman. 2006a. Improving the use of research evidence in guideline development: Group composition and consultation process. *Health Research Policy and Systems* 4:15.

Fretheim, A., H. J. Schünemann, and A. D. Oxman. 2006b. Improving the use of research evidence in guideline development: Group processes. *Health Research Policy and Systems* 4:17.

Guyatt, G., E. A. Akl, J. Hirsh, C. Kearon, M. Crowther, D. Gutterman, S. Z. Lewis, I. Nathanson, R. Jaeschke, and H. Schünemann. 2010. The vexing problem of guidelines and conflict of interest: A potential solution. *Annals of Internal Medicine* 152(11):738–741.

Harris, R. P., M. Helfand, S. H. Woolf, K. N. Lohr, C. D. Mulrow, S. M. Teutsch, D. Atkins, and Methods Work Group Third U. S. Preventive Services Task Force. 2001. Current methods of the U.S. Preventive Services Task Force: A review of the process. *American Journal of Preventive Medicine* 20(Suppl 3): 21–35.

Helfand, M., and H. Balshem. 2010. AHRQ Series Paper 2: Principles for developing guidance: AHRQ and the Effective Health-Care Program. *Journal of Clinical Epidemiology* 63(5):484–490.

HHS (Department of Health and Human Services). 2010. Request for Information on development of an inventory of comparative effectiveness research. *Federal Register* 75 (137):41867–41868.

Higgins, J. P. T., and S. Green, eds. 2008. *Cochrane handbook for systematic reviews of interventions.* Chichester, UK: John Wiley & Sons.

Hutchings, A., and R. Raine. 2006. A systematic review of factors affecting the judgments produced by formal consensus development methods in health care. *Journal of Health Services Research & Policy* 11(3):172–179.

ICMJE (International Committee of Medical Journal Editors). 2007. *Sponsorship, authorship, and accountability.* http://www.icmje.org/update_sponsor.html (accessed September 8, 2010).

ICMJE. 2010. *ICMJE uniform disclosure form for potential conflicts of interest.* http://www.icmje.org/coi_disclosure.pdf (accessed January 11, 2011).

IOM (Institute of Medicine). 2005. *Getting to know the committee process.* Washington, DC: The National Academies Press.

IOM. 2008. *Knowing what works in health care: A roadmap for the nation.* Edited by J. Eden, B. Wheatley, B. McNeil, and H. Sox. Washington, DC: The National Academies Press.

IOM. 2009a. *Conflict of interest in medical research, education, and practice.* Edited by B. Lo and M. Field. Washington, DC: The National Academies Press.

IOM. 2009b. *Initial national priorities for comparative effectiveness research.* Washington, DC: The National Academies Press.

Joanna Briggs Institute. 2010. *Protocols and works in progress.* Adelaide, Australia: The Joanna Briggs Institute. http://www.joannabriggs.edu.au/pubs/systematic_reviews_prot.php (accessed June 17, 2010).

Kahan, J. P., R. E. Park, L. L. Leape, S. J. Bernstein, L. H. Hilborne, L. Parker, C. J. Kamberg, D. J. Ballard, and R. H. Brooke. 1996. Variations in specialty in physician ratings of the appropriateness and necessity of indications for procedures. *Medical Care* 34(6):512–523.

KDIGO (Kidney Disease: Improving Global Outcomes). 2010. *Clinical practice guidelines.* http://www.kdigo.org/clinical_practice_guidelines/guideline_development_process.php (accessed July 16, 2010).

Lavis, J., H. Davies, A. Oxman, J. L. Denis, K. Golden-Biddle, and E. Ferlie. 2005. Towards systematic reviews that inform health care management and policy-making. *Journal of Health Services Research & Policy* 10(Suppl 1):35–48.

Liberati, A., D. G. Altman, J. Tetzlaff, C. Mulrow, P. C. Gotzsche, J. Ioannidis, M. Clarke, P. J. Devereaux, J. Kleijnen, and D. Moher. 2009. The PRISMA statement for reporting systematic reviews and meta-analyses of studies that evaluate health care interventions: Explanation and elaboration. *Annals of Internal Medicine* 151(4):W1–W30.

McPartland, J. M. 2009. Obesity, the endocannabinoid system, and bias arising from pharmaceutical sponsorship. *PLoS One* 4(3):e5092.

Moher, D., J. Tetzlaff, A. C. Tricco, M. Sampson, and D. G. Altman. 2007. Epidemiology and reporting characteristics of systematic reviews. *PLoS Medicine* 4(3): 447–455.

Mulrow, C., P. Langhorne, and J. Grimshaw. 1997. Integrating heterogeneous pieces of evidence in systematic reviews. *Annals of Internal Medicine* 127(11):989–995.

Murphy, M. K., N. A. Black, D. L. Lamping, C. M. McKee, C. F. Sanderson, J. Askham, and T. Marteur. 1998. Consensus development methods, and their use in clinical guideline development. *Health Technology Assessment* 2(3):1–88.

NIH (National Institutes of Health). 2010. *The NIH Consensus Development Program.* Kensington, MD: NIH Consensus Development Program Information Center. http://consensus.nih.gov/aboutcdp.htm (accessed July 16, 2010).

NPAF (National Patient Advocate Foundation). 2011. *National Patient Advocate Foundation launches Comparative Effectiveness Research (CER) Database.* http://www.npaf.org/images/pdf/news/NPAF_CER_010611.pdf (accessed February 1, 2011).

Oxman, A., and G. Guyatt. 1993. The science of reviewing research. *Annals of the New York Academy of Sciences* 703:125–133.

Pagliari, C., and J. Grimshaw. 2002. Impact of group structure and process on multidisciplinary evidence-based guideline development: An observational study. *Journal of Evaluation in Clinical Practice* 8(2):145–153.

PIPC (Partnership to Improve Patient Care). 2011. *Welcome to the CER Inventory.* http://www.cerinventory.org/ (accessed February 1, 2011).

Richardson, W. S., M. S. Wilson, J. Mishikawa, and R. S. A. Hayward. 1995. The well-built clinical question: A key to evidence based decisions. *ACP Journal Club* 123(3):A12–A13.

Rockey, S. J., and F. S. Collins. 2010. Managing financial conflict of interest in biomedical research. *JAMA* 303(23):2400–2402.

Roundtree, A. K., M. A. Kallen, M. A. Lopez-Olivo, B. Kimmel, B. Skidmore, Z. Ortiz, V. Cox, and M. E. Suarez-Almazor. 2008. Poor reporting of search strategy and conflict of interest in over 250 narrative and systematic reviews of two biologic agents in arthritis: A systematic review. *Journal of Clinical Epidemiology* 62(2):128–137.

Sacks, H. S., J. Berrier, D. Reitman, V. A. Ancona-Berk, and T. C. Chalmers. 1987. Metaanalyses of randomized controlled trials. *New England Journal of Medicine* 316(8):450–455.

Sawaya, G. F., J. Guirguis-Blake, M. LeFevre, R. Harris, D. Petitti, and for the U.S. Preventive Services Task Force. 2007. Update on the methods of the U.S. Preventive Services Task Force: Estimating certainty and magnitude of net benefit. *Annals of Internal Medicine* 147(12):871–875.

Schünemann, H. J., A. Fretheim, and A. D. Oxman. 2006. Improving the use of research evidence in guideline development: Grading evidence and recommendations. *Health Research Policy Systems* 4:21.

Shrier, I., J. Boivin, R. Platt, R. Steele, J. Brophy, F. Carnevale, M. Eisenberg, A. Furlan, R. Kakuma, M. Macdonald, L. Pilote, and M. Rossignol. 2008. The interpretation of systematic reviews with meta-analyses: An objective or subjective process? *BMC Medical Informatics and Decision Making* 8(1):19.

Silagy, C. A., P. Middelton, and S. Hopewell. 2002. Publishing protocols of systematic reviews: Comparing what was done to what was planned. *JAMA* 287(21):2831–2834.

Slutsky, J., D. Atkins, S. Chang, and B. Collins Sharp. 2010. AHRQ Series Paper 1: Comparing medical interventions: AHRQ and the Effective Health-Care Program. *Journal of Clinical Epidemiology* 63(5):481–483.

Srivastava, R., C. Norlin, B. C. James, S. Muret-Wagstaff, P. C. Young, and A. Auerbach. 2005. Community and hospital-based physicians' attitudes regarding pediatric hospitalist systems. *Pediatrics* 115(1):34–38.

Sun, X., M. Briel, S. Walter, and G. Guyatt. 2010. Is a subgroup effect believable? Updating criteria to evaluate the credibility of subgroup analyses. *BMJ* 340:c117.

Tunis, S., D. Stryer, and C. M. Clancy. 2003. Practical clinical trial: Increasing the value of clinical research for decision making in clinical and health policy. *JAMA* 290(12):1624–1632.

Whitlock, E. P., C. T. Orleans, N. Pender, and J. Allan. 2002. Evaluating primary care behavioral counseling interventions: An evidence-based approach. *American Journal of Preventive Medicine* 22(4):267–284.

Whitlock, E. P., S. A. Lopez, S. Chang, M. Helfand, M. Eder, and N. Floyd. 2010. AHRQ Series Paper 3: Identifying, selecting, and refining topics for comparative effectiveness systematic reviews: AHRQ and the Effective Health-Care Program. *Journal of Clinical Epidemiology* 63(5):491–501.

Woolf, S. H., C. G. DiGuiseppi, D. Atkins, and D. B. Kamerow. 1996. Developing evidence-based clinical practice guidelines: Lessons learned by the U.S. Preventive Services Task Force. *Annual Review of Public Health* 17:511–538.

3

Standards for Finding and Assessing Individual Studies

Abstract: *This chapter addresses the identification, screening, data collection, and appraisal of the individual studies that make up a systematic review's (SR's) body of evidence. The committee recommends six related standards. The search should be comprehensive and include both published and unpublished research. The potential for bias to enter the selection process is significant and well documented. Without appropriate measures to counter the biased reporting of primary evidence from clinical trials and observational studies, SRs will reflect and possibly exacerbate existing distortions in the biomedical literature. The review team should document the search process and keep track of the decisions that are made for each article. Quality assurance and control are critical during data collection and extraction because of the substantial potential for errors. At least two review team members, working independently, should screen and select studies and extract quantitative and other critical data from included studies. Each eligible study should be systematically appraised for risk of bias; relevance to the study's populations, interventions, and outcomes measures; and fidelity of the implementation of the interventions.*

The search for evidence and critical assessment of the individual studies identified are the core of a systematic review (SR).

These SR steps require meticulous execution and documentation to minimize the risk of a biased synthesis of evidence. Current practice falls short of recommended guidance and thus results in a meaningful proportion of reviews that are of poor quality (Golder et al., 2008; Moher et al., 2007a; Yoshii et al., 2009). An extensive literature documents that many SRs provide scant, if any, documentation of their search and screening methods. SRs often fail to acknowledge or address the risk of reporting biases, neglect to appraise the quality of individual studies included in the review, and are subject to errors during data extraction and the meta-analysis (Cooper et al., 2006; Delaney et al., 2007; Edwards et al., 2002; Golder et al., 2008; Gøtzsche et al., 2007; Horton et al., 2010; Jones et al., 2005; Lundh et al., 2009; Moher et al., 2007a; Roundtree et al., 2008; Tramer et al., 1997). The conduct of the search for and selection of evidence may have serious implications for patients' and clinicians' decisions. An SR might lead to the wrong conclusions and, ultimately, the wrong clinical recommendations, if relevant data are missed, errors are uncorrected, or unreliable research is used (Dickersin, 1990; Dwan et al., 2008; Glanville et al., 2006; Gluud, 2006; Kirkham et al., 2010; Turner et al., 2008).

In this chapter, the committee recommends methodological standards for the steps involved in identifying and assessing the individual studies that make up an SR's body of evidence: planning and conducting the search for studies, screening and selecting studies, managing data collection from eligible studies, and assessing the quality of individual studies. The committee focused on steps to minimize bias and to promote scientifically rigorous SRs based on evidence (when available), expert guidance, and thoughtful reasoning. The recommended standards set a high bar that will be challenging for many SR teams. However, the available evidence does not suggest that it is safe to cut corners if resources are limited. These best practices should be thoughtfully considered by anyone conducting an SR. It is especially important that the SR is transparent in reporting what methods were used and why.

Each standard consists of two parts: first, a brief statement describing the related SR step and, second, one or more elements of performance that are fundamental to carrying out the step. Box 3-1 lists all of the chapter's recommended standards.

Note that, as throughout this report, the chapter's references to "expert guidance" refer to the published methodological advice of the Agency for Healthcare Research and Quality (AHRQ) Effective Health Care Program, the Centre for Reviews and Dissemination (CRD) (University of York), and the Cochrane Collaboration.

Appendix E contains a detailed summary of expert guidance on this chapter's topics.

THE SEARCH PROCESS

When healthcare decision makers turn to SRs to learn the potential benefits and harms of alternative health care therapies, it is with the expectation that the SR will provide a complete picture of all that is known about an intervention. Research is relevant to individual decision making, whether it reveals benefits, harms, or lack of effectiveness of a health intervention. Thus, the overarching objective of the SR search for evidence is to identify all the studies (and all the relevant data from the studies) that may pertain to the research question and analytic framework. The task is a challenging one. Hundreds of thousands of research articles are indexed in bibliographic databases each year. Yet despite the enormous volume of published research, a substantial proportion of effectiveness data are never published or are not easy to access. For example, approximately 50 percent of studies appearing as conference abstracts are never fully published (Scherer et al., 2007), and some studies are not even reported as conference abstracts. Even when there are published reports of effectiveness studies, the studies often report only a subset of the relevant data. Furthermore, it is well documented that the data reported may not represent all the findings on an intervention's effectiveness because of pervasive reporting bias in the biomedical literature. Moreover, crucial information from the studies is often difficult to locate because it is kept in researchers' files, government agency records, or manufacturers' proprietary records.

The following overview further describes the context for the SR search process: the nature of the reporting bias in the biomedical literature; key sources of information on comparative effectiveness; and expert guidance on how to plan and conduct the search. The committee's related standards are presented at the end of the section.

Planning the Search

The search strategy should be an integral component of the research protocol[1] that specifies procedures for finding the evidence directly relevant to the SR. Items described in the protocol include,

---

[1] See Chapter 2 for the committee's recommended standards for establishing the research protocol.

BOX 3-1
Recommended Standards for Finding and
Assessing Individual Studies

Standard 3.1 Conduct a comprehensive systematic search for evidence
  Required elements:
    3.1.1 Work with a librarian or other information specialist trained
           in performing systematic reviews (SRs) to plan the search
           strategy
    3.1.2 Design the search strategy to address each key research
           question
    3.1.3 Use an independent librarian or other information special-
           ist to peer review the search strategy
    3.1.4 Search bibliographic databases
    3.1.5 Search citation indexes
    3.1.6 Search literature cited by eligible studies
    3.1.7 Update the search at intervals appropriate to the pace of
           generation of new information for the research question
           being addressed
    3.1.8 Search subject-specific databases if other databases are
           unlikely to provide all relevant evidence
    3.1.9 Search regional bibliographic databases if other data-
           bases are unlikely to provide all relevant evidence

Standard 3.2 Take action to address potentially biased reporting of
research results
  Required elements:
    3.2.1 Search grey-literature databases, clinical trial registries,
           and other sources of unpublished information about
           studies
    3.2.2 Invite researchers to clarify information related to study
           eligibility, study characteristics, and risk of bias
    3.2.3 Invite all study sponsors to submit unpublished data, in-
           cluding unreported outcomes, for possible inclusion in the
           systematic review
    3.2.4 Handsearch selected journals and conference abstracts
    3.2.5 Conduct a web search
    3.2.6 Search for studies reported in languages other than En-
           glish if appropriate

Standard 3.3 Screen and select studies
  Required elements:
    3.3.1 Include or exclude studies based on the protocol's pre-
           specified criteria

3.3.2 Use observational studies in addition to randomized clinical trials to evaluate harms of interventions

3.3.3 Use two or more members of the review team, working independently, to screen and select studies

3.3.4 Train screeners using written documentation; test and re-test screeners to improve accuracy and consistency

3.3.5 Use one of two strategies to select studies: (1) read all full-text articles identified in the search or (2) screen titles and abstracts of all articles and then read the full text of articles identified in initial screening.

3.3.6 Taking account of the risk of bias, consider using observational studies to address gaps in the evidence from randomized clinical trials on the benefits of interventions

Standard 3.4 Document the search

Required elements:

3.4.1 Provide a line-by-line description of the search strategy, including the date of every search for each database, web browser, etc.

3.4.2 Document the disposition of each report identified including reasons for their exclusion if appropriate

Standard 3.5 Manage data collection

Required elements:

3.5.1 At a minimum, use two or more researchers, working independently, to extract quantitative and other critical data from each study. For other types of data, one individual could extract the data while the second individual independently checks for accuracy and completeness. Establish a fair procedure for resolving discrepancies—do not simply give final decision-making power to the senior reviewer

3.5.2 Link publications from the same study to avoid including data from the same study more than once

3.5.3 Use standard data extraction forms developed for the specific systematic review

3.5.4 Pilot-test the data extraction forms and process

Standard 3.6 Critically appraise each study

Required elements:

3.6.1 Systematically assess the risk of bias, using predefined criteria

3.6.2 Assess the relevance of the study's populations, interventions, and outcome measures

3.6.3 Assess the fidelity of the implementation of interventions

but are not limited to, the study question; the criteria for a study's inclusion in the review (including language and year of report, publication status, and study design restrictions, if any); the databases, journals, and other sources to be searched for evidence; and the search strategy (e.g., sequence of database thesaurus terms, text words, methods of handsearching).

Expertise in Searching

A librarian or other qualified information specialist with training or experience in conducting SRs should work with the SR team to design the search strategy to ensure appropriate translation of the research question into search concepts, correct choice of Boolean operators and line numbers, appropriate translation of the search strategy for each database, relevant subject headings, and appropriate application and spelling of terms (Sampson and McGowan, 2006). The Cochrane Collaboration includes an Information Retrieval Methods Group[2] that provides a valuable resource for information specialists seeking a professional group with learning opportunities.

Expert guidance recommends that an experienced librarian or information specialist with training in SR search methods should also be involved in performing the search (CRD, 2009; Lefebvre et al., 2008; McGowan and Sampson, 2005; Relevo and Balshem, 2011). Navigating through the various sources of research data and publications is a complex task that requires experience with a wide range of bibliographic databases and electronic information sources, and substantial resources (CRD, 2009; Lefebvre et al., 2008; Relevo and Balshem, 2011).

Ensuring an Accurate Search

An analysis of SRs published in the *Cochrane Database of Systematic Reviews* found that 90.5 percent of the MEDLINE searches contained at least one search error (Sampson and McGowan, 2006). Errors included spelling errors, the omission of spelling variants and truncations, the use of incorrect Boolean operators and line numbers, inadequate translation of the search strategy for different databases,

---

[2] For more information on the Cochrane Information Retrieval Methods Group, go to http://irmg.cochrane.org/.

misuse of MeSH[3] and free-text terms, unwarranted explosion of MeSH terms, and redundancy in search terms. Common sense suggests that these errors affect the accuracy and overall quality of SRs. AHRQ and CRD SR experts recommend peer review of the electronic search strategy to identify and prevent these errors from occurring (CRD, 2009; Relevo and Balshem, 2011). The peer reviewer should be independent from the review team in order to provide an unbiased and scientifically rigorous review, and should have expertise in information retrieval and SRs. In addition, the peer review process should take place prior to the search process, rather than in conjunction with the peer review of the final report, because the search process will provide the data that are synthesized and analyzed in the SR.

Sampson and colleagues (2009) recently surveyed individuals experienced in SR searching and identified aspects of the search process that experts agree are likely to have a large impact on the sensitivity and precision of a search: accurate translation of each research question into search concepts; correct choice of Boolean and proximity operators; absence of spelling errors; correct line numbers and combination of line numbers; accurate adaptation of the search strategy for each database; and inclusion of relevant subject headings. Then they developed practice guidelines for peer review of electronic search strategies. For example, to identify spelling errors in the search they recommended that long strings of terms be broken into discrete search statements in order to make null or misspelled terms more obvious and easier to detect. They also recommended cutting and pasting the search into a spell checker. As these guidelines and others are implemented, future research needs to be conducted to validate that peer review does improve the search quality.

Reporting Bias

Reporting biases (Song et al., 2010), particularly publication bias (Dickersin, 1990; Hopewell et al., 2009a) and selective reporting of trial outcomes and analyses (Chan et al., 2004a, 2004b; Dwan et al., 2008; Gluud, 2006; Hopewell et al., 2008; Turner et al., 2008; Vedula et al., 2009), present the greatest obstacle to obtaining a complete collection of relevant information on the effectiveness of healthcare interventions. Reporting biases have been identified across many health fields and interventions, including treatment, prevention, and diagnosis. For example, McGauran and colleagues (2010) identified

---

[3] MeSH (Medical Subject Headings) is the National Library of Medicine's controlled vocabulary thesaurus.

instances of reporting bias spanning 40 indications and 50 different pharmacological, surgical, diagnostic, and preventive interventions and selective reporting of study data as well as efforts by manufacturers to suppress publication. Furthermore, the potential for reporting bias exists across the entire research continuum—from before completion of the study (e.g., investigators' decisions to register a trial or to report only a selection of trial outcomes), to reporting in conference abstracts, selection of a journal for submission, and submission of the manuscript to a journal or other resource, to editorial review and acceptance.

The following describes the various ways in which reporting of research findings may be biased. Table 3-1 provides definitions of the types of reporting biases.

Publication Bias

The term *publication bias* refers to the likelihood that publication of research findings depends on the nature and direction of

TABLE 3-1 Types of Reporting Biases

Type of Reporting Bias	Definition
Publication bias	The publication or nonpublication of research findings, depending on the nature and direction of the results
Selective outcome reporting bias	The selective reporting of some outcomes but not others, depending on the nature and direction of the results
Time-lag bias	The rapid or delayed publication of research findings, depending on the nature and direction of the results
Location bias	The publication of research findings in journals with different ease of access or levels of indexing in standard databases, depending on the nature and direction of results.
Language bias	The publication of research findings in a particular language, depending on the nature and direction of the results
Multiple (duplicate) publications	The multiple or singular publication of research findings, depending on the nature and direction of the results
Citation bias	The citation or noncitation of research findings, depending on the nature and direction of the results

SOURCE: Sterne et al. (2008).

a study's results. More than two decades of research have shown that positive findings are more likely to be published than null or negative results. At least four SRs have assessed the association between study results and publication of findings (Song et al., 2009). These investigations plus additional individual studies indicate a strong association between statistically significant or positive results and likelihood of publication (Dickersin and Chalmers, 2010).

Investigators (not journal editors) are believed to be the major reason for failure to publish research findings (Dickersin and Min, 1993; Dickersin et al., 1992). Studies examining the influence of editors on acceptance of submitted manuscripts have not found an association between results and publication (Dickersin et al., 2007; Lynch et al., 2007; Okike et al., 2008; Olson et al., 2002).

Selective Outcome Reporting Bias

To avert problems introduced by *post hoc* selection of study outcomes, a randomized controlled trial's (RCT's) primary outcome should be stated in the research protocol *a priori*, before the study begins (Kirkham et al., 2010). Statistical testing of the effect of an intervention on multiple possible outcomes in a study can lead to a greater probability of statistically significant results obtained by chance. When primary or other outcomes of a study are selected and reported *post hoc* (i.e., after statistical testing), the reader should be aware that the published results for the "primary outcome" may be only a subset of relevant findings, and may be selectively reported because they are statistically significant.

Outcome reporting bias refers to the selective reporting of some outcomes but not others because of the nature and direction of the results. This can happen when investigators rely on hypothesis testing to prioritize research based on the statistical significance of an association. In the extreme, if only positive outcomes are selectively reported, we would not know that an intervention is ineffective for an important outcome, even if it had been tested frequently (Chan and Altman, 2005; Chan et al., 2004a,b; Dwan et al., 2008; Turner et al., 2008; Vedula et al., 2009).

Recent research on selective outcome reporting bias has focused on industry-funded trials, in part because internal company documents may be available, and in part because of evidence of biased reporting that favors their test interventions (Golder and Loke, 2008; Jorgensen et al., 2008; Lexchin et al., 2003; Nassir Ghaemi et al., 2008; Ross et al., 2009; Sismondo 2008; Vedula et al., 2009).

Mathieu and colleagues (2009) found substantial evidence of selective outcome reporting. The researchers reviewed 323 RCTs with results published in high-impact journals in 2008. They found that only 147 had been registered before the end of the trial with the primary outcome specified. Of these 147, 46 (31 percent) were published with different primary outcomes than were registered, with 22 introducing a new primary outcome. In 23 of the 46 discrepancies, the influence of the discrepancy could not be determined. Among the remaining 23 discrepancies, 19 favored a statistically significant result (i.e. a new statistically significant primary outcome was introduced in the published article or a nonsignificant primary outcome was omitted or not defined as primary in the published article).

In a study of 100 trials published in high-impact journals between September 2006 and February 2007 and also registered in a trial registry, Ewart and colleagues found that in 34 cases (31 percent) the primary outcome had changed (10 by addition of a new primary outcome; 3 by promotion from a secondary outcome; 20 by deletion of a primary outcome; and 6 by demotion to a secondary outcome); and in 77 cases (70 percent) the secondary outcome changed (54 by addition of a new secondary outcome; 5 by demotion from a primary outcome; 48 by deletion; 3 by promotion to a primary outcome) (Ewart et al., 2009).

Acquiring unpublished data from industry can be challenging. However, when available, unpublished data can change an SR's conclusions about the benefits and harms of treatment. A review by Eyding and colleagues demonstrates both the challenge of acquiring all relevant data from a manufacturer and how acquisition of those data can change the conclusion of an SR (Eyding et al., 2010). In their SR, which included both published and unpublished data acquired from the drug manufacturer, Eyding and colleagues found that published data overestimated the benefit of the antidepressant reboxetine over placebo by up to 115 percent and over selective serotonin reuptake inhibitors (SSRIs) by up to 23 percent. The addition of unpublished data changed the superiority of reboxetine vs. placebo to a nonsignificant difference and the nonsignificant difference between reboxetine and SSRIs to inferiority for reboxetine. For patients with adverse events and rates of withdrawals from adverse events inclusion of unpublished data changed nonsignificant difference between reboxetine and placebo to inferiority of reboxetine; while for rates of withdrawals for adverse events inclusion of unpublished data changed the nonsignificant difference between reboxetine and fluoxetine to an inferiority of fluoxetine.

Although there are many studies documenting the problem of publication bias and selective outcome reporting bias, few studies have examined the effect of such bias on SR findings. One recent study by Kirkham and colleagues assessed the impact of outcome reporting bias in individual trials on 81 SRs published in 2006 and 2007 by Cochrane review groups (Kirkham et al., 2010). More than one third of the reviews (34 percent) included at least one RCT with suspected outcome reporting bias. The authors assessed the potential impact of the bias and found that meta-analyses omitting trials with presumed selective outcome reporting for the primary outcome could overestimate the treatment effect. They also concluded that trials should not be excluded from SRs simply because outcome data appear to be missing when in fact the missing data may be due to selective outcome reporting. The authors suggest that in such cases the trialists should be asked to provide the outcome data that were analyzed, but not reported.

Time-lag Bias

In an SR of the literature, Hopewell and her colleagues (2009a) found that trials with positive results (statistically significant in favor of the experimental arm) were published about a year sooner than trials with null or negative results (not statistically significant or statistically significant in favor of the control arm). This has implications for both systematic review teams and patients. If positive findings are more likely to be available during the search process, then SRs may provide a biased view of current knowledge. The limited evidence available implies that publication delays may be caused by the investigator rather than by journal editors (Dickersin et al., 2002b; Ioannidis et al., 1997, 1998).

Location Bias

The location of published research findings in journals with different ease of access or levels of indexing is also correlated with the nature and direction of results. For example, in a Cochrane methodology review, Hopewell and colleagues identified five studies that assessed the impact of including trials published in the grey literature in an SR (Hopewell et al., 2009a). The studies found that trials in the published literature tend to be larger and show an overall larger treatment effect than those trials found in the grey literature (primarily abstracts and unpublished data, such as data from trial registries, "file drawer data," and data from individual trialists).

The researchers suggest that, by excluding grey literature, an SR or meta-analysis is likely to artificially inflate the benefits of a health care intervention.

Language Bias

As in other types of reporting bias, language bias refers to the publication of research findings in certain languages, depending on the nature and direction of the findings. For example, some evidence shows that investigators in Germany may choose to publish their negative RCT findings in non-English language journals and their positive RCT findings in English-language journals (Egger and Zellweger-Zahner, 1997; Heres et al., 2004). However, there is no definitive evidence on the impact of excluding articles in languages other than English (LOE), nor is there evidence that non-English language articles are of lower quality (Moher et al., 1996); the differences observed appear to be minor (Moher et al., 2003).

Some studies suggest that, depending on clinical specialty or disease, excluding research in LOE may not bias SR findings (Egger et al., 2003; Gregoire et al., 1995; Moher et al., 2000, 2003; Morrison et al., 2009). In a recent SR, Morrison and colleagues examined the impact on estimates of treatment effect when RCTs published in LOE are excluded (Morrison et al., 2009).[4] The researchers identified five eligible reports (describing three unique studies) that assessed the impact of excluding articles in LOE on the results of a meta-analysis. None of the five reports found major differences between English-only meta-analyses and meta-analyses that included trials in LOE (Egger et al., 2003; Jüni et al., 2002; Moher et al., 2000, 2003; Pham et al., 2005; Schulz et al., 1995).

Many SRs do not include articles in LOE, probably because of the time and cost involved in obtaining and translating them. The committee recommends that the SR team consider whether the topic of the review might require searching for studies not published in English.

Multiple (Duplicate) Publication Bias

Investigators sometimes publish the same findings multiple times, either overtly or what appears to be covertly. When two or more articles are identical, this constitutes plagiarism. When the articles are not identical, the systematic review team has difficulty

---

[4]The Morrison study excluded complementary and alternative medicine interventions.

discerning whether the articles are describing the findings from the same or different studies. von Elm and colleagues described four situations that may suggest duplicate publication; these include articles with the following features: (1) identical samples and outcomes; (2) identical samples and different outcomes; (3) samples that are larger or smaller, yet with identical outcomes; and (4) different samples and different outcomes (von Elm et al., 2004). The World Association of Medical Editors (WAME, 2010) and the International Committee of Medical Journal Editors (ICMJE, 2010) have condemned duplicate or multiple publication when there is no clear indication that the article has been published before.

Von Elm and colleagues (2004) identified 141 SRs in anesthesia and analgesia that included 56 studies that had been published two or more times. Little overlap occurred among authors on the duplicate publications, with no cross-referencing of the articles. Of the duplicates, 33 percent were funded by the pharmaceutical industry. Most of the duplicate articles (63 percent) were published in journal supplements soon after the "main" article. Positive results appear to be published more often in duplicate, which can lead to overestimates of a treatment effect if the data are double counted (Tramer et al., 1997).

Citation Bias

Searches of online databases of cited articles are one way to identify research that has been cited in the references of published articles. However, many studies show that, across a broad array of topics, authors tend to cite selectively only the positive results of other studies (omitting the negative or null findings) (Gøtzsche, 1987; Kjaergard and Als-Nielsen, 2002; Nieminen et al., 2007; Ravnskov, 1992, 1995; Schmidt and Gøtzsche, 2005;). Selective pooling of results, that is, when the authors perform a meta-analysis of studies they have selected without a systematic search for all evidence, could be considered both a non-SR and a form of citation bias. Because a selective meta-analysis or pooling does not reflect the true state of research evidence, it is prone to selection bias and may even reflect what the authors want us to know, rather than the totality of knowledge.

Addressing Reporting Bias

Reporting bias clearly presents a fundamental obstacle to the scientific integrity of SRs on the effectiveness of healthcare interventions. However, at this juncture, important, unresolved questions remain on how to overcome the problem. No empirically-based techniques have been developed that can predict which topics or research questions are most vulnerable to reporting bias. Nor can one determine when reporting bias will lead to an "incorrect" conclusion about the effectiveness of an intervention. Moreover, researchers have not yet developed a low-cost, effective approach to identifying a complete, unbiased literature for SRs of comparative effectiveness research (CER).

SR experts recommend a prespecified, systematic approach to the search for evidence that includes not only easy-to-access bibliographic databases, but also other information sources that contain grey literature, particularly trial data, and other unpublished reports. The search should be comprehensive and include both published and unpublished research. The evidence on reporting bias (described above) is persuasive. Without appropriate measures to counter the biased reporting of primary evidence from clinical trials and observational studies, SRs may only reflect—and could even exacerbate—existing distortions in the biomedical literature. The implications of developing clinical guidance from incomplete or biased knowledge may be serious (Moore, 1995; Thompson et al., 2008). Yet, many SRs fail to address the risk of bias during the search process.

Expert guidance also suggests that the SR team contact the researchers and sponsors of primary research to clarify unclear reports or to obtain unpublished data that are relevant to the SR. See Table 3-2 for key techniques and information sources recommended by AHRQ, CRD, and the Cochrane Collaboration. Appendix E provides further details on expert guidance.

Key Information Sources

Despite the imperative to conduct an unbiased search, many SRs use abbreviated methods to search for the evidence, often because of resource limitations. A common error is to rely solely on a limited number of bibliographic databases. Large databases, such as MEDLINE and Embase (Box 3-2), are relatively easy to use, but they often lack research findings that are essential to answering questions of comparative effectiveness (CRD, 2009; Hopewell et al., 2009b; Lefebvre et al., 2008; Scherer et al., 2007; Song et al., 2010). The appropriate sources of information for an SR depend on the research question, analytic framework, patient outcomes of interest, study population, research design (e.g., trial data vs. observational

TABLE 3-2 Expert Suggestions for Conducting the Search Process and Addressing Reporting Bias

	AHRQ	CRD	Cochrane
Expertise required for the search:			
• Work with a librarian or other information specialist with SR training to plan the search strategy	√	√	√
• Use an independent librarian or other information specialist to peer review the search strategy		√	
Search:			
• Bibliographic databases	√	√	√
• Citation indexes	√	√	√
• Databases of unpublished and ongoing studies	√	√	√
• Grey-literature databases	√	√	√
• Handsearch selected and conference abstracts	√	√	
• Literature cited by eligible studies	√	√	√
• Regional bibliographic databases	√	√	√
• Studies reported in languages other than English	√	√	√
• Subject-specific databases	√	√	√
• Web/Internet		√	
Contact:			
• Researchers to clarify study eligibility, study characteristics, and risk of bias		√	√
• Study sponsors and researchers to submit unpublished data	√	√	√

NOTE: See Appendix E for further details on guidance for searching for evidence from AHRQ, CRD, and Cochrane Collaboration.

data), likelihood of publication, authors, and other factors (Egger et al., 2003; Hartling et al., 2005; Helmer et al., 2001; Lemeshow et al., 2005). Relevant research findings may reside in a large, well-known bibliographic databases, subject-specific or regional databases, or in the grey literature.

The following summarizes the available evidence on the utility of key data sources—such as bibliographic databases, grey literature, trial registries, and authors or sponsors of relevant research—primarily for searching for results from RCTs. While considerable research has been done to date on finding relevant randomized trials (Dickersin et al., 1985; Dickersin et al., 1994; McKibbon et al., 2009; Royle and Milne, 2003; Royle and Waugh, 2003), less work has been done on methods for identifying qualitative (Flemming and Briggs,

---

BOX 3-2
Bibliographic Databases

- **Cochrane Central Register of Controlled Trials (CENTRAL)**—A database of more than 500,000 records of controlled trials and other healthcare interventions including citations published in languages other than English and conference proceedings.
- **Database of Abstracts of Reviews of Effect (DARE)**—A database, managed by the Centre for Reviews and Dissemination (York University), with 15,000 abstracts of systematic reviews including more than 6,000 Cochrane reviews and protocols. DARE focuses on the effects of health interventions including diagnostic and prognostic studies, rehabilitation, screening, and treatment.
- **Embase**—A biomedical and pharmaceutical database indexing 20 million records from over 3,500 international journals in drug research, pharmacology, pharmaceutics, toxicology, clinical and experimental human medicine, health policy and management, public health, occupational health, environmental health, drug dependence and abuse, psychiatry, forensic medicine, and biomedical engineering/ instrumentation.
- **MEDLINE**—The National Library of Medicine's (NLM's) bibliographic database with more than 18 million references to journals covering the fields of medicine, nursing, dentistry, veterinary medicine, the health care system, and the preclinical sciences.

Regional Databases
- African Index Medicus (AIM)—An index of African health literature and information sources. AIM was established by the World Health Organization in collaboration with the Association for Health Information and Libraries in Africa.
- Latin American and Caribbean Health Sciences Literature (LILACS)—A database for health scientific-technique literature published by Latin American and Caribbean authors missing from international databases. It covers the description and indexing of theses, books, books chapters, congresses or conferences annals, scientific-technical reports, and journal articles.

SOURCES: BIREME (2010); Cochrane Collaboration (2010a); CRD (2010); Dickersin et al. (2002a); Embase (2010); National Library of Medicine (2008); WHO (2006).

2007) and observational data for a given topic (Booth 2006; Furlan et al., 2006; Kuper et al., 2006; Lemeshow et al., 2005). The few electronic search strategies that have been evaluated to identify studies of harms, for example, suggest that further methodological research is needed to find an efficient balance between sensitivity[5] and precision in conducting electronic searches (Golder and Loke, 2009).

Less is known about the consequences of including studies missed in these searches. For example, one SR of the literature on search methods found that adverse effects information was included more frequently in unpublished sources, but also concluded that there was insufficient evidence to determine how including unpublished studies affects an SR's pooled risk estimates of adverse effects (Golder and Loke, 2010). Nevertheless, one must assume that the consequences of missing relevant articles may be clinically significant especially if the search fails to identify data that might alter conclusions about the risks and benefits of an intervention.

Bibliographic Databases

Unfortunately, little empirical evidence is available to guide the development of an SR bibliographic search strategy. As a result, the researcher has to scrutinize a large volume of articles to identify the relatively small proportion that are relevant to the research question under consideration. At present, no one database or information source is sufficient to ensure an unbiased, balanced picture of what is known about the effectiveness, harms, and benefits of health interventions (Betran et al., 2005; Crumley et al., 2005; Royle et al., 2005; Tricco et al., 2008). Betran and colleagues, for example, assessed the utility of different databases for identifying studies for a World Health Organization (WHO) SR of maternal morbidity and mortality (Betran et al., 2005). After screening more than 64,000 different citations, they identified 2,093 potentially eligible studies. Several databases were sources of research not found elsewhere; 20 percent of citations were found only in MEDLINE, 7.4 percent in Embase, and 5.6 percent in LILACS and other topic specific databases.

Specialized databases   Depending on the subject of the SR, specialized topical databases such as POPLINE and PsycINFO may provide research findings not available in other databases (Box 3-3). POPLINE is a specialized database of abstracts of scientific articles, reports, books, and unpublished reports in the field of population, family planning, and related health issues. PsycINFO, a database of psychological literature, contains journal articles, book chapters,

---

[5] In literature searching, "sensitivity" is the proportion of relevant articles that are identified using a specific search strategy; "precision" refers to the proportion of articles identified by a search strategy that are relevant (CRD 2009).

BOX 3-3
Subject-Specific Databases

- **Campbell Collaboration Social, Psychological, Educational & Criminological Trials Register (C2-SPECTR)**—A registry of more than 10,000 trials in education, social work and welfare, and criminal justice. The primary purpose of C2-SPECTR is to provide support for the Campbell Collaboration systematic reviews (SRs), but the registry is open to the public.
- **Cumulative Index to Nursing and Allied Health Literature (CINAHL)**— CINAHL indexes nearly 3,000 journals as well as healthcare books, nursing dissertations, selected conference proceedings, standards of practice, educational software, audiovisuals, and book chapters from nursing and allied health. It includes more than 2 million records dating from 1981.
- **POPLINE**—A database on reproductive health with nearly 370,000 records of abstracts of scientific articles, reports, books, and unpublished reports in the fields of population, family planning, and related health issues. POPLINE is maintained by the K4Health Project at the Johns Hopkins Bloomberg School of Public Health and is funded by the U.S. Agency for International Development.
- **PsycINFO**—A database of psychological literature, including journal articles, book chapters, books, technical reports, and dissertations. PsycINFO has more than 2.8 million records and over 2,450 titles and is maintained by the American Psychological Association.

SOURCES: APA (2010); Campbell Collaboration (2000); EBSCO Publishing (2010); Knowledge for Health (2010).

---

books, technical reports, and dissertations related to behavioral health interventions.

Citation indexes   Scopus, Web of Science, and other citation indexes are valuable for finding cited reports from journals, trade publications, book series, and conference papers from the scientific, technical, medical, social sciences, and arts and humanities fields (Bakkalbasi et al., 2006; Chapman et al., 2010; Falagas et al., 2008; ISI Web of Knowledge, 2009; Kuper et al., 2006; Scopus, 2010). Searching the citations of previous SRs on the same topic could be particularly fruitful.

Grey literature   Grey literature includes trial registries (discussed below), conference abstracts, books, dissertations, monographs, and reports held by the Food and Drug Administration (FDA) and other government agencies, academics, business, and industry.

BOX 3-4
Grey-Literature Databases

- **New York Academy of Medicine Grey Literature Report**—A bimonthly publication of the New York Academy of Medicine Library that includes grey literature in health services research and selected public health topics.
- **OAIster**—An archive of digital resources worldwide with more than 23 million records from over 1,100 contributors, including digitized books and journal articles, digital text, audio files, video files, photographic images, data sets, and theses and research papers.
- **ProQuest Dissertations & Theses Database (PQDT)**—A database with 2.7 million searchable citations for dissertations and theses from around the world dating from 1861. More than 70,000 new full-text dissertations and theses are added each year.
- **System for Information on Grey Literature in Europe (OpenSIGLE)**—A multidisciplinary database that includes technical or research reports, doctoral dissertations, some conference papers, some official publications, and other types of grey literature in pure and applied science and technology, economics, other sciences, and humanities.

SOURCES: New York Academy of Medicine (2010); Online Computer Library Center (2010); OpenSIGLE (2010); ProQuest (2010).

Grey-literature databases, such as those described in Box 3-4, are important sources for technical or research reports, doctoral dissertations, conference papers, and other research.

Handsearching Handsearching is when researchers manually examine—page by page—each article, abstract, editorial, letter to the editor, or other items in journals to identify reports of RCTs or other relevant evidence (Hopewell et al., 2009b). No empirical research shows how an SR's conclusions might be affected by adding trials identified through a handsearch. However, for some CER topics and circumstances, handsearching may be important (CRD, 2009; Hopewell et al., 2009a; Lefebvre et al., 2008; Relevo and Balshem, 2011). The first or only appearance of a trial report, for example, may be in the nonindexed portions of a journal.

Contributors to the Cochrane Collaboration have handsearched literally thousands of journals and conference abstracts to identify controlled clinical trials and studies that may be eligible for Cochrane reviews (Dickersin et al., 2002a). Using a publicly available resource, one can identify which journals, abstracts, and years have been or are being searched by going to the Cochrane Master List of Journals Being Searched.[6] If a subject area has been well covered by Cochrane, then it is probably reasonable to forgo handsearching and to rely on the Cochrane Central Register of Controlled Trials (CENTRAL), which should contain the identified articles and abstracts. It is always advisable to check with the relevant Cochrane review group to confirm the journals/conference abstracts that have been searched and how they are indexed in CENTRAL. The CENTRAL database is available to all subscribers to the Cochrane Library. For example, if the search topic was eye trials, numerous years of journals and conference abstracts have been searched, and included citations have been MeSH coded if they were from a source not indexed on MEDLINE. Because of the comprehensive searching and indexing available for the eyes and vision field, one would not need to search beyond CENTRAL.

Clinical Trials Data

Clinical trials produce essential data for SRs on the therapeutic effectiveness and adverse effects of health care interventions. However, the findings for a substantial number of clinical trials are never published (Bennett and Jull, 2003; Hopewell et al., 2009b; MacLean et al., 2003; Mathieu et al., 2009; McAuley et al., 2000; Savoie et al., 2003; Turner et al., 2008). Thus, the search for trial data should include trial registries (ClinicalTrials.gov, Clinical Study Results, Current Controlled Trials, and WHO International Clinical Trials Registry), FDA medical and statistical reviews records (MacLean et al., 2003; Turner et al., 2008), conference abstracts (Hopewell et al., 2009b; McAuley et al., 2000), non-English literature, and outreach to investigators (CRD, 2009; Golder et al., 2010; Hopewell et al., 2009b; Lefebvre et al., 2008; Miller, 2010; O'Connor, 2009; Relevo and Balshem, 2011; Song et al., 2010).

Trial registries Trial registries have the potential to address the effects of reporting bias if they provide complete data on both ongoing and completed trials (Boissel, 1993; Dickersin, 1988; Dickersin and Rennie, 2003; Hirsch, 2008; NLM, 2009; Ross et al., 2009; Savoie et al., 2003; Song et al., 2010; WHO, 2010; Wood, 2009). One can access a large proportion of international trials registries using the WHO International Clinical Trials Registry Platform (WHO, 2010).

---

[6] Available at http://uscc. cochrane. org/en/newPage1.html.

ClinicalTrials.gov is the most comprehensive public registry. It was established in 2000 by the National Library of Medicine as required by the *FDA Modernization Act of 1997*[7] (NLM, 2009). At its start, ClinicalTrials.gov had minimal utility for SRs because the required data were quite limited, industry compliance with the mandate was poor, and government enforcement of sponsors' obligation to submit complete data was lax (Zarin, 2005). The International Committee of Medical Journal Editors (ICMJE), among others, spurred trial registration overall by requiring authors to enroll trials in a public trials registry at or before the beginning of patient enrollment as a precondition for publication in member journals (DeAngelis et al., 2004). The implementation of this policy is associated with a 73 percent increase in worldwide trial registrations at ClinicalTrials.gov for all intervention types (Zarin et al., 2005).

The FDA Amendments Act of 2007[8] significantly expanded the potential depth and breadth of the ClinicalTrials.gov registry. The act mandates that sponsors of any ongoing clinical trial involving a drug, biological product, or device approved for marketing by the FDA, not only register the trial,[9] but also submit data on the trial's research protocol and study results (including adverse events).[10] As of October 2010, 2,300 results records are available. Much of the required data have not yet been submitted (Miller, 2010), and Congress has allowed sponsors to delay posting of results data until after the product is granted FDA approval. New regulations governing the scope and timing of results posting are pending (Wood, 2009).

Data gathered as part of the FDA approval process The FDA requires sponsors to submit extensive data about efficacy and safety as part of the New Drug Application (NDA) process. FDA analysts— statisticians, physicians, pharmacologists, and chemists—examine and analyze these data.

Although the material submitted by the sponsor is confidential, under the *Freedom of Information Act*, the FDA is required to make its analysts' reports public after redacting proprietary or sensitive information. Since 1998, selected, redacted copies of reports conducted by FDA analysts have been publicly available (see Drugs@

---

[7] Public Law 105-115 sec. 113.

[8] Public Law 110-85.

[9] Phase I trials are excluded.

[10] Required data include demographic and baseline characteristics of the patients, the number of patients lost to follow-up, the number excluded from the analysis, and the primary and secondary outcomes measures (including a table of values with appropriate tests of the statistical significance of the values) (Miller 2010).

FDA[11]). When available, these are useful for obtaining clinical trials data, especially when studies are not otherwise reported.[12,13] For example, as part of an SR of complications from nonsteroidal anti-inflammatory drugs (NSAIDs), MacLean and colleagues identified trials using the FDA repository. They compared two groups of studies meeting inclusion criteria for the SR: published reports of trials and studies included in submissions to the FDA. They identified 20 published studies on the topic and 37 studies submitted to the FDA that met their inclusion criteria. Only one study was in both the published and FDA groups (i.e., only 1 of 37 studies submitted to the FDA was published) (MacLean et al., 2003). The authors found no meaningful differences in the information reported in the FDA report and the published report on sample size, gender distribution, indication for drug use, and components of study methodological quality. This indicated, at least in this case, there is no reason to omit unpublished research from an SR for reasons of study quality.

Several studies have demonstrated that the FDA repository provides opportunities for finding out about unpublished trials, and that reporting biases exist such that unpublished studies are associated more often with negative findings. Lee and colleagues examined 909 trials supporting 90 approved drugs in FDA reviews, and found that 43 percent (394 of 909) were published 5 years post-approval and that positive results were associated with publication (Lee et al., 2008).

Rising and colleagues (2008) conducted a study of all efficacy trials found in approved NDAs for new molecular entities from 2001 to 2002 and all published clinical trials corresponding to trials within those NDAs. The authors found that trials in NDAs with favorable primary outcomes were nearly five times more likely to be published than trials with unfavorable primary outcomes. In addition, for those 99 cases in which conclusions were provided in both the NDA and the published paper, in 9 (9 percent) the conclusion was different in the NDA and the publication and all changes favored the test drug. Published papers included more outcomes favoring the test drug than the NDAs. The authors also found that, excluding outcomes with unknown significance, 43 outcomes in the NDAs did not favor the test drug (35 were nonsignificant and 8

---

[11] Available at http://www.accessdata.fda.gov/scripts/cder/drugsatfda/.

[12] NDA data were not easily accessed at the time of the MacLean study; the investigators had to collect the data through a Freedom of Information Act request.

[13] NDAs are available at http://www.accessdata.fda.gov/scripts/cder/drugsatfda/index.cfm?fuseaction=Search.Search_Drug_Name.

favored the comparator). Of these 20 (47 percent) were not included in the published papers and of the 23 that were published 5 changed between the NDA-reported outcome and the published outcome with 4 changed to favor the test drug in the published results.

Turner and his colleagues (2008) examined FDA submissions for 12 antidepressants, and identified 74 clinical trials, of which 31 percent had not been reported. The researchers compared FDA review data of each drug's effects with the published trial data. They found that the published data suggested that 94 percent of the antidepressant trials were positive. In contrast, the FDA data indicated that only 51 percent of trials were positive. Moreover, when meta-analyses were conducted with and without the FDA data, the researchers found that the published reports overstated the effect size from 11 to 69 percent for the individual drugs. Overall studies judged positive by the FDA were 12 times as likely to be published in a way that agreed with the FDA than studies not judged positive by the FDA.

FDA material can also be useful for detecting selective outcome reporting bias and selective analysis bias. For example, Turner and colleagues (2008) found that the conclusions for 11 of 57 published trials did not agree between the FDA review and the publication. In some cases, the journal publication reported different p values than the FDA report of the same study, reflecting preferential reporting of comparisons or analyses that had statistically significant p values.

The main limitation of the FDA files is that they may remain unavailable for several years after a drug is approved. Data on older drugs within a class are often missing. For example, of the 9 atypical antipsychotic drugs marketed in the United States in 2010, the FDA material is available for 7 of them. FDA reviews are not available for the 2 oldest drugs—clozapine (approved in 1989) and risperidone (approved in 1993) (McDonagh et al., 2010).

Contacting Authors and Study Sponsors for Missing Data

As noted earlier in the chapter, more than half of all trial findings may never be published (Hopewell et al., 2009b; Song et al., 2009). If a published report on a trial is available, key data are often missing. When published reports do not contain the information needed for the SR (e.g., for the assessment of bias, description of study characteristics), the SR team should contact the author to clarify and obtain missing data and to clear up any other uncertainties such as possible duplicate publication (CRD, 2009; Glasziou et al., 2008; Higgins and Deeks, 2008; Relevo and Balshem, 2011). Several studies have documented that collecting some, if not all, data needed for a meta-analysis is feasible by directly contacting the relevant author and Principal Investigators (Devereaux et al., 2004; Kelley et al., 2004; Kirkham et al., 2010; Song et al., 2010). For example, in a study assessing outcome reporting bias in Cochrane SRs, Kirkham and colleagues (2010) e-mailed the authors of the RCTs that were included in the SRs to clarify whether a trial measured the SR's primary outcome. The researchers were able to obtain missing trial data from more than a third of the authors contacted (39 percent). Of these, 60 percent responded within a day and the remainder within 3 weeks.

Updating Searches

When patients, clinicians, clinical practice guideline (CPG) developers, and others look for SRs to guide their decisions, they hope to find the most current information available. However, in the Rising study described earlier, the researchers found that 23 percent of the efficacy trials submitted to the FDA for new molecular entities from 2001–2002 were still not published 5 years after FDA approval (Rising et al., 2008). Moher and colleagues (2007b) cite a compelling example—treatment of traumatic brain injury (TBI)—of how an updated SR can change beliefs about the risks and benefits of an intervention. Corticosteroids had been used routinely over three decades for TBI when a new clinical trial suggested that patients who had TBI and were treated with corticosteroids were at higher risk of death compared with placebo (CRASH Trial Collaborators, 2004). When Alderson and Roberts incorporated the new trial data in an update of an earlier SR on the topic, findings about mortality risk dramatically reversed—leading to the conclusion that steroids should no longer be routinely used in patients with TBI (Alderson and Roberts, 2005).

Two opportunities are available for updating the search and the SR. The first opportunity for updating is just before the review's initial publication. Because a meaningful amount of time is likely to have elapsed since the initial search, SRs are at risk of being outdated even before they are finalized (Shojania et al., 2007). Among a cohort of SRs on the effectiveness of drugs, devices, or procedures published between 1995 and 2005 and indexed in the ACP Journal Club[14] database, on average more than 1 year (61 weeks) elapsed

---

[14] The ACP Journal Club, once a stand-alone bimonthly journal, is now a monthly feature of the *Annals of Internal Medicine*. The club's purpose is to feature structured abstracts (with commentaries from clinical experts) of the best original and review articles in internal medicine and other specialties. For more information go to www.acpjc.org.

between the final search and publication and 74 weeks elapsed between the final search and indexing in MEDLINE (when findings are more easily accessible) (Sampson et al., 2008). AHRQ requires Evidence-Based Practice Centers (EPCs) to update SR searches at the time of peer review.[15] CRD and the Cochrane Collaboration recommend that the search be updated before the final analysis but do not specify an exact time period (CRD, 2009; Higgins et al., 2008).

The second opportunity for updating is post-publication, and occurs periodically over time, to ensure a review is kept up-to-date. In examining how often reviews need updating, Shojania and colleagues (2007) followed 100 meta-analyses, published between 1995 and 2005 and indexed in the *ACP Journal Club*, of the comparative effectiveness of drugs, devices, or procedures. Within 5.5 years, half of the reviews had new evidence that would have substantively changed conclusions about effectiveness, and within 2 years nearly 25 percent had such evidence.

Updating also provides an opportunity to identify and incorporate studies with negative findings that may have taken longer to be published than those with positive findings (Hopewell et al., 2009b) and larger scale confirmatory trials that can appear in publications after smaller trials (Song et al., 2010).

According to the Cochrane Handbook, an SR may be out-of-date under the following scenarios:

- A change is needed in the research question or selection criteria for studies. For example, a new intervention (e.g., a newly marketed drug within a class) or a new outcome of the interventions may have been identified since the last update;
- New studies are available;
- Methods are out-of-date; or
- Factual statements in the introduction and discussion sections of the review are not up-to-date.

Identifying reasons to change the research question and searching for new studies are the initial steps in updating. If the questions are still up-to-date, and searches do not identify relevant new studies, the SR can be considered up-to-date (Moher and Tsertsvadze, 2006). If new studies are identified, then their results must be incorporated into the existing SR.

---

[15] Personal communication, Stephanie Chang, Medical Officer, AHRQ (March 12, 2010).

A typical approach to updating is to consider the need to update the research question and conduct a new literature search every 2 years. Because some reviews become out-of-date sooner than this, several recent investigations have developed and tested strategies to identify SRs that need updating earlier (Barrowman et al., 2003; Garritty et al., 2009; Higgins et al., 2008; Louden et al., 2008; Sutton et al., 2009; Voisin et al., 2008). These strategies use the findings that some fields move faster than others; large studies are more likely to change conclusions than small ones; and both literature scans and consultation with experts can help identify the need for an update. In the best available study of an updating strategy, Shojania and colleagues sought signals that an update would be needed sooner rather than later after publication of an SR (Shojania et al., 2007). Fifty-seven percent of reviews had one or more of these signals for updating. Cardiovascular medicine, heterogeneity in the original review, and publication of a new trial larger than the previous largest trial were associated with shorter survival times, while inclusion of more than 13 studies in the original review was associated with increased time before an update was needed. In 23 cases the signal occurred within 2 years of publication. The median survival of a review without any signal that an update was needed was 5.5 years.

RECOMMENDED STANDARDS FOR THE SEARCH PROCESS

The committee recommends the following standards and elements of performance for identifying the body of evidence for an SR:

Standard 3.1—Conduct a comprehensive systematic search for evidence
> Required elements:
> 3.1.1   Work with a librarian or other information specialist trained in performing systematic reviews to plan the search strategy
> 3.1.2   Design the search strategy to address each key research question
> 3.1.3   Use an independent librarian or other information specialist to peer review the search strategy
> 3.1.4   Search bibliographic databases
> 3.1.5   Search citation indexes
> 3.1.6   Search literature cited by eligible studies
> 3.1.7   Update the search at intervals appropriate to the pace of generation of new information for the research question being addressed

3.1.8   Search subject-specific databases if other databases are unlikely to provide all relevant evidence

3.1.9   Search regional bibliographic databases if other databases are unlikely to provide all relevant evidence

Standard 3.2—Take action to address reporting biases of research results

Required elements:

3.2.1   Search grey-literature databases, clinical trial registries, and other sources of unpublished information about studies

3.2.2   Invite researchers to clarify information related to study eligibility, study characteristics, and risk of bias

3.2.3   Invite all study sponsors to submit unpublished data, including unreported outcomes, for possible inclusion in the systematic review

3.2.4   Handsearch selected journals and conference abstracts

3.2.5   Conduct a web search

3.2.6   Search for studies reported in languages other than English if appropriate

Rationale

In summary, little evidence directly addresses the influence of each search step on the final outcome of the SR (Tricco et al., 2008). Moreover, the SR team cannot judge in advance whether reporting bias will be a threat to any given review. However, evidence shows the risks of conducting a nonsystematic, incomplete search. Relying solely on mainstream databases and published reports may misinform clinical decisions. Thus, the search should include sources of unpublished data, including grey-literature databases, trial registries, and FDA submissions such as NDAs.

The search to identify a body of evidence on comparative effectiveness must be systematic, prespecified, and include an array of information sources that can provide both published and unpublished research data. The essence of CER and patient-centered health care is an accurate and fair accounting of the evidence in the research literature on the effectiveness and potential benefits and harms of health care interventions (IOM, 2008, 2009). Informed health care decision making by consumers, patients, clinicians, and others, demands unbiased and comprehensive information. Developers of clinical practice guidelines cannot produce sound advice without it.

SRs are most useful when they are up-to-date. Assuming a field is active, initial searches should be updated when the SR is finalized for publication, and studies ongoing at the time the review was undertaken should be checked for availability of results. In addition, notations of ongoing trials (e.g., such as those identified by searching trials registries) is important to notify the SR readers when new information can be expected in the future.

Some of the expert search methods that the committee endorses are resource intensive and time consuming. The committee is not suggesting an exhaustive search using all possible methods and all available sources of unpublished studies and grey literature. For each SR, the researcher must determine how best to identify a comprehensive and unbiased set of the relevant studies that might be included in the review. The review team should consider what information sources are appropriate given the topic of the review and review those sources. Conference abstracts and proceedings will rarely provide useful unpublished data but they may alert the reviewer to otherwise unpublished trials. In the case of drug studies, FDA reviews and trial registries are likely sources of unpublished data that, when included, may change an SR's outcomes and conclusions from a review relying only on published data. Searches of these sources and requests to manufacturers should always be conducted. With the growing body of SRs being performed on behalf of state and federal agencies, those reviews should also be considered as a potential source of otherwise unpublished data and a search for such reports is also warranted. The increased burden on reviewers, particularly with regard to the inclusion of FDA reviews, will likely decrease over time as reviewers gain experience in using those sources and in more efficiently and effectively abstracting the relevant data. The protection against potential bias brought about by inclusion of these data sources makes the development of that expertise critical.

The search process is also likely to become less resource intensive as specialized databases of comprehensive article collections used in previous SRs are developed, or automated search and retrieval methods are tested and implemented.

SCREENING AND SELECTING STUDIES

Selecting which studies should be included in the SR is a multi-step, labor-intensive process. EPC staff have estimated that the SR search, review of abstracts, and retrieval and review of selected full-text papers takes an average of 332 hours (Cohen et al., 2008). If the search is conducted appropriately, it is likely to yield hundreds—if not thousands—of potential studies (typically in the form of citations and abstracts). The next step—the focus of this section of the chapter—is to screen the collected studies to determine which ones are actually relevant to the research question under consideration.

The screening and selection process requires careful, sometimes subjective, judgments and meticulous documentation. Decisions on which studies are relevant to the research question and analytic framework are among the most significant judgments made during the course of an SR. If the study inclusion criteria are too narrow, critical data may be missed. If the inclusion criteria are too broad, irrelevant studies may overburden the process.

The following overview summarizes the available evidence on how to best screen, select, and document this critical phase of an SR. The focus is on unbiased selection of studies, inclusion of observational studies, and documentation of the process. The committee's related standards are presented at the end of the section.

See Table 3-3 for steps recommended by AHRQ, CRD, and the Cochrane Collaboration for screening publications and extracting data from eligible studies. Appendix E provides additional details.

Ensuring an Unbiased Selection of Studies

Use Prespecified Inclusion and Exclusion Criteria

Using prespecified inclusion and exclusion criteria to choose studies is the best way to minimize the risk of researcher biases influencing the ultimate results of the SR (CRD, 2009; Higgins and Deeks, 2008; Liberati et al., 2009; Silagy et al., 2002). The SR research protocol should make explicit which studies to include or exclude

TABLE 3-3 Expert Suggestions for Screening Publications and Extracting Data from Eligible Studies

	AHRQ	CRD	Cochrane
Use two or more members of the review team, working independently, to screen studies	√	√	√
Train screeners			√
Use two or more researchers, working independently, to extract data from each study		√	√
Use standard data extraction forms developed for the specific systematic review	√	√	√
Pilot-test the data extraction forms and process	√	√	√

NOTE: See Appendix E for further details on guidance on screening and extracting data from AHRQ, CRD, and the Cochrane Collaboration.

based on the patient population and patient outcomes of interest, the healthcare intervention and comparators, clinical settings (if relevant), and study designs (e.g., randomized vs. observational research) that are appropriate for the research question. Only studies that meet all of the criteria and none of the exclusion criteria should be included in the SR. Box 3-5 provides an example of selection criteria from a recent EPC research protocol for an SR of therapies for children with an autism spectrum disorder.

Although little empirical evidence informs the development of the screening criteria, numerous studies have shown that, too often, SRs allow excessive subjectivity into the screening process (Cooper et al., 2006; Delaney et al., 2007; Dixon et al., 2005; Edwards et al., 2002; Linde and Willich, 2003; Lundh et al., 2009; Mrkobrada et al., 2008; Peinemann et al., 2008; Thompson et al., 2008). Mrkobrada and colleagues, for example, assessed the quality of all the nephrology-related SRs published in 2005 (Mrkobrada et al., 2008). Of the 90 SRs, 51 did not report efforts to minimize bias during the selection process, such as using prespecified inclusion criteria and having more than one person select eligible studies. An assessment of critical care meta-analyses published between 1994 and 2003 yielded similar findings. Delaney and colleagues (2007) examined 139 meta-analyses related to critical care medicine in journals or the Cochrane Database of Systematic Reviews. They found that a substantial proportion of the papers did not address potential biases in the selection of studies; 14 of the 36 Cochrane reviews (39 percent) and 69 of the 92 journal articles (75 percent).

Reviewing the full-text papers for all citations identified in the original search is time consuming and expensive. Expert guidance recommends that a two-stage approach to screening citations for inclusion in an SR is acceptable in minimizing bias or producing quality work (CRD, 2009; Higgins and Deeks, 2008). The first step is to screen the titles and abstracts against the inclusion criteria. The second step is to screen the full-text papers passing the first screen. Selecting studies based solely on the titles and abstracts requires judgment and experience with the literature (Cooper et al., 2006; Dixon et al., 2005; Liberati et al., 2009).

Minimize Subjectivity

Even when the selection criteria are prespecified and explicit, decisions on including particular studies can be subjective. AHRQ, CRD, and the Cochrane Collaboration recommend that more than one individual independently screens and selects studies in order to

---

BOX 3-5
Study Selection Criteria for a Systematic
Review of Therapies for Children with
Autism Spectrum Disorders (ASD)

Review questions: Among children ages 2–12 with ASD, what are the short- and long-term effects of available behavioral, educational, family, medical, allied health, or complementary or alternative treatment approaches? Specifically,

   a. What are the effects on core symptoms (e.g. social deficits, communication deficits, and repetitive behaviors), in the short term (≤6 months)?
   b. What are the effects on commonly associated symptoms (e.g. motor, sensory, medical, mood/anxiety, irritability, and hyperactivity) in the short term (≤6 months)?
   c. What are the longer-term effects (>6 months) on core symptoms (e.g. social deficits, communication deficits, and repetitive behaviors)?
   d. What are the longer-term effects (>6 months) on commonly associated symptoms (e.g. motor, sensory, medical, mood/anxiety, irritability, and hyperactivity)?

Category	Selection criteria
Population	Children ages 2–12 who are diagnosed with a ASD and children under age 2 at risk for diagnosis of a ASD
Interventions	Treatment modalities aimed at modifying the core symptoms of ASD
Study settings	Developed nations/regions including the United States, Canada, United Kingdom, Western Europe, Japan, Australia, New Zealand, Israel, or South America
Time period	1980–present
Outcomes	Short- and long-term outcomes, harms, and quality of life related to treatment for core symptoms
Study design	• Controlled trials, prospective trials with historical controls, prospective or retrospective cohort studies, and medium to large case series. • N ≥ 10 • Original research studies that provide sufficient detail regarding methods and results to enable use and adjustment of the data and results

SOURCE: Adapted from the AHRQ EPC Research Protocol, Therapies for Children with ASD (AHRQ EHC, 2009).

---

minimize bias and human error and to help ensure that the selection process is reproducible (Table 3-3) (CRD, 2009; Higgins and Deeks, 2008; Khan, 2001; Relevo and Balshem, 2011). Although doubling the number of screeners is costly, the committee agrees that the additional expense is justified because of the extent of errors and bias that occur when only one individual does the screening. With-out two screeners, SRs may miss relevant data that might affect conclusions about the effectiveness of an intervention. Edwards and colleagues (2002), for example, found that using two review-ers may reduce the likelihood that relevant studies are discarded. The researchers increased the number of eligible trials by up to 32 percent (depending on the reviewer).

Experience, screener training, and pilot-testing of screening crite-ria are key to an accurate search and selection process. The Cochrane Collaboration recommends that screeners be trained by pilot testing the eligibility criteria on a sample of studies and assessing reliability (Higgins and Deeks, 2008), and certain Cochrane groups require that screeners take the Cochrane online training for handsearchers and pass a test on identification of clinical trials before they become involved (Cochrane Collaboration, 2010b).

Use Observational Studies, as Appropriate

In CER, observational studies should be considered complemen-tary to RCTs (Dreyer and Garner, 2009; Perlin and Kupersmith, 2007). Both can provide useful information for decision makers. Observa-tional studies are critical for evaluating the harms of interventions (Chou and Helfand, 2005). RCTs often lack prespecified hypotheses regarding harms; are not adequately powered to detect serious, but uncommon events (Vandenbroucke, 2004); or exclude patients who are more susceptible to adverse events (Rothwell, 2005). Well-conducted, observational evaluations of harms, particularly those based on large registries of patients seen in actual practice, can help to validate estimates of the severity and frequency of adverse events derived from RCTs, identify subgroups of patients at higher or lower susceptibility, and detect important harms not identified in RCTs (Chou et al., 2010).

The proper role of observational studies in evaluating the ben-efits of interventions is less clear. RCTs are the gold standard for determining efficacy and effectiveness. For this reason they are the preferred starting place for determining intervention effectiveness. Even if they are available, however, trials may not provide data on outcomes that are important to patients, clinicians, and developers of CPGs. When faced with treatment choices, decision makers want to know who is most likely to benefit from a treatment and what the potential tradeoffs are. Some trials are designed to fulfill regu-latory requirements (e.g., for FDA approval) rather than to inform everyday treatment decisions and these studies may address narrow patient populations and intervention options. For example, study populations may not represent the population affected by the condition of interest; patients could be younger or not as ill (Norris et al., 2010). As a result, a trial may leave unanswered certain important questions about the treatment's effects in different clinical settings and for different types of patients (Nallamothu et al., 2008).

Thus, although RCTs are subject to less bias, when the available RCTs do not examine how an intervention works in everyday practice or evaluate patient-important outcomes, observational studies may provide the evidence needed to address the SR team's questions. Deciding to extend eligibility of study designs to observational studies represents a fundamental challenge because the suitability of observational studies for assessment of effectiveness depends heavily on a number of clinical and contextual factors. The likelihood of selection bias, recall bias, and other biases are so high in certain clinical situations that no observational study could address the question with an acceptable risk of bias (Norris et al., 2010).

An important note is that in CER, observational studies of benefits are intended to complement, rather than substitute for, RCTs. Most literature about observational studies of effectiveness has examined whether observational studies can be relied on to make judgments about effectiveness when there are no high-quality RCTs on the same research question (Concato et al., 2000; Deeks et al., 2003; Shikata et al., 2006). The committee did not find evidence to support a recommendation about substituting observational data in the absence of data from RCTs. Reasonable criteria for relying on observational studies in the absence of RCT data have been proposed (Glasziou et al., 2007), but little empiric data support these criteria.

The decision to include or exclude observational studies in an SR should be justifiable, explicit and well-documented (Atkins, 2007; Chambers et al., 2009; Chou et al., 2010; CRD, 2009; Goldsmith et al., 2007). Once this decision has been made, authors of SRs of CER should search for observational research, such as cohort and case-control studies, to supplement RCT findings. Less is known about searching for observational studies than for RCTs (Golder and Loke, 2009; Kuper et al., 2006; Wieland and Dickersin, 2005; Wilczynski et al., 2004). The SR team should work closely with a librarian with training and experience in this area and should consider peer review of the search strategy (Sampson et al., 2009).

Documenting the Screening and Selection Process

SRs rarely document the screening and selection process in a way that would allow anyone to either replicate it or to appraise the appropriateness of the selected studies (Golder et al., 2008; Moher et al., 2007a). In light of the subjective nature of study selection and the large volume of possible citations, the importance of maintaining a detailed account of study selection cannot be understated. Yet, years after reporting guidelines have been disseminated and updated, documentation remains inadequate in most published SRs (Liberati et al., 2009).

Clearly, the search, screening, and selection process is complex and highly technical. The effort required in keeping track of citations, search strategies, full-text articles, and study data is daunting. Experts recommend using reference management software, such as EndNote, RefWorks, or RevMan, to document the process and keep track of the decisions that are made for each article (Cochrane IMS, 2010; CRD, 2009; Elamin et al., 2009; Hernandez et al., 2008; Lefebvre et al., 2008; RefWorks, 2009; Relevo and Balshem, 2011; Thomson Reuters, 2010). Documentation should occur in real time—not retrospectively, but as the search, screening, and selection are carried out. This will help ensure accurate recordkeeping and adherence to protocol.

The SR final report should include a flow chart that shows the number of studies that remain after each stage of the selection process.[16] Figure 3-1 provides an example of an annotated flow chart. The flow chart documents the number of records identified through electronic databases searched, whether additional records were identified through other sources, and the reasons for excluding articles. Maintaining a record of excluded as well as selected articles is important.

RECOMMENDED STANDARDS FOR SCREENING AND SELECTING STUDIES

The committee recommends the following standards for screening and selecting studies for an SR:

Standard 3.3—Screen and select studies
   Required elements:
      3.3.1   Include or exclude studies based on the protocol's prespecified criteria
      3.3.2   Use observational studies in addition to randomized clinical trials to evaluate harms of interventions
      3.3.3   Use two or more members of the review team, working independently, to screen and select studies

---

[16] See Chapter 5 for a complete review of SR reporting issues.

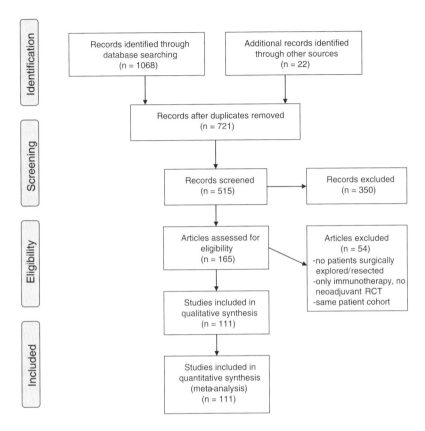

FIGURE 3-1 Example of a flow chart.
SOURCE: Gillen et al. (2010).

3.3.4 Train screeners using written documentation; test and retest screeners to improve accuracy and consistency

3.3.5 Use one of two strategies to select studies: (1) read all full-text articles identified in the search or (2) screen titles and abstracts of all articles and then read the full-text of articles identified in initial screening

3.3.6 Taking account of the risk of bias, consider using observational studies to address gaps in the evidence from randomized clinical trials on the benefits of interventions

Standard 3.4—Document the search
Required elements:
    3.4.1   Provide a line-by-line description of the search strategy, including the date of search for each database, web browser, etc.
    3.4.2   Document the disposition of each report identified including reasons for their exclusion if appropriate

Rationale

The primary purpose of CER is to generate reliable, scientific information to guide the real-world choices of patients, clinicians, developers of clinical practice guidelines, and others. The committee recommends the above standards and performance elements to address the pervasive problems of bias, errors, and inadequate documentation of the study selection process in SRs. While the evidence base for these standards is sparse, these common-sense standards draw from the expert guidance of AHRQ, CRD, and the Cochrane Collaboration. The recommended performance elements will help ensure scientific rigor and promote transparency—key committee criteria for judging possible SR standards.

The potential for bias to enter the selection process is significant and well documented. SR experts recommend a number of techniques and information sources that can help protect against an incomplete and biased collection of evidence. For example, the selection of studies to include in an SR should be prespecified in the research protocol. The research team must balance the imperative for a thorough search with constraints on time and resources. However, using only one screener does not sufficiently protect against a biased selection of studies. Experts agree that using two screeners can reduce error and subjectivity. Although the associated cost may be substantial, and representatives of several SR organizations did tell the committee and IOM staff that dual screening is too costly, the committee concludes that SRs may not be reliable without two screeners. A two-step process will save the time and expense of obtaining full-text articles until after initial screening of citations and abstracts.

Observational studies are important inputs for SRs of comparative effectiveness. The plan for using observational research should be clearly outlined in the protocol along with other selection criteria. Many CER questions cannot be fully answered without observational data on the potential harms, benefits, and long-term effects. In many instances, trial findings are not generalizable to individual patients. Neither experimental nor observational research should be used in an SR without strict methodological scrutiny.

Finally, detailed documentation of methods is essential to scientific inquiry. It is imperative in SRs. Study methods should be reported in sufficient detail so that searches can be replicated and appraised.

MANAGING DATA COLLECTION

Many but not all SRs on the comparative effectiveness of health interventions include a quantitative synthesis (meta-analysis) of the findings of RCTs. Whether or not a quantitative or qualitative synthesis is planned, the assessment of what is known about an intervention's effectiveness should begin with a clear and systematic description of the included studies (CRD, 2009; Deeks et al., 2008). This requires extracting both qualitative and quantitative data from each study, then summarizing the details on each study's methods, participants, setting, context, interventions, outcomes, results, publications, and investigators. Data extraction refers to the process that researchers use to collect and transcribe the data from each individual study. Which data are extracted depends on the research question, types of data that are available, and whether meta-analysis is appropriate.[17] Box 3-6 lists the types of data that are often collected.

The first part of this chapter focused on key methodological judgments regarding the search for and selection of all relevant high-quality evidence pertinent to a research question. Data collection is just as integral to ensuring an accurate and fair accounting of what is known about the effectiveness of a health care intervention. Quality assurance and control are especially important because of the substantial potential for errors in data handling (Gøtzsche et al., 2007). The following section focuses on how standards can help minimize common mistakes during data extraction and concludes with the committee's recommended standard and performance elements for managing data collection.

Preventing Errors

Data extraction errors are common and have been documented in numerous studies (Buscemi et al., 2006; Gøtzsche et al., 2007; Horton et al., 2010; Jones et al., 2005; Tramer et al., 1997). Gøtzsche

---

[17] Qualitative and quantitative synthesis methods are the subject of Chapter 4.

BOX 3-6
Types of Data Extracted from Individual Studies

General Information
1. Researcher performing data extraction
2. Date of data extraction
3. Identification features of the study:
   - Record number (to uniquely identify study)
   - Author
   - Article title
   - Citation
   - Type of publication (e.g., journal article, conference abstract)
   - Country of origin
   - Source of funding

Study Characteristics
1. Aim/objectives of the study
2. Study design
3. Study inclusion and exclusion criteria
4. Recruitment procedures used (e.g., details of randomization, blinding)
5. Unit of allocation (e.g., participant, general practice, etc.)

Participant Characteristics
1. Characteristics of participants at the beginning of the study, such as:
   - Age
   - Gender
   - Race/ethnicity
   - Socioeconomic status
   - Disease characteristics
   - Comorbidities
2. Number of participants in each characteristic category for intervention and comparison group(s) or mean/median characteristic values (record whether it is the number eligible, enrolled, or randomized that is reported in the study)

Intervention and Setting
1. Setting in which the intervention is delivered
2. Description of the intervention(s) and control(s) (e.g. dose, route of administration, number of cycles, duration of cycle, care

and colleagues, for example, examined 27 meta-analyses published in 2004 on a variety of topics, including the effectiveness of acetaminophen for pain in patients with osteoarthritis, antidepressants for mood in trials with active placebos, physical and chemical methods to reduce asthma symptoms from house dust-mite allergens,

provider, how the intervention was developed, theoretical basis [where relevant])

3. Description of cointerventions

Outcome Data/Results

1. Unit of assessment/analysis
2. Statistical techniques used
3. For each prespecified outcome:
   - Whether reported
   - Definition used in study
   - Measurement tool or method used
   - Unit of measurement (if appropriate)
   - Length of follow-up, number and/or times of follow-up measurements
4. For all intervention group(s) and control group(s):
   - Number of participants enrolled
   - Number of participants included in the analysis
   - Number of withdrawals and exclusions lost to follow-up
   - Summary outcome data, e.g., dichotomous (number of events, number of participants), continuous (mean and standard deviation)
5. Type of analysis used in study (e.g. intention to treat, per protocol)
6. Results of study analysis, e.g., dichotomous (odds ratio, risk ratio and confidence intervals, p-value), continuous (mean difference, confidence intervals)
7. If subgroup analysis is planned, the above information on outcome data or results will need to be extracted for each patient subgroup
8. Additional outcomes
9. Record details of any additional relevant outcomes reported
10. Costs
11. Resource use
12. Adverse events

SOURCE: CRD (2009).

and inhaled corticosteroids for asthma symptoms (Gøtzsche et al., 2007). The study focused on identifying the extent of errors in the meta-analyses that used a specific statistical technique (standardized mean difference). The researchers randomly selected two trials from each meta-analysis and extracted outcome data from each related trial report. They found numerous errors and were unable to replicate the results of more than a third of the 27 meta-analyses (37 percent). The studies had used the incorrect number of patients in calculations, incorrectly calculated means and standard deviations, and even got the direction of treatment effect wrong. The impact of the mistakes was not trivial; in some cases, correcting errors negated findings of effectiveness and, in other cases, actually reversed the direction of the measured effect.

In another study, Jones and colleagues (2005) found numerous errors in 42 reviews conducted by the Cochrane Cystic Fibrosis and Genetic Disorders Group. The researchers documented data extraction errors in 20 reviews (48 percent), errors in interpretation in 7 reviews (17 percent), and reporting errors in 18 reviews (43 percent). All the data-handling errors changed the summary results but, in contrast with the Gøtzsche study, the errors did not affect the overall conclusions.

Using Two Data Extractors

Data extraction is an understudied process. Little is known about how best to optimize accuracy and efficiency. One study found that SR experience appears to have little impact on error rates (Horton et al., 2010). In 2006, Horton and colleagues conducted a prospective cross-sectional study to assess whether experience improves accuracy. The researchers assigned data extractors to three different groups based on SR and data extraction experience. The most experienced group had more than 7 years of related experience. The least experienced group had less than 2 years of experience. Surprisingly, error rates were high regardless of experience, ranging from 28.3 percent to 31.2 percent.

The only known effective means of reducing data extraction errors is to have at least two individuals independently extract data (Buscemi et al., 2006). In a pilot study sponsored by AHRQ, Buscemi and colleagues compared the rate of errors that occurred when only one versus two individuals extracted the data from 30 RCTs on the efficacy and safety of melatonin for the management of sleep disorders (Buscemi et al., 2006). When only one reviewer extracted the data, a second reviewer checked the extracted data for accuracy and completeness. The two reviewers resolved discrepancies by mutual consensus. With two reviewers, each individual independently extracted the data, then resolved discrepancies through discussion or in consultation with a third party. Single extraction was faster, but resulted in 21.7 percent more mistakes.

Experts recommend that two data extractors should be used whenever possible (CRD, 2009; Higgins and Deeks, 2008; Van de Voorde and Leonard, 2007). The Cochrane Collaboration advises that more than one person extract data from every study (Higgins and Deeks, 2008). CRD concurs but also suggests that, at a minimum, one individual could extract the data if a second individual independently checks for accuracy and completeness (CRD, 2009).

Addressing Duplicate Publication

Duplicate publication is another form of reporting bias with the potential to distort the findings of an SR. The ICMJE defines redundant (or duplicate) publication as publication of a paper that overlaps substantially with one already published in print or electronic media (ICMJE, 2010). When this occurs, perceptions of the safety and effectiveness of a treatment may be incorrect because it appears that the intervention was tested in more patients than in reality (Tramer et al., 1997). If meta-analyses double count data, the findings obviously will be incorrect.

There have been reports of redundant publication of effectiveness research since at least the 1980s (Arrivé et al., 2008; Bailey, 2002; Bankier et al., 2008; DeAngelis, 2004; Gøtzsche, 1989; Huston and Moher, 1996; Huth, 1986; Mojon-Azzi et al., 2004; Rosenthal et al., 2003; Schein and Paladugu, 2001). Tramer and colleagues, for example, searched for published findings of trials on the effectiveness of the antinausea drug ondansetron to determine the extent of redundant publications (Tramer et al., 1997). The researchers found that the most commonly duplicated RCT reports were those papers that showed the greatest benefit from ondansetron. Twenty-eight percent of patient data were duplicated. As a result, the drug's effectiveness as an antiemetic was overestimated by 23 percent. Gøtszche and colleagues reached similar conclusions in a study of controlled trials on the use of NSAIDs for rheumatoid arthritis (Gøtzsche, 1989).

Linking publications from the same study Detecting multiple publications of the same data is difficult particularly when the data are published in different places or at different times without proper attribution to previous or simultaneous publications (Song et al., 2010). The Cochrane Collaboration recommends electronically linking citations from the same studies so that they are not treated as separate studies and that data from each study are included only once in the SR analyses.

Data Extraction Forms

Data extraction forms are common-sense tools for collecting and documenting the data that will be used in the SR analysis. Numerous formats have been developed, but there is no evidence to support any particular form. Elamin and colleagues (2009) surveyed expert systematic reviewers to describe their experiences with various data extraction tools including paper and pencil formats, spreadsheets, web-based surveys, electronic databases, and special web-based software. The respondents did not appear to favor one type of form over another, and the researchers concluded that no one tool is appropriate for all SRs. AHRQ, CRD, and the Cochrane Collaboration all recommend that the form be pilot-tested to help ensure that the appropriate data are collected (Table 3-3).

RECOMMENDED STANDARD FOR EXTRACTING DATA

The committee recommends the following standard to promote accurate and reliable data extraction:

Standard 3.5—Manage data collection
Required elements:
    3.5.1   At a minimum, use two or more researchers, working independently, to extract quantitative and other critical data from each study. For other types of data, one individual could extract the data while the second individual independently checks for accuracy and completeness. Establish a fair procedure for resolving discrepancies; do not simply give final decision-making power to the senior reviewer
    3.5.2   Link publications from the same study to avoid including data from the same study more than once
    3.5.3   Use standard data extraction forms developed for the specific systematic review
    3.5.4   Pilot-test the data extraction forms and process

Rationale

Quality assurance (e.g., double data extraction) and quality control (e.g., asking a third person to check the primary outcome data entered into the data system) are essential when data are extracted from individual studies from the collected body of evidence. Neither peer reviewers of the SR draft report nor journal editors can detect these kinds of errors. The committee recommends the above performance elements to maximize the scientific rigor of the SR. Consumers, patients, clinicians, and clinical practice guideline developers should not have to question the credibility or accuracy of SRs on the effectiveness of healthcare interventions. Using two researchers to extract data may be costly, but currently, there is no alternative way to ensure that the correct data are used in the synthesis of the collected body of evidence. The committee also recommends that the review team should use a standard data extraction form to help minimize data entry errors. The particular circumstances of the SR—such as the complexity or unique data needs of the project—should guide the selection of the form.

CRITICAL APPRAISAL OF INDIVIDUAL STUDIES

If an SR is to be based on the best available evidence on the comparative effectiveness of interventions, it should include a systematic, critical assessment of the individual eligible studies. The SR should assess the strengths and limitations of the evidence so that decision makers can judge whether the data and results of the included studies are valid. Yet, an extensive literature documents that SRs—across a wide range of clinical specialties—often either fail to appraise or fail to report the appraisal of the individual studies included in the review (Delaney et al., 2007; Dixon et al., 2005; Lundh et al., 2009; Moher et al., 2007a; Moja et al., 2005; Mrkobrada et al., 2008; Roundtree et al., 2008), This includes SRs in general surgery (Dixon et al., 2005), critical care (Delaney et al., 2007), nephrology (Mrkobrada et al., 2008), pediatric oncology (Lundh et al., 2009), and rheumatology (Roundtree et al., 2008).

Methodological studies have demonstrated that problems in the design, conduct, and analysis of clinical studies lead to biased findings. Table 3-4 describes types of bias and some of the measures clinical researchers use to avoid them. The systematic reviewer examines whether the study incorporates these measures to protect against these biases and whether or not the measures were effective. For example, in considering selection bias, the reviewer would note whether the study uses random assignment of participants to treatments and concealment of allocation,[18] because studies that employ these measures are less susceptible to selection bias than those that do not. The reviewer would also note whether there were baseline

---

[18] Allocation concealment is a method used to prevent selection bias in clinical trials by concealing the allocation sequence from those assigning participants to intervention groups. Allocation concealment prevents researchers from (unconsciously or otherwise) influencing the intervention group to which each participant is assigned.

TABLE 3-4 Types of Bias in Individual Studies

Potential Bias	Goal	Relevant Domains in the Cochrane Risk of Bias Tool (for RCTs)	Other Potentially Relevant Domains (Including Observational Studies)
Allocation bias or selection bias: One or more baseline characteristic(s) of individuals is associated with prognosis	At inception, groups being compared are similar in all respects other than the treatment they get	• Sequence generation • Allocation concealment	• Adequate sample size • Similarity of groups at baseline • Use of an inception cohort (e.g., new user designs) • Use of analytical methods to classify subjects into groups (instrumental variable, matching, or other)
Attrition bias: Differences among groups in withdrawal from a study associated with outcome	Maintain follow-up of all enrolled participant groups throughout study	• Sequence generation • Blinding of participants, study personnel, health care providers, and outcome assessors • Incomplete outcome data	• Overall rates of loss to follow-up • Measures to obtain complete follow-up information on all, even those who move, discontinue treatment, etc.
Performance bias: Differences in treatment or care given to comparison groups during the study affects observed results	Maintain comparable conditions throughout study period	• Blinding of participants, personnel, and outcome assessors	• Comparable intensity of services and cointerventions in the compared groups • Other measures as appropriate
Detection bias: Differences among groups in how outcomes are assessed is associated with outcome	Use valid, reliable measures of outcome and assess them in the same manner for all groups being compared	• Blinding of participants, healthcare providers. and outcome assessors	• Measures to ensure equal and accurate ascertainment of exposures and outcomes across groups
Reporting biases: Differences between planned and reported results is associated with nature and direction of findings	Measure and report all preplanned outcomes	• Selective outcome reporting • Selective analysis reporting	

SOURCE: Higgins and Altman (2008).

differences in the assembled groups, because the presence of such differences may indicate that potential flaws in the study design indeed resulted in observable bias.

This section of the chapter describes the concepts and related issues that are fundamental to assessing the individual studies in an SR. The committee's related standards are presented at the end of the section.

Key Concepts

Internal Validity

An internally valid study is conducted in a manner that minimizes bias so that the results are likely due to a real effect of the intervention being tested. By examining features of each study's design and conduct, systematic reviewers arrive at a judgment about the level of confidence one may place in each study, that is, the extent to which the study results can be believed. Assessing internal validity is concerned primarily (but not exclusively) with an examination of the risk of bias. When there are no or few flaws in the design, conduct, and reporting of a study, the results are more likely to be a true indicator of the effects of the compared treatments. When serious flaws are present, the results of a study are likely to be due to biases, rather than to real differences in the treatments that are compared.

Relevance

The need to consider features of a study that might affect its relevance to decision makers is a key principle of CER. SRs use the "applicability," "relevance," "directness," or "external validity" to capture this idea (Rothwell, 1995, 2005). In the context of SRs of CER, "applicability" has been defined as "the extent to which the effects observed in published studies are likely to reflect the expected results when a specific intervention is applied to the population of interest under 'real-world' conditions" (Atkins et al., 2010).

Because applicability is not an inherent characteristic of a study, it is not possible to devise a uniform system for assessing applicability of individual studies (Jüni et al., 2001). However, an SR can describe study characteristics that are likely to affect applicability. In the initial steps in the SR process, by consulting users and stakeholders, the review team should seek to understand the situations to which the findings of the review will be applied (see Chapter 2,

Standards 2.3–2.5). The review team should then decide whether to incorporate relevance into the design of the inclusion criteria and into the protocol for extracting data from included studies.

For a particular review, the review team should develop *a priori* hypotheses about characteristics that are likely to be important and plan to include them when extracting data from studies (Green and Higgins, 2008). Across clinical topics, some study characteristics are likely to affect users' perceptions of an individual study's applicability in practice (Rothwell, 2006). These characteristics can be classified using the PICO(TS)[19] framework and should be considered candidates for abstraction in most SRs of effectiveness (Table 3-5). Among RCTs of drug treatments, for example, some characteristics affecting the *patients* include whether eligibility criteria were narrow or broad, whether there was a run-in period in which some participants were excluded prior to randomization, and what the rates of outcomes were in the control or placebo group.

Fidelity and Quality of Interventions

Users of SRs often need detailed information about interventions and comparators to judge the relevance and validity of the results. Fidelity and quality refer to two dimensions of carrying out an intervention that should be documented to allow meaningful comparisons between studies.

The fidelity of an intervention refers to the extent to which the intervention has been delivered as planned (CRD, 2009). In the context of an SR, an assessment of fidelity requires *a priori* identification of these key features and abstraction of how they were implemented in each study. Frameworks to assess fidelity in individual studies exist, although there has been little experience of their use in SRs (Carroll et al., 2007; Glasgow, 2006; Glasgow et al., 1999).

Fidelity is particularly important for complex interventions. A complex intervention is usually defined as one that has multiple components. For example, a program intended to help people lose weight might include counseling about diet and exercise, access to peers, education, community events, and other components (Craig et al., 2008). Many behavioral interventions, as well as interventions in the organization of care, are complex. Individual studies may

---

[19] "PICOTS" is a commonly used mnemonic for guiding the formulation of an SR's research question. The acronym refers to: Population, Intervention, Comparator, Outcomes, Timing, and Setting. Some systematic review teams use an abbreviated form such as PICO or PICOS.

TABLE 3-5 Characteristics of Individual Studies That May Affect Applicability

Characteristic	Condition That May Limit Applicability	Example	Feature That Should Be Abstracted into Evidence Tables
Population	Narrow eligibility criteria and exclusion of those with co-morbidities	In the Fracture Intervention Trial (FIT) trial (Cummings et al., 1998), the trial randomized only 4000 of 54,000 originally screened. Participants were healthier, younger, thinner, and more adherent than typical women with osteoporosis.	Eligibility criteria and proportion of screened patients enrolled; presence of co-morbidities
	Large differences between demographics of study population and community patients	Cardiovascular clinical trials used to inform Medicare coverage enrolled patients who were significantly younger (60.1 vs. 74.7 years) and more likely to be male (75% vs. 42%) than Medicare patients with cardiovascular disease (Dhruva and Redberg, 2008).	Demographic characteristics: age, sex, race, and ethnicity
	Narrow or unrepresentative severity, stage of illness, or comorbidities	Two-thirds of patients treated for congestive heart failure (CHF) would have been ineligible for major trials. Community patients had less severe CHF and more comorbidities, and were more likely to have had a recent cardiac event or procedure (Dhruva and Redberg, 2008).	Severity or stage of illness; co-morbidities; referral or primary care population; volunteers vs. population-based recruitment strategies
	Run in period with high-exclusion rate for nonadherence or side effects	Trial of etanercept for juvenile arthritis used an active run-in phase and excluded children who had side effects, resulting in a study with a low rate of side effects.	Run-in period; include attrition before randomization and reasons (nonadherence, side effects, nonresponse) (Bravata et al., 2007; Dhruva and Redberg, 2008)
	Event rates much higher or lower than observed in population-based studies	In the Women's Health Initiative trial of post-menopausal hormone therapy, the relatively healthy volunteer participants had a lower rate of heart disease (by up to 50%) than expected for a similar population in the community (Anderson et al., 2004).	Event rates in treatment and control groups

continued

TABLE 3-5 Continued

Characteristic	Condition That May Limit Applicability	Example	Feature That Should Be Abstracted into Evidence Tables
Intervention	Doses or schedules not reflected in current practice	Duloxetine is usually prescribed at 40–60 mg/d. Most published trials, however, used up to 120 mg/d (Gartlehner et al., 2007).	Dose, schedule, and duration of medication
	Intensity and delivery of behavioral interventions that may not be feasible for routine use	Studies of behavioral interventions to promote healthy diet employed high number and longer duration of visits than are available to most community patients (Whitlock et al., 2008).	Hours, frequency, delivery mechanisms (group vs. individual), and duration
	Monitoring practices or visit frequency not used in typical practice	Efficacy studies with strict pill counts and monitoring for antiretroviral treatment does not always translate to effectiveness in real-world practice (Fletcher, 2007).	Interventions to promote adherence (e.g., monitoring, frequent contact). Incentives given to study participants
	Older versions of an intervention no longer in common use	Only one of 23 trials comparing coronary artery bypass surgery with percutaneous coronary angioplasty used the type of drug-eluting stent that is currently used in practice (Bravata et al., 2007).	Specific product and features for rapidly changing technology
	Cointerventions that are likely to modify effectiveness of therapy	Supplementing zinc with iron reduces the effectiveness of iron alone on hemoglobin outcomes. (Walker et al., 2005). Recommendations for iron are based on studies examining iron alone, but patients most often take vitamins in a multivitamin form.	Cointerventions
	Highly selected intervention team or level of training/proficiency not widely available	Trials of carotid endarterectomy selected surgeons based on operative experience and low complication rates and are not representative of community experience of vascular surgeons (Wennberg et al., 1998).	Selection process, training, and skill of intervention team

Comparator	Inadequate dose of comparison therapy	A fixed-dose study (Walker et al., 2005) by the makers of duloxetine compared 80 and 120 mg/d of duloxetine (high dose) with 20 mg of paroxetine (low dose) (Detke et al., 2004).	Dose and schedule of comparator, if applicable
	Use of substandard alternative therapy	In early trials of magnesium in acute myocardial infarction, standard of treatment did not include many current practices including thrombolysis and beta-blockade (Li et al., 2007).	Relative comparability to the treatment option
Outcomes	Composite outcomes that mix outcomes of different significance	Cardiovascular trials frequently use composite outcomes that mix outcomes of varying importance to patients (Ferreira-Gonzalez et al., 2007).	Effects of intervention on most important benefits and harms, and how they are defined
	Short-term or surrogate outcomes	Trials of biologics for rheumatoid arthritis used radiographic progression rather than symptoms (Ioannidis and Lau, 1997). Trials of Alzheimer's disease drugs primarily looked at changes in scales of cognitive function over 6 months, which may not reflect their ability to produce clinically important changes such as institutionalization rates (Hansen et al., 2006).	How outcome defined and at what time

continued

TABLE 3-5 Continued

Characteristic	Condition That May Limit Applicability	Example	Feature That Should Be Abstracted into Evidence Tables
Setting	Standards of care differ markedly from setting of interest	Studies conducted in China and Russia examined the effectiveness of self-breast exams on reducing breast cancer mortality, but these countries do not routinely have concurrent mammogram screening as is available in the United States (Humphrey et al., 2002).	Geographic setting
	Specialty population or level of care differs from that seen in community	Early studies of open surgical repair for abdominal aortic aneurysms found an inverse relationship between hospital volume and short-term mortality (Wilt, 2006).	Clinical setting (e.g., referral center vs. community)

SOURCE: Atkins et al. (2011).

differ widely in how they implement these components. For example, among specialized clinic programs to reduce complications from anticoagulant therapy, decisions about dosing might be made by pharmacists, nurses, physicians, or a computerized algorithm.

Assessing the quality of the intervention is particularly important in reviews of interventions that require technical skill, such as surgical procedures or physical therapy, and in reviews of evolving technologies, such as new devices. The effectiveness and safety of such interventions may vary, depending on the skill of the practitioners, and may change rapidly as practitioners gain experience with them or as modifications are made to correct problems encountered in development.

Variation in the implementation of key elements or features of a complex intervention can influence their effectiveness. The features of a complex intervention may reflect how it is modified to accommodate different practice settings and patients' circumstances (Cohen et al., 2008). In these circumstances it can be difficult to distinguish between an ineffective intervention and a failed implementation.

Risk of Bias in Individual Studies

The committee chose the term "risk of bias" to describe the focus of the assessment of individual studies and the term "quality" to describe the focus of the assessment of a body of evidence (the subject of Chapter 4). The risk of bias terminology has been used and evaluated for assessing individual RCTs for more than two decades. A similar tool for observational studies has yet to be developed and validated.

As alternatives to "risk of bias," many systematic reviewers and organizations that develop practice guidelines use terms such as "study quality," "methodological quality," "study limitations," or "internal validity" to describe the critical appraisal of individual studies. Indeed, reviewers may assign a quality score to a study based on criteria assumed to relate to a study's internal and sometimes external validity. "Study quality" is a broader concept than risk of bias, however, and might include choice of outcome measures, statistical tests, intervention (i.e., dosing, frequency, and intensity of treatments), and reporting. The term "quality" also encompasses errors attributable to chance (e.g., because of inadequate sample size) or erroneous inference (e.g., incorrect interpretation of the study results) (Lohr and Carey, 1999).

Analysis at the level of a group or body of studies can often verify and quantify the direction and magnitude of bias caused by methodological problems.[20] For an individual study, however, one cannot be certain how specific flaws have influenced the estimate of effect; that is, one cannot be certain about the presence, magnitude, and direction of the bias. For this reason, for individual studies, systematic reviewers assess the risk of bias rather than assert that a particular bias is present. A study with a high risk of bias is not credible and may overestimate or underestimate the true effect of the treatment under study. This judgment is based on methodologic research examining the relationship among study characteristics, such as the appropriate use of randomization, allocation concealment, or masking, in relation to estimation of the "true" effect. When an SR has a sufficient number of studies, the authors should attempt to verify and quantify the direction and magnitude of bias caused by methodological problems directly using meta-analysis methods.

In recent years, systematic review teams have moved away from scoring systems to assess the quality of individual studies toward a focus on the components of quality and risk of bias (Jüni, 1999). Quality scoring systems have not been validated. Studies assessed as excellent quality using one scoring method may be subsequently assessed as lower quality using another scoring method (Moher et al., 1996). Moreover, with an emphasis on risk of bias, the SR more appropriately assesses the quality of study design and conduct rather than the quality of reporting.

The committee chose the term "risk of bias" to describe the focus of the assessment of individual studies and the term "quality" to describe the focus of the assessment of a body of evidence (the subject of Chapter 4). The risk of bias terminology has been used and evaluated for assessing individual RCTs for more than two decades. A similar tool for observational studies has yet to be developed and validated.

Risk of Bias in Randomized Controlled Trials

As a general rule, randomized trials, without question, have more protections against bias than observational studies and are less likely to produce biased or misleading results. Even among randomized trials, however, study design features influence the observed results. In the 1980s, for example, Chalmers and colleagues reviewed 145 RCTs of treatments for acute myocardial infarction to assess how blinding treatment assignment affected the results (Chalmers et al., 1981, 1983). Trials that allowed participants to know what treat-

---

[20] Chapter 4 addresses the assessment of a body of evidence.

ment they were assigned had greater treatment effects than studies that masked treatment assignment. The effect of masking was dramatic: Statistically significant differences in case-fatality rates were reported in 24.4 percent of the trials that did not blind participants versus 8.8 percent of the RCTs that masked treatment assignment.

Methodological research conducted in the past 15 years has sought to identify additional features of controlled trials that make them more or less susceptible to bias. This research on the empiric evidence of bias forms the basis of current recommendations for assessing the risk of bias in SRs of RCTs. Much of this research takes the form of meta-epidemiological studies that examine the association of individual study characteristics and estimates of the magnitude of effect among trials included in a set of meta-analyses. In a review published in 1999, Moher and colleagues found strong, consistent empiric evidence of bias for three study design features: allocation concealment, double blinding, and type of randomized trial (Moher et al., 1999). In two separate reviews, allocation concealment and double blinding were shown to be associated with study findings. Pildal and colleagues showed that trials that are inadequately concealed and not double blinded are more likely to show a statistically significant treatment effect (Pildal et al., 2008). Yet Wood and colleagues showed that this effect may be confined to subjective, as opposed to objective, outcome measures and outcomes other than all-cause mortality (Wood et al., 2008).

Since 1999, other trial features, such as stopping early (Montori et al., 2005), handling of missing outcome data (Wood et al., 2004), trial size (Nüesch et al., 2010), and use of intention-to-treat analysis have been evaluated empirically. A study conducted by the Cochrane Back Pain Review Group found empiric evidence of bias for 11 study design features (van Tulder et al., 2009) (Box 3-7).

A recent reanalysis confirmed this finding in Moher and colleagues' (1998) original dataset (effect sizes were smaller for trials that met the criterion for 10 of the 11 items) and in back pain trials (11 of 11 items), but not in trials included in a sample of EPC reports (Hempell et al., 2011). The influence of certain factors, such as allocation concealment, appears to vary depending on the clinical area (Balk et al., 2002) and the type of outcome measured (Wood et al., 2008).

The implication is that systematic review teams should always assess the details of each study's design to determine how potential biases associated with the study design may have influenced the observed results, because ignoring the possibility could be hazardous (Light and Pillemer, 1984).

BOX 3-7
Cochrane Back Pain Group Criteria for
Internal Validity of Randomized Trials of Back Pain

1. Was the method of randomization adequate?
2. Was the treatment allocation concealed?
3. Were the groups similar at baseline regarding the most important prognostic indicators?
4. Was the outcome assessor blinded?
5. Was the care provider blinded?
6. Were patients blinded?
7. Was the drop-out rate acceptable and the reasons given?
8. Were all randomized participants analyzed in the group to which they were originally assigned?
9. Were cointerventions avoided or similar?
10. Was the compliance acceptable in all groups?
11. Was the timing of the outcome assessment similar in all groups?

SOURCE: Adapted from van Tulder et al. (2009).

Risk of Bias in Observational Studies

In the 1970s and 1980s, several thorough scientific reviews of medical or educational interventions established that the positive results of uncontrolled or poorly controlled studies did not always hold up in well-controlled studies. The discrepancy was most dramatic when randomized trials were compared with observational studies of the same intervention (Chalmers, 1982; DerSimonian and Laird, 1986; Glass and Smith, 1979; Hoaglin et al., 1982; Miller et al., 1989; Wortman and Yeaton, 1983).

The likelihood and magnitude of bias is often greater in observational studies because they lack randomization and concealment of allocation. Even when feasible, many observational studies fail to use appropriate steps to address the risk of bias, such as publication of a detailed protocol and blinding of outcome assessors. For example, observational studies commonly report the outcomes of patients who choose treatments based on their own preferences and the advice of their provider. However, factors that influence treatment choices can also influence outcomes (e.g., sicker patients may tend to choose more extreme interventions); thus, such studies often fail to meet the goal of initially comparable groups. This type of bias—called selection bias—produces imbalances in factors associated with prognosis and the outcomes of interest. Although a variety of statistical methods can be used to attempt to reduce the impact of selection bias, there is no way that analysis can be used to correct for unknown factors that may be associated with prognosis. Thus, it is generally acknowledged that "adjustment" in the analysis cannot be viewed as a substitute for a study design that minimizes this bias.

While selection bias is a widely recognized concern, observational studies are also particularly subject to detection bias, performance bias, and information biases.

Tools for Assessing Study Design

Tools for assessing study design have been used for over two decades (Atkins et al., 2001; Coles 2008; Cook et al., 1993; Frazier et al., 1987; Gartlehner et al., 2004; Lohr, 1998; Mulrow and Oxman, 1994). Although a large number of instruments or tools can be used to assess the quality of individual studies, they are all based on the principle that, whenever possible, clinical researchers conducting a comparative clinical study should use several strategies to avoid error and bias.

Instruments vary in clinical and methodological scope. For example, the Cochrane risk of bias tool (Box 3-8) pertains to randomized trials, whereas the U.S. Preventive Services Task Force (USPSTF) tool includes observational studies as well as randomized trials. Some instruments, such as the one in Box 3-7, are designed to be used in a specific clinical area. This instrument was validated in a set of trials related to back pain treatments (van Tulder et al., 2009).

BOX 3-8
Cochrane Risk of Bias Tool Domains

- Sequence generation
- Allocation concealment
- Blinding of participants, personnel, and outcome assessors
- Incomplete outcome data
- Selecting outcome reporting
- Other sources of bias

SOURCE: Adapted from Higgins and Altman (2008).

Instruments also differ in whether they are domain based or goal based. The Cochrane Risk of Bias Tool is an example of a domain-based instrument in which the author assesses the risk of bias in each of five domains. Using detailed criteria for making each judgment, the author must answer a specific question for each domain with "Yes" (low risk of bias) or "No" (high risk of bias.) Then, the author must make judgments about which domains are most important in the particular circumstances of the study, taking into account the likely direction and magnitude of the bias and empirical evidence that it is influential in similar studies. For example, in a study of mortality rates for severely ill patients taking different types of medications for heart disease, the investigators might decide that differential loss to follow-up among treatment groups is critical, but lack of blinding of outcome assessors is not likely to be an important cause of bias (Wood et al., 2008).

Like other tools, the Cochrane tool includes an "other" category to take account of biases that arise from aspects of study design, conduct, and reporting in specific circumstances. Examples include carry-over effects in cross-over trials, recruitment bias in cluster-randomized trials, and biases introduced by trials stopped early for benefit (Bassler et al., 2010).

Other instruments are goal based (criteria based). For example, in the USPSTF criteria (Box 3-9), the criterion "initial assembly of groups" refers to the Table 3-4 goal: "At inception, groups being compared [should be] similar in all respects other than the treatment they get." This criterion is related to the first two domains in the Cochrane Risk of Bias tool (sequence generation and allocation concealment). However, instead of rating the study on these two domains, the review author using the USPSTF tool must integrate information about the method of allocating subjects (sequence generation and allocation concealment) with baseline information about the groups, and consider the magnitude and direction of bias, if any, in order to make a judgment about whether the goal of similar groups at inception of the study was met.

Although the existence and consequences of these biases are widely acknowledged, tools to assess the risk of bias in observational studies of comparative effectiveness are poorly developed (Deeks et al., 2003). There is no agreed-on set of critical elements for a tool and few data on how well they perform when used in the context of an SR (Sanderson et al., 2007). The lack of validated tools is a major limitation for judging how much confidence to put in the results of observational studies, particularly for beneficial effects.

BOX 3-9
USPSTF Criteria for Grading the Internal
Validity of Individual Studies (Randomized
Controlled Trials [RCTs] and Cohort Studies)*

- Initial assembly of comparable groups
- For RCTs: Adequate randomization, including concealment and whether potential confounders were distributed equally among groups
- For cohort studies: Consideration of potential confounders with either restriction or measurement for adjustment in the analysis; consideration of inception cohorts
- Maintenance of comparable groups
- Important differential loss to follow-up or overall high loss to follow-up
- Measurements: Equal, reliable, and valid
- Clear definition of interventions
- All important outcomes considered
- Analysis: Adjustment for potential confounders for cohort studies, or intention-to-treat analysis for RCTs

---

*Criteria for case-control studies, systematic reviews, and diagnostic accuracy studies are omitted.
SOURCE: Harris et al. (2001).

RECOMMENDED STANDARDS FOR ASSESSING THE QUALITY AND RELEVANCE OF INDIVIDUAL STUDIES

The committee recommends the following standard and elements of performance for assessing individual studies.

Standard 3.6—Critically appraise each study
Required elements:

    3.6.1 Systematically assess the risk of bias, using predefined criteria

    3.6.2 Assess the relevance of the study's populations, interventions, and outcome measures

    3.6.3 Assess the fidelity of the implementation of interventions

Rationale

SRs of CER should place a high value on highly applicable, highly reliable evidence about effectiveness (Helfand and Balshem 2010). The standards draw from the expert guidance of AHRQ, CRD, and the Cochrane Collaboration. The recommended performance elements will help ensure scientific rigor and promote transparency—key committee criteria for judging possible SR standards.

Many types of studies can be used to assess the effects of interventions. The first step in assessing the validity of a particular study is to consider its design in relation to appropriateness to the question(s) addressed in the review. Both components of "validity"—applicability and risk of bias—should be examined. For questions about effectiveness, when there are gaps in the evidence from RCTs, reviewers should consider whether observational studies could provide useful information, taking into account that, in many circumstances, observational study designs will not be suitable, either because the risk of bias is very high, or because observational studies that address the populations, comparisons, and outcomes that are not adequately addressed in RCTs are not available.

A well-designed, well-conducted RCT is the most reliable method to compare the effects of different interventions. Validated instruments to assess the risk of bias in RCTs are available. The committee does not recommend a specific tool or set of criteria for assessing risk of bias. Nevertheless, it is essential that at the outset of the SR—during the development of the research protocol—the review team choose and document its planned approach to critically appraising individual studies.[21] The appraisal should then follow the prespecified approach. Any deviation from the planned approach should be clearly explained and documented in the final report.

REFERENCES

AHRQ EHC (Agency for Healthcare Research and Quality, Effective Health Care Program). 2009. *Therapies for children with autism spectrum disorders:Research protocol document*. http://effectivehealthcare.ahrq.gov/index.cfm/search-for-guides-reviews-and-reports/?pageaction=displayproduct&productid=366#953 (accessed June 25, 2010).

Alderson, P., and I. Roberts. 2005. Corticosteroids for acute traumatic brain injury. *Cochrane Database of Systematic Reviews* 2005(1):CD000196.

---

[21] See Chapter 2, Standard 2.6 (Develop a systematic review protocol).

Anderson, G. L., M. Limacher, A. R. Assaf, T. Bassford, S. A. A. Beresford, H. Black, D. Bonds, R. Brunner, R. Brzyski, B. Caan, R. Chlebowski, D. Curb, M. Gass, J. Hays, G. Heiss, S. Hendrix, B. V. Howard, J. Hsia, A. Hubbell, R. Jackson, K. C. Johnson, H. Judd, J. M. Kotchen, L. Kuller, A. Z. LaCroix, D. Lane, R. D. Langer, N. Lasser, C. E. Lewis, J. Manson, K. Margolis, J. Ockene, M. J. O'Sullivan, L. Phillips, R. L. Prentice, C. Ritenbaugh, J. Robbins, J. E. Rossouw, G. Sarto, M. L. Stefanick, L. Van Horn, J. Wactawski-Wende, R. Wallace, S. Wassertheil-Smoller, and the Women's Health Initiative Steering Committee. 2004. Effects of conjugated, equine estrogen in postmenopausal women with hysterectomy: The Women's Health Initiative randomized controlled trial. *JAMA* 291(14):1701–1712.

APA (American Psychological Association). 2010. *PsychINFO*. http://www.apa.org/pubs/databases/psycinfo/index.aspx (accessed June 1, 2010).

Arrivé, L., M. Lewin, P. Dono, L. Monnier-Cholley, C. Hoeffel, and J. M. Tubiana. 2008. Redundant publication in the journal *Radiology*. *Radiology* 247(3):836–840.

Atkins, D. 2007. Creating and synthesizing evidence with decision makers in mind: Integrating evidence from clinical trials and other study designs. *Medical Care* 45(10 Suppl 2):S16–S22.

Atkins, D., R. Harris, C. D. Mulrow, H. Nelson, M. Pignone, S. Saha, and H. C. Sox. 2001. Workshops: New recommendations and reviews from the U.S. Preventive Services Task Force. *Journal of General Internal Medicine* 16(Suppl 1):11–16.

Atkins, D., S. Chang, G. Gartlehner, D. I. Buckley, E. P. Whitlock, E. Berliner, and D. Matchar. 2010. Assessing the applicability of studies when comparing medical interventions. In *Methods guide for comparative effectiveness reviews*, edited by Agency for Healthcare Research and Quality. http://www.effectivehealthcare.ahrq.gov/index.cfm/search-for-guides-reviews-and-reports/?productid=603&pageaction=displayproduct (accessed January 19, 2011).

Bailey, B. J. 2002. Duplicate publication in the field of otolaryngology–head and neck surgery. *Otolaryngology–Head and Neck Surgery* 126(3):211–216.

Bakkalbasi, N., K. Bauer, J. Glover, and L. Wang. 2006. Three options for citation tracking: Google Scholar, Scopus and Web of Science. *Biomedical Digital Libraries* 3(1):7.

Balk, E. M., P. A. L. Bonis, H. Moskowitz, C. H. Schmid, J. P. A. Ioannidis, C. Wang, and J. Lau. 2002. Correlation of quality measures with estimates of treatment effect in meta-analyses of randomized controlled trials. *JAMA* 287(22):2973–2982.

Bankier, A. A., D. Levine, R. G. Sheiman, M. H. Lev, and H. Y. Kressel. 2008. Redundant publications in *Radiology*: Shades of gray in a seemingly black-and-white issue. *Radiology* 247(3):605–607.

Barrowman, N. J., M. Fang, M. Sampson, and D. Moher. 2003. Identifying null metaanalyses that are ripe for updating. *BMC Medical Research Methodology* 3(1):13.

Bassler, D., M. Briel, V. M. Montori, M. Lane, P. Glasziou, Q. Zhou, D. Heels-Ansdell, S. D. Walter, G. H. Guyatt, Stopit-Study Group, D. N. Flynn, M. B. Elamin, M. H. Murad, N. O. Abu Elnour, J. F. Lampropulos, A. Sood, R. J. Mullan, P. J. Erwin, C. R. Bankhead, R. Perera, C. Ruiz Culebro, J. J. You, S. M. Mulla, J. Kaur, K. A. Nerenberg, H. Schunemann, D. J. Cook, K. Lutz, C. M. Ribic, N. Vale, G. Malaga, E. A. Akl, I. Ferreira-Gonzalez, P. Alonso-Coello, G. Urrutia, R. Kunz, H. C. Bucher, A. J. Nordmann, H. Raatz, S. A. da Silva, F. Tuche, B. Strahm, B. Djulbegovic, N. K. Adhikari, E. J. Mills, F. Gwadry-Sridhar, H. Kirpalani, H. P. Soares, P. J. Karanicolas, K. E. Burns, P. O. Vandvik, F. Coto-Yglesias, P. P. Chrispim, and T. Ramsay. 2010. Stopping randomized trials early for benefit and estimation of treatment effects: Systematic review and meta-regression analysis. *JAMA* 303(12):1180–1187.

Bennett, D. A., and A. Jull. 2003. FDA: Untapped source of unpublished trials. *Lancet* 361(9367):1402–1403.

Betran, A., L. Say, M. Gulmezoglu, T. Allen, and L. Hampson. 2005. Effectiveness of different databases in identifying studies for systematic reviews: Experience from the WHO systematic review of maternal morbidity and mortality. *BMC Medical Research Methodology* 5(1):6.

BIREME (Latin American and Caribbean Center on Health Sciences).2010. *LILACS database*. http://bvsmodelo.bvsalud.org/site/lilacs/I/ililacs.htm (accessed June 7, 2010).

Boissel, J. P. 1993. International Collaborative Group on Clinical Trial Registries: Position paper and consensus recommendations on clinical trial registries. *Clinical Trials and Meta-analysis* 28(4–5):255–266.

Booth, A. 2006. "Brimful of STARLITE": Toward standards for reporting literature searches. *Journal of the Medical Library Association* 94(4):421–429.

Bravata, D. M., K. McDonald, A. Gienger, V. Sundaram, D. K. Owens, and M. A. Hlatky. 2007. Comparative effectiveness of percutaneous coronary interventions and coronary artery bypass grafting for coronary artery disease. *Journal of General Internal Medicine* 22(Suppl 1):47.

Buscemi, N., L. Hartling, B. Vandermeer, L. Tjosvold, and T. P. Klassen. 2006. Single data extraction generated more errors than double data extraction in systematic reviews. *Journal of Clinical Epidemiology* 59(7):697–703.

Campbell Collaboration. 2000. *About the C2-SPECTR Database*. http://geb9101.gse.upenn.edu/ (accessed June 1, 2010).

Carroll, C., M. Patterson, S. Wood, A. Booth, J. Rick, and S. Balain. 2007. A conceptual framework for implementation fidelity. *Implementation Science* 2(1):Article No. 40.

Chalmers, T. C. 1982. The randomized controlled trial as a basis for therapeutic decisions. In *The randomized clinical trial and therapeutic decisions*, edited by J. M. Lachin, N. Tygstrup, and E. Juhl. New York: Marcel Dekker.

Chalmers, T. C., H. Smith, B. Blackburn, B. Silverman, B. Schroeder, D. Reitman, and A. Ambroz. 1981. A method for assessing the quality of a randomized control trial. *Controlled Clinical Trials* 2(1):31–49.

Chalmers, T. C., P. Celano, H. S. Sacks, and H. Smith, Jr. 1983. Bias in treatment assignment in controlled clinical trials. *New England Journal of Medicine* 309(22):1358–1361.

Chambers, D., M. Rodgers, and N. Woolacott. 2009. Not only randomized controlled trials, but also case series should be considered in systematic reviews of rapidly developing technologies. *Journal of Clinical Epidemiology* 62(12):1253–1260.

Chan, A. W., and D. G. Altman. 2005. Identifying outcome reporting bias in randomised trials on PubMed: Review of publications and survey of authors. *BMJ* 330(7494):753.

Chan, A., K. Krleza-Jeric, I. Schmid, and D. G. Altman. 2004a. Outcome reporting bias in randomized trials funded by the Canadian Institutes of Health Research. *Canadian Medical Association Journal* 171(7):735–740.

Chan, A. W., A. Hrobjartsson, M. T. Haahr, P. C. Gøtzsche, and D. G. Altman. 2004b. Empirical evidence for selective reporting of outcomes in randomized trials: Comparison of protocols to published articles. *JAMA* 291(20):2457–2465.

Chapman, A. L., L. C. Morgan, and G. Gartlehner. 2010. Semi-automating the manual literature search for systematic reviews increases efficiency. *Health Information and Libraries Journal* 27(1):22–27.

Chou, R., and M. Helfand. 2005. Challenges in systematic reviews that assess treatment harms. *Annals of Internal Medicine* 142(12):1090–1099.

Chou, R., N. Aronson, D. Atkins, A. S. Ismaila, P. Santaguida, D. H. Smith, E. Whitlock, T. J. Wilt, and D. Moher. 2010. AHRQ series paper 4: Assessing harms when comparing medical interventions: AHRQ and the Effective Health Care Program. *Journal of Clinical Epidemiology* 63(5):502–512.

Cochrane Collaboration. 2010a. *Cochrane Central Register of Controlled Trials.* http://onlinelibrary.wiley.com/o/cochrane/cochrane_clcentral_articles_fs.html (accessed June 7, 2010).

Cochrane Collaboration. 2010b. *Cochrane training.* http://www.cochrane.org/training (accessed January 29, 2011).

Cochrane IMS. 2010. *About RevMan 5.* http://ims.cochrane.org/revman (accessed November 11, 2010).

Cohen, D. J., B. F. Crabtree, R. S. Etz, B. A. Balasubramanian, K. E. Donahue, L. C. Leviton, E. C. Clark, N. F. Isaacson, K. C. Stange, and L. W. Green. 2008. Fidelity versus flexibility: Translating evidence-based research into practice. *American Journal of Preventive Medicine* 35(5, Supplement 1):S381–S389.

Coles, B. 2008. Cochrane information retrieval methods group. *About the Cochrane Collaboration (methods groups)* 3: Article No. CE000145.

Concato, J., N. Shah, and R. I. Horwitz. 2000. Randomized, controlled trials, observational studies, and the hierarchy of research designs. *New England Journal of Medicine* 342(25):1887–1892.

Cook, D. J., G. H. Guyatt, G. Ryan, J. Clifton, L. Buckingham, A. Willan, W. McIlroy, and A. D. Oxman. 1993. Should unpublished data be included in meta-analyses? Current convictions and controversies. *JAMA* 269(21):2749–2753.

Cooper, M., W. Ungar, and S. Zlotkin. 2006. An assessment of inter-rater agreement of the literature filtering process in the development of evidence-based dietary guidelines. *Public Health Nutrition* 9(4):494–500.

Craig, P., P. Dieppe, S. Macintyre, S. Michie, I. Nazareth, and M. Petticrew. 2008. Developing and evaluating complex interventions: The new Medical Research Council guidance. *BMJ* 337(7676):979–983.

CRASH Trial Collaborators. 2004. Effect of intravenous corticosteroids on death within 14 days in 10,008 adults with clinically significant head injury (MRC CRASH trial): Randomised placebo-controlled trial. *Lancet* 364(9442):1321–1328.

CRD (Centre for Reviews and Dissemination). 2009. *Systematic reviews: CRD's guidance for undertaking reviews in health care.* York, UK: York Publishing Services, Ltd.

CRD. 2010. *Database of Abstracts of Reviews of Effects (DARE).* http://www.crd.york.ac.uk/crdweb/html/help.htm (accessed May 28, 2010).

Crumley, E. T., N. Wiebe, K. Cramer, T. P. Klassen, and L. Hartling. 2005. Which resources should be used to identify RCT/CCTs for systematic reviews: A systematic review. *BMC Medical Research Methodology* 5:24.

Cummings, S. R., D. M. Black, D. E. Thompson, W. B. Applegate, E. Barrett-Connor, T. A. Musliner, L. Palermo, R. Prineas, S. M. Rubin, J. C. Scott, T. Vogt, R. Wallace, A. J. Yates, and A. Z. LaCroix. 1998. Effect of alendronate on risk of fracture in women with low bone density but without vertebral fractures: Results from the fracture intervention trial. *JAMA* 280(24):2077–2082.

DeAngelis, C. D., J. M. Drazen, F. A. Frizelle, C. Haug, J. Hoey, R. Horton, S. Kotzin, C. Laine, A. Marusic, A. J. Overbeke, T. V. Schroeder, H. C. Sox, and M. B. Van der Weyden. 2004. Clinical trial registration: A statement from the International Committee of Medical Journal Editors. *JAMA* 292(11):1363–1364.

Deeks, J. J., J. Dinnes, R. D'Amico, A. J. Sowden, C. Sakarovitch, F. Song, M. Petticrew, and D. G. Altman. 2003. Evaluating non-randomised intervention studies. *Health Technology Assessment* 7(27):1–173.

Deeks, J., J. Higgins, and D. Altman, eds. 2008. Analysing data and undertaking meta-analyses. In *Cochrane Handbook for Systematic Reviews of Interventions*, edited by J. P. T. Higgins and S. Green, Chichester, UK: John Wiley & Sons.

Delaney, A., S. M. Bagshaw, A. Ferland, K. Laupland, B. Manns, and C. Doig. 2007. The quality of reports of critical care meta-analyses in the Cochrane Database of Systematic Reviews: An independent appraisal. *Critical Care Medicine* 35(2):589–594.

DerSimonian, R., and N. Laird. 1986. Meta-analysis in clinical trials. *Controlled Clinical Trials* 7(3):177–188.

Detke, M. J., C. G. Wiltse, C. H. Mallinckrodt, R. K. McNamara, M. A. Demitrack, and I. Bitter. 2004. Duloxetine in the acute and long-term treatment of major depressive disorder: A placebo- and paroxetine-controlled trial. *European Neuropsychopharmacology* 14(6):457–470.

Devereaux, P. J., P. T. L. Choi, S. El-Dika, M. Bhandari, V. M. Montori, H. J. Schünemann, A. Garg, J. W. Busse, D. Heels-Ansdell, W. A. Ghali, B. J. Manns, and G. H. Guyatt. 2004. An observational study found that authors of randomized controlled trials frequently use concealment of randomization and blinding, despite the failure to report these methods. *Journal of Clinical Epidemiology* 57(12):1232–1236.

Dhruva, S. S., and R. F. Redberg. 2008. Variations between clinical trial participants and Medicare beneficiaries in evidence used for Medicare national coverage decisions. *Archives of Internal Medicine* 168(2):136–140.

Dickersin, K. 1988. Report from the panel on the case for registers of clinical trials at the eighth annual meeting of the Society for Clinical Trials. *Controlled Clinical Trials* 9(1):76–80.

Dickersin, K. 1990. The existence of publication bias and risk factors for its occurrence. *JAMA* 263(10):1385–1389.

Dickersin, K., and I. Chalmers. 2010. *Recognising, investigating and dealing with incomplete and biased reporting of clinical research: From Francis Bacon to the World Health Organisation*. http://www.jameslindlibrary.org (accessed June 11, 2010).

Dickersin, K., and Y. I. Min. 1993. NIH clinical trials and publication bias. *Online Journal of Current Clinical Trials* April 28:Document no. 50.

Dickersin, K., and D. Rennie. 2003. Registering clinical trials. *JAMA* 290(4):516–523.

Dickersin, K., P. Hewitt, L. Mutch, I. Chalmers, and T. C. Chalmers. 1985. Perusing the literature: Comparison of MEDLINE searching with a perinatal trials database. *Controlled Clinical Trials* 6(4):306–317.

Dickersin, K., Y. I. Min, and C. L. Meinert. 1992. Factors influencing publication of research results: Follow-up of applications submitted to two institutional review boards. *JAMA* 267(3):374–378.

Dickersin, K., R. Scherer, and C. Lefebvre. 1994. Identifying relevant studies for systematic reviews. *BMJ* 309(6964):1286–1291.

Dickersin, K., E. Manheimer, S. Wieland, K. A. Robinson, C. Lefebvre, S. McDonald, and the Central Development Group. 2002a. Development of the Cochrane Collaboration's Central Register of Controlled Clinical Trials. *Evaluation and the Health Professions* 25(1):38–64.

Dickersin, K., C. M. Olson, D. Rennie, D. Cook, A. Flanagin, Q. Zhu, J. Reiling, and B. Pace. 2002b. Association between time interval to publication and statistical significance. *JAMA* 287(21):2829–2831.

Dickersin, K., E. Ssemanda, C. Mansell, and D. Rennie. 2007. What do the *JAMA* editors say when they discuss manuscripts that they are considering for publication? Developing a schema for classifying the content of editorial discussion. *BMC Medical Research Methodology* 7: Article no. 44.

Dixon, E., M. Hameed, F. Sutherland, D. J. Cook, and C. Doig. 2005. Evaluating meta-analyses in the general surgical literature: A critical appraisal. *Annals of Surgery* 241(3):450–459.

Dreyer, N. A., and S. Garner. 2009. Registries for robust evidence. *JAMA* 302(7):790–791.

Dwan, K., D. G. Altman, J. A. Arnaiz, J. Bloom, A. Chan, E. Cronin, E. Decullier, P. J. Easterbrook, E. Von Elm, C. Gamble, D. Ghersi, J. P. A. Ioannidis, J. Simes, and P. R. Williamson. 2008. Systematic review of the empirical evidence of study publication bias and outcome reporting bias. *PLoS ONE* 3(8):e3081.

EBSCO Publishing. 2010. *The CINAHL database*. http://www.ebscohost.com/thisTopic.php?marketID=1&topicID=53 (accessed June 1, 2010).

Edwards, P., M. Clarke, C. DiGuiseppi, S. Pratap, I. Roberts, and R. Wentz. 2002. Identification of randomized controlled trials in systematic reviews: Accuracy and reliability of screening records. *Statistics in Medicine* 21(11):1635–1640.

Egger, M., and T. Zellweger-Zahner. 1997. Language bias in randomised controlled trials published in English and German. *Lancet* 350(9074):326.

Egger, M., P. Jüni, C. Bartlett, F. Holenstein, and J. Sterne. 2003. How important are comprehensive literature searches and the assessment of trial quality in systematic reviews? Empirical study. *Health Technology Assessment* 7(1):1–76.

Elamin, M. B., D. N. Flynn, D. Bassler, M. Briel, P. Alonso-Coello, P. J. Karanicolas, G. H. Guyatt, G. Malaga, T. A. Furukawa, R. Kunz, H. Schünemann, M. H. Murad, C. Barbui, A. Cipriani, and V. M. Montori. 2009. Choice of data extraction tools for systematic reviews depends on resources and review complexity. *Journal of Clinical Epidemiology* 62(5):506–510.

Embase. 2010. *What is Embase?* http://www.info.embase.com/what-is-embase (accessed May 28, 2010).

Ewart, R., H. Lausen, and N. Millian. 2009. Undisclosed changes in outcomes in randomized controlled trials: An observational study. *Annals of Family Medicine* 7(6):542–546.

Eyding, D., M. Lelgemann, U. Grouven, M. Härter, M. Kromp, T. Kaiser, M. F. Kerekes, M. Gerken, and B. Wieseler. 2010. Reboxetine for acute treatment of major depression: Systematic review and meta-analysis of published and unpublished placebo and selective serotonin reuptake inhibitor controlled trials. *BMJ* 341:c4737.

Falagas, M. E., E. I. Pitsouni, G. A. Malietzis, and G. Pappas. 2008. Comparison of PubMed, Scopus, Web of Science, and Google Scholar: Strengths and weaknesses. *Journal of the Federation of American Societies for Experimental Biology* 22(2):338–342.

Ferreira-Gonzalez, I., J. W. Busse, D. Heels-Ansdell, V. M. Montori, E. A. Akl, D. M. Bryant, J. Alonso, R. Jaeschke, H. J. Schunemann, G. Permanyer-Miralda, A. Domingo-Salvany, and G. H. Guyatt. 2007. Problems with use of composite end points in cardiovascular trials: Systematic review of randomised controlled trials. *BMJ* 334(7597):786–788.

Flemming, K., and M. Briggs. 2007. Electronic searching to locate qualitative research: Evaluation of three strategies. *Journal of Advanced Nursing* 57(1):95–100.

Fletcher, C. V. 2007. Translating efficacy into effectiveness in antiretroviral therapy. *Drugs* 67(14):1969–1979.

Frazier, L. M., C. D. Mulrow, and L. T. Alexander, Jr. 1987. Need for insulin therapy in type II diabetes mellitus: A randomized trial. *Archives of Internal Medicine* 147(6):1085–1089.

Furlan, A. D., E. Irvin, and C. Bombardier. 2006. Limited search strategies were effective in finding relevant nonrandomized studies. *Journal of Clinical Epidemiology* 59(12):1303–1311.

Garritty, C., A. C. Tricco, M. Sampson, A. Tsertsvadze, K. Shojania, M. P. Eccles, J. Grimshaw, and D. Moher. 2009. A framework for updating systematic reviews. In *Updating systematic reviews: The policies and practices of health care organizations involved in evidence synthesis.* Garrity, C. M.Sc. thesis. Toronto, ON: University of Toronto.

Gartlehner, G., S. West, K. N. Lohr, L. Kahwati, J. Johnson, R. Harris, L. Whitener, C. Voisin, and S. Sutton. 2004. Assessing the need to update prevention guidelines: A comparison of two methods. *International Journal for Quality in Health Care* 16(5):399–406.

Gartlehner, G., R. A. Hansen, P. Thieda, A. M. DeVeaugh-Geiss, B. N. Gaynes, E. E. Krebs, L. J. Lux, L. C. Morgan, J. A. Shumate, L. G. Monroe, and K. N. Lohr. 2007. *Comparative effectiveness of second-generation antidepressants in the pharmacologic treatment of adult depression.* Rockville, MD: Agency for Healthcare Research and Quality.

Gillen, S., T. Schuster, C. Meyer zum Büschenfelde, H. Friess, and J. Kleeff. 2010. Preoperative/neoadjuvant therapy in pancreatic cancer: A systematic review and meta-analysis of response and resection percentages. *PLoS Med* 7(4):e1000267.

Glanville, J. M., C. Lefebvre, J. N. V. Miles, and J. Camosso-Stefinovic. 2006. How to identify randomized controlled trials in MEDLINE: Ten years on. *Journal of the Medical Library Association* 94(2):130–136.

Glasgow, R. E. 2006. RE-AIMing research for application: Ways to improve evidence for family medicine. *Journal of the American Board of Family Medicine* 19(1):11–19.

Glasgow, R. E., T. M. Vogt, and S. M. Boles. 1999. Evaluating the public health impact of health promotion interventions: The RE-AIM framework. *American Journal of Public Health* 89(9):1322–1327.

Glass, G. V., and M. L. Smith. 1979. Meta-analysis of research on class size and achievement. *Educational Evaluation and Policy Analysis* 1(1):2–16.

Glasziou, P., I. Chalmers, M. Rawlins, and P. McCulloch. 2007. When are randomised trials unnecessary? Picking signal from noise. *BMJ* 334(7589):349–351.

Glasziou, P., E. Meats, C. Heneghan, and S. Shepperd. 2008. What is missing from descriptions of treatment in trials and reviews? *BMJ* 336(7659):1472–1474.

Gluud, L. L. 2006. Bias in clinical intervention research. *American Journal of Epidemiology* 163(6):493–501.

Golder, S., and Y. K. Loke. 2008. Is there evidence for biased reporting of published adverse effects data in pharmaceutical industry-funded studies? *British Journal of Clinical Pharmacology* 66(6):767–773.

Golder, S., and Y. Loke. 2009. Search strategies to identify information on adverse effects: A systematic review. *Journal of the Medical Library Association* 97(2):84–92.

Golder, S., and Y. K. Loke. 2010. Sources of information on adverse effects: A systematic review. *Health Information & Libraries Journal* 27(3):176–190.

Golder, S., Y. Loke, and H. M. McIntosh. 2008. Poor reporting and inadequate searches were apparent in systematic reviews of adverse effects. *Journal of Clinical Epidemiology* 61(5):440–448.

Goldsmith, M. R., C. R. Bankhead, and J. Austoker. 2007. Synthesising quantitative and qualitative research in evidence-based patient information. *Journal of Epidemiology & Community Health* 61(3):262–270.

Gøtzsche, P. C. 1987. Reference bias in reports of drug trials. *BMJ (Clinical Research Ed.)* 295(6599):654–656.

Gøtzsche, P. C. 1989. Multiple publication of reports of drug trials. *European Journal of Clinical Pharmacology* 36(5):429–432.

Gøtzsche, P. C., A. Hrobjartsson, K. Maric, and B. Tendal. 2007. Data extraction errors in meta-analyses that use standardized mean differences. *JAMA* 298(4):430–437.

Green, S., and J. P. T. Higgins. 2008. Preparing a Cochrane review. In *Cochrane handbook for systematic reviews of interventions*, edited by J. P. T. Higgins and S. Green. Chichester, UK: John Wiley & Sons.

Gregoire, G., F. Derderian, and J. Le Lorier. 1995. Selecting the language of the publications included in a meta-analysis: Is there a Tower of Babel bias? *Journal of Clinical Epidemiology* 48(1):159–163.

Hansen, R. A., G. Gartlehner, D. Kaufer, K. N. Lohr, and T. Carey. 2006. *Drug class review of Alzheimer's drugs: Final report*. http://www.ohsu.edu/drugeffectiveness/reports/final.cfm (accessed November 12, 2010).

Harris, R. P., M. Helfand, S. H. Woolf, K. N. Lohr, C. D. Mulrow, S. M. Teutsch, D. Atkins, and Methods Work Group, Third U.S. Preventive Services Task Force. 2001. Current methods of the U.S. Preventive Services Task Force: A review of the process. *American Journal of Preventive Medicine* 20(3 Suppl):21–35.

Hartling, L., F. A. McAlister, B. H. Rowe, J. Ezekowitz, C. Friesen, and T. P. Klassen. 2005. Challenges in systematic reviews of therapeutic devices and procedures. *Annals of Internal Medicine* 142(12 Pt 2):1100–1111.

Helfand, M., and H. Balshem. 2010. AHRQ series paper 2: Principles for developing guidance: AHRQ and the Effective Health Care Program. *Journal of Clinical Epidemiology* 63(5):484–490.

Helmer, D., I. Savoie, C. Green, and A. Kazanjian. 2001. Evidence-based practice: Extending the search to find material for the systematic review. *Bulletin of the Medical Library Association* 89(4):346–352.

Hempell, S., M. Suttorp, J. Miles, Z. Wang, M. Maglione, S. Morton, B. Johnsen, D. Valentine, and P. Shekelle. 2011. Assessing the empirical evidence of associations between internal validity and effect sizes in randomized controlled trials. Evidence Report/Technology Assessment No. HHSA 290 2007 10062 I (prepared by the Southern California Evidence-based Practice Center under Contract No. 290-2007-10062-I), Rockville, MD: AHRQ.

Heres, S., S. Wagenpfeil, J. Hamann, W. Kissling, and S. Leucht. 2004. Language bias in neuroscience: Is the Tower of Babel located in Germany? *European Psychiatry* 19(4):230–232.

Hernandez, D. A., M. M. El-Masri, and C. A. Hernandez. 2008. Choosing and using citation and bibliographic database software (BDS). *Diabetic Education* 34(3):457–474.

Higgins, J. P. T., and D. G. Altman. 2008. Assessing risk of bias in included studies. In *Cochrane handbook for systematic reviews of interventions*, edited by J. P. T. Higgins and S. Green. Chichester, U.: The Cochrane Collaboration.

Higgins, J. P. T., and J. J. Deeks. 2008. Selecting studies and collecting data. In *Cochrane handbook for systematic reviews of interventions*, edited by J. P. T. Higgins and S. Green. Chichester, UK: The Cochrane Collaboration.

Higgins, J. P. T., S. Green, and R. Scholten. 2008. Maintaining reviews: Updates, amendments and feedback. In *Cochrane handbook for systematic reviews of interventions*, edited by J. P. T. Higgins and S. Green. Chichester, UK: The Cochrane Collaboration.

Hirsch, L. 2008. Trial registration and results disclosure: Impact of U.S. legislation on sponsors, investigators, and medical journal editors. *Current Medical Research and Opinion* 24(6):1683–1689.

Hoaglin, D. C., R. L. Light, B. McPeek, F. Mosteller, and M. A. Stoto. 1982. *Data for decisions*. Cambridge, MA: Abt Books.

Hopewell, S., L. Wolfenden, and M. Clarke. 2008. Reporting of adverse events in systematic reviews can be improved: Survey results. *Journal of Clinical Epidemiology* 61(6):597–602.

Hopewell, S., K. Loudon, and M. J. Clarke et al. 2009a. Publication bias in clinical trials due to statistical significance or direction of trial results. *Cochrane Database of Systematic Reviews* 1:MR000006.pub3.

Hopewell, S., M. J. Clarke, C. Lefebvre, and R. W. Scherer. 2009b. Handsearching versus electronic searching to identify reports of randomized trials. *Cochrane Database of Systematic Reviews* 4: MR000001.pub2.

Horton, J., B. Vandermeer, L. Hartling, L. Tjosvold, T. P. Klassen, and N. Buscemi. 2010. Systematic review data extraction: Cross-sectional study showed that experience did not increase accuracy. *Journal of Clinical Epidemiology* 63(3):289–298.

Humphrey, L., B. K. S. Chan, S. Detlefsen, and M. Helfand. 2002. Screening for breast cancer. Edited by Oregon Health & Science University Evidence-based Practice Center under Contract No. 290-97-0018. Rockville, MD: Agency for Healthcare Research and Quality.

Huston, P., and D. Moher. 1996. Redundancy, disaggregation, and the integrity of medical research. *Lancet* 347(9007):1024–1026.

Huth, E. J. 1986. Irresponsible authorship and wasteful publication. *Annals of Internal Medicine* 104(2):257–259.

ICMJE (International Committee of Medical Journal Editors). 2010. *Uniform requirements for manuscripts submitted to biomedical journals: Writing and editing for biomedical publication*. http://www.icmje.org/urm_full.pdf (accessed July 8, 2010).

Ioannidis, J. P. A., J. C. Cappelleri, H. S. Sacks, and J. Lau. 1997. The relationship between study design, results, and reporting of randomized clinical trials of HIV infection. *Controlled Clinical Trials* 18(5):431–444.

Ioannidis, J. 1998. Effect of the statistical significance of results on the time to completion and publication of randomized efficacy trials. *JAMA* 279:281–286.

IOM (Institute of Medicine). 2008. *Knowing what works in health care: A roadmap for the nation*. Edited by J. Eden, B. Wheatley, B. McNeil, and H. Sox. Washington, DC: The National Academies Press.

IOM. 2009. *Initial national priorities for comparative effectiveness research*. Washington, DC: The National Academies Press.

ISI Web of Knowledge. 2009. *Web of science*. http://images.isiknowledge.com/WOKRS49B3/help/WOS/h_database.html (accessed May 28, 2010).

Jones, A. P., T. Remmington, P. R. Williamson, D. Ashby, and R. S. Smyth. 2005. High prevalence but low impact of data extraction and reporting errors were found in Cochrane systematic reviews. *Journal of Clinical Epidemiology* 58(7):741–742.

Jorgensen, A. W., K. L. Maric, B. Tendal, A. Faurschou, and P. C. Gotzsche. 2008. Industry-supported meta-analyses compared with meta-analyses with nonprofit or no support: Differences in methodological quality and conclusions. *BMC Medical Research Methodology* 8: Article no. 60.

Jüni, P. 1999. The hazards of scoring the quality of clinical trials for meta-analysis. *JAMA* 282:1054–1060.

Jüni, P., M. Egger, D. G. Altman, and G. D. Smith. 2001. Assessing the quality of randomised controlled trials. In *Systematic review in health care: Meta-analysis in context*, edited by M. Egger, G. D. Smith, and D. G. Altman. London, UK: BMJ Publishing Group.

Jüni, P., F. Holenstein, J. Sterne, C. Bartlett, and M. Egger. 2002. Direction and impact of language bias in meta-analyses of controlled trials: Empirical study. *International Journal of Epidemiology* 31(1):115–123.

Kelley, G., K. Kelley, and Z. Vu Tran. 2004. Retrieval of missing data for meta-analysis: A practical example. *International Journal of Technology Assessment in Health Care* 20(3):296.

Khan, K. S., and J. Kleijnen. 2001. Stage II Conducting the review: Phase 4 Selection of studies. In *CRD Report No. 4*, edited by K. S. Khan, G. ter Riet, H. Glanville, A. J. Sowden and J. Kleijnen. York, U.K.: NHS Centre for Reviews and Dissemination, University of York.

Kirkham, J. J., K. M. Dwan, D. G. Altman, C. Gamble, S. Dodd, R. S. Smyth, and P. R. Williamson. 2010. The impact of outcome reporting bias in randomised controlled trials on a cohort of systematic reviews. *BMJ* 340(7747):637–640.

Kjaergard, L. L., and B. Als-Nielsen. 2002. Association between competing interests and authors' conclusions: Epidemiological study of randomised clinical trials published in the *BMJ*. *BMJ* 325(7358):249.

Knowledge for Health. 2010. *About POPLINE.* http://www.popline.org/aboutpl.html (accessed June 1, 2010).

Kuper, H., A. Nicholson, and H. Hemingway. 2006. Searching for observational studies: What does citation tracking add to PubMed? A case study in depression and coronary heart disease. *BMC Medical Research Methodology* 6:4.

Lee, K., P. Bacchetti, and I. Sim. 2008. Publication of clinical trials supporting successful new drug applications: A literature analysis. *PLoS Medicine* 5(9):1348–1356.

Lefebvre, C., E. Manheimer, and J. Glanville. 2008. Searching for studies. In *Cochrane handbook for systematic reviews of interventions*, edited by J. P. T. Higgins and S. Green. Chichester, U.K.: The Cochrane Collaboration.

Lemeshow, A. R., R. E. Blum, J. A. Berlin, M. A. Stoto, and G. A. Colditz. 2005. Searching one or two databases was insufficient for meta-analysis of observational studies. *Journal of Clinical Epidemiology* 58(9):867–873.

Lexchin, J., L. A. Bero, B. Djulbegovic, and O. Clark. 2003. Pharmaceutical industry sponsorship and research outcome and quality: Systematic review. *BMJ* 326(7400):1167–1170.

Li, J., Q. Zhang, M. Zhang, and M. Egger. 2007. Intravenous magnesium for acute myocardial infarction. *Cochrane Database of Systematic Reviews* 2:CD002755.

Liberati, A., D. G. Altman, J. Tetzlaff, C. Mulrow, P. C. Gotzsche, J. P. A. Ioannidis, M. Clarke, P. J. Devereaux, J. Kleijnen, and D. Moher. 2009. The PRISMA statement for reporting systematic reviews and meta-analyses of studies that evaluate health care interventions: Explanation and elaboration. *Annals of Internal Medicine* 151(4):W1–W30.

Light, R. L., and D. Pillemer. 1984. *Summing up: The science of reviewing research*. Cambridge, MA: Harvard University Press.

Linde, K., and S. N. Willich. 2003. How objective are systematic reviews? Differences between reviews on complementary medicine. *Journal of the Royal Society of Medicine* 96(1):17–22.

Lohr, K. 1998. *Grading articles and evidence: Issues and options*. Research Triangle Park, NC: RTI-UNC Evidence-based Practice Center.

Lohr, K. N., and T. S. Carey. 1999. Assessing "best evidence": Issues in grading the quality of studies for systematic reviews. *Joint Commission Journal on Quality Improvement* 25(9):470–479.

Louden, K., S. Hopewell, M. Clarke, D. Moher, R. Scholten, A. Eisinga, and S. D. French. 2008. A decision tree and checklist to guide decisions on whether, and when, to update Cochrane reviews. In *A decision tool for updating Cochrane reviews*. Chichester, U.K.: The Cochrane Collaboration.

Lundh, A., S. L. Knijnenburg, A. W. Jorgensen, E. C. van Dalen, and L. C. M. Kremer. 2009. Quality of systematic reviews in pediatric oncology: A systematic review. *Cancer Treatment Reviews* 35(8):645–652.

Lynch, J. R., M. R. A. Cunningham, W. J. Warme, D. C. Schaad, F. M. Wolf, and S. S. Leopold. 2007. Commercially funded and United States-based research is more likely to be published: Good-quality studies with negative outcomes are not. *Journal of Bone and Joint Surgery* (American Volume) 89A(5):1010–1018.

MacLean, C. H., S. C. Morton, J. J. Ofman, E. A. Roth, P. G. Shekelle, and Center Southern California Evidence-Based Practice. 2003. How useful are unpublished data from the Food and Drug Administration in meta-analysis? *Journal of Clinical Epidemiology* 56(1):44–51.

Mathieu, S., I. Boutron, D. Moher, D. G. Altman, and P. Ravaud. 2009. Comparison of registered and published primary outcomes in randomized controlled trials. *JAMA* 302(9):977–984.

McAuley, L., B. Pham, P. Tugwell, and D. Moher. 2000. Does the inclusion of grey literature influence estimates of intervention effectiveness reported in meta-analyses? *Lancet* 356(9237):1228–1231.

McDonagh, M. S., K. Peterson, S. Carson, R. Fu, and S. Thakurta. 2010. *Drug class review: Atypical antipsychotic drugs. Update 3.* http://derp.ohsu.edu/final/AAP_final_report_update%203_version%203_JUL_10.pdf (accessed November 4, 2010).

McGauran, N., B. Wieseler, J. Kreis, Y. Schuler, H. Kolsch, and T. Kaiser. 2010. Reporting bias in medical research: A narrative review. *Trials* 11:37.

McGowan, J., and M. Sampson. 2005. Systematic reviews need systematic searchers. *Journal of the Medical Library Association* 93(1):74–80.

McKibbon, K. A., N. L. Wilczynski, R. B. Haynes, and T. Hedges. 2009. Retrieving randomized controlled trials from Medline: A comparison of 38 published search filters. *Health Information and Libraries Journal* 26(3):187–202.

Miller, J. 2010. Registering clinical trial results: The next step. *JAMA* 303(8):773–774.

Miller, J. N., G. A. Colditz, and F. Mosteller. 1989. How study design affects outcomes in comparisons of therapy II: Surgical. *Statistics in Medicine* 8(4):455–466.

Moher, D., and A. Tsertsvadze. 2006. Systematic reviews: When is an update an update? *Lancet* 367(9514):881–883.

Moher, D., P. Fortin, A. R. Jadad, P. Jüni, T. Klassen, J. LeLorier, A. Liberati, K. Linde, and A. Penna. 1996. Completeness of reporting of trials published in languages other than English: Implications for conduct and reporting of systematic reviews. *Lancet* 347(8998):363–366.

Moher, D., B. Pham, A. Jones, D. J. Cook, A. R. Jadad, M. Moher, P. Tugwell, and T. P. Klassen. 1998. Does quality of reports of randomised trials affect estimates of intervention efficacy reported in meta-analyses? *Lancet* 352(9128):609–613.

Moher, D., D. J. Cook, S. Eastwood, I. Olkin, D. Rennie, and D. F. Stroup. 1999. Improving the quality of reports of mega-analyses of randomised controlled trials: The QUOROM statement. *Lancet* 354(9193):1896–1900.

Moher, D., B. Pham, T. P. Klassen, K. F. Schulz, J. A. Berlin, A. R. Jadad, and A. Liberati. 2000. What contributions do languages other than English make on the results of meta-analyses? *Journal of Clinical Epidemiology* 53(9):964–972.

Moher, D., B. Pham, M. L. Lawson, and T. P. Klassen. 2003. The inclusion of reports of randomised trials published in languages other than English in systematic reviews. *Health Technology Assessment* 7(41):1–90.

Moher, D., J. Tetzlaff, A. C. Tricco, M. Sampson, and D. G. Altman. 2007a. Epidemiology and reporting characteristics of systematic reviews. *PLoS Medicine* 4(3):447–455.

Moher, D., A. Tsertsvadze, A. C. Tricco, M. Eccles, J. Grimshaw, M. Sampson, and N. Barrowman. 2007b. A systematic review identified few methods and strategies describing when and how to update systematic reviews. *Journal of Clinical Epidemiology* 60(11):1095–1104.

Moja, L., E. Telaro, R. D'Amico, I. Moschetti, L. Coe, and A. Liberati. 2005. Assessment of methodological quality of primary studies by systematic reviews: results of the metaquality cross sectional study. *BMJ* 330:1053.

Mojon-Azzi, S. M., X. Jiang, U. Wagner, and D. S. Mojon. 2004. Redundant publications in scientific ophthalmologic journals: The tip of the iceberg? *Ophthalmology* 111(5):863–866.

Montori, V. M., P. J. Devereaux, N. K. Adhikari, K. E. A. Burns, C. H. Eggert, M. Briel, C. Lacchetti, T. W. Leung, E. Darling, D. M. Bryant, H. C. Bucher, H. J. Schünemann, M. O. Meade, D. J. Cook, P. J. Erwin, A. Sood, R. Sood, B. Lo, C. A. Thompson, Q. Zhou, E. Mills, and G. Guyatt. 2005. Randomized trials stopped early for benefit: A systematic review. *JAMA* 294(17):2203–2209.

Moore, T. 1995. *Deadly medicine: Why tens of thousands of hearts died in America's worst drug disaster*. New York: Simon & Schuster.

Morrison, A., K. Moulton, M. Clark, J. Polisena, M. Fiander, M. Mierzwinski-Urban, S. Mensinkai, T. Clifford, and B. Hutton. 2009. English-language restriction when conducting systematic review-based meta-analyses: Systematic review of published studies. Ottawa, CA: Canadian Agency for Drugs and Technologies in Health.

Mrkobrada, M., H. Thiessen-Philbrook, R. B. Haynes, A. V. Iansavichus, F. Rehman, and A. X. Garg. 2008. Need for quality improvement in renal systematic reviews. *Clinical Journal of the American Society of Nephrology* 3(4):1102–1114.

Mulrow, C. D., and A. D. Oxman. 1994. *Cochrane Collaboration handbook, The Cochrane Library*. Chichester, U.K.: The Cochrane Collaboration.

Nallamothu, B. K., R. A. Hayward, and E. R. Bates. 2008. Beyond the randomized clinical trial: The role of effectiveness studies in evaluating cardiovascular therapies. *Circulation* 118(12):1294–1303.

Nassir Ghaemi, S., A. A. Shirzadi, and M. Filkowski. 2008. Publication bias and the pharmaceutical industry: The case of lamotrigine in bipolar disorder. *Medscape Journal of Medicine* 10(9):211.

National Library of Medicine. 2008. *MEDLINE fact sheet*. http://www.nlm.nih.gov/pubs/factsheets/medline.html (accessed May 28, 2010).

New York Academy of Medicine. 2010. *Grey literature report*. http://www.nyam.org/library/pages/grey_literature_report (accessed June 2, 2010).

Nieminen, P., G. Rucker, J. Miettunen, J. Carpenter, and M. Schumacher. 2007. Statistically significant papers in psychiatry were cited more often than others. *Journal of Clinical Epidemiology* 60(9):939–946.

NLM (National Library of Medicine). 2009. *Fact sheet: ClinicalTrials.gov*. http://www.nlm.nih.gov/pubs/factsheets/clintrial.html (accessed June 16, 2010).

Norris, S., D. Atkins, W. Bruening, S. Fox, E. Johnson, R. Kane, S. C. Morton, M. Oremus, M. Ospina, G. Randhawa, K. Schoelles, P. Shekelle, and M. Viswanathan. 2010. Selecting observational studies for comparing medical interventions. In *Methods guide for comparative effectiveness reviews*, edited by Agency for Healthcare Research and Quality. http://www.effectivehealthcare.ahrq.gov/index.cfm/search-for-guides-reviews-and-reports/?pageaction=displayProduct&productID=454 (accessed January 19, 2011).

Nüesch, E., S. Trelle, S. Reichenbach, A. W. S. Rutjes, B. Tschannen, D. G. Altman, M. Egger, and P. Jüni. 2010. Small study effects in meta-analyses of osteoarthritis trials: Meta-epidemiological study. *BMJ* 341(7766):241.

O'Connor, A. B. 2009. The need for improved access to FDA reviews. *JAMA* 302(2):191–193.

Okike, K., M. S. Kocher, C. T. Mehlman, J. D. Heckman, and M. Bhandari. 2008. Publication bias in orthopedic research: An analysis of scientific factors associated with publication in the *Journal of Bone and Joint Surgery* (American Volume). 90A(3):595–601.

Olson, C. M., D. Rennie, D. Cook, K. Dickersin, A. Flanagin, J. W. Hogan, Q. Zhu, J. Reiling, and B. Pace. 2002. Publication bias in editorial decision making. *JAMA* 287(21):2825–2828.

Online Computer Library Center. 2010. *The OAIster® database*. http://www.oclc.org/oaister/ (accessed June 3, 2010).

OpenSIGLE. 2010. *OpenSIGLE*. http://opensigle.inist.fr/ (accessed June 2, 2010).

Peinemann, F., N. McGauran, S. Sauerland, and S. Lange. 2008. Disagreement in primary study selection between systematic reviews on negative pressure wound therapy. *BMC Medical Research Methodology* 8:41.

Perlin, J. B., and J. Kupersmith. 2007. Information technology and the inferential gap. *Health Affairs* 26(2):W192–W194.

Pham, B., T. P. Klassen, M. L. Lawson, and D. Moher. 2005. Language of publication restrictions in systematic reviews gave different results depending on whether the intervention was conventional or complementary. *Journal of Clinical Epidemiology* 58(8):769–776.

Pildal, J., A. Hrobjartsson, K. J. Jorgensen, J. Hilden, D. G. Altman, and P. C. Gøtzsche. 2007. Impact of allocation concealment on conclusions drawn from meta-analyses of randomized trials (2007) vol. 36 (847–857). *International Journal of Epidemiology* 36(4):847–857.

ProQuest. 2010. *ProQuest dissertations & theses database*. http://www.proquest.com/en-US/catalogs/databases/detail/pqdt.shtml (accessed June 2, 2010).

Ravnskov, U. 1992. Cholesterol lowering trials in coronary heart disease: Frequency of citation and outcome. *BMJ* 305(6844):15–19.

Ravnskov, U. 1995. Quotation bias in reviews of the diet–heart idea. *Journal of Clinical Epidemiology* 48(5):713–719.

RefWorks. 2009. *RefWorks*. http://refworks.com/content/products/content.asp (accessed July 2, 2010).

Relevo, R., and H. Balshem. 2011. Finding evidence for comparing medical interventions. In *Methods guide for comparative effectiveness reviews*, edited by Agency for Healthcare Research and Quality. http://www.effectivehealthcare.ahrq.gov/index.cfm/search-for-guides-reviews-and-reports/?pageaction=displayProduct&productID=605 (accessed January 19, 2011).

Rising, K., P. Bacchetti, and L. Bero. 2008. Reporting bias in drug trials submitted to the Food and Drug Administration: Review of publication and presentation. *PLoS Medicine* 5(11):1561–1570.

Rosenthal, E. L., J. L. Masdon, C. Buckman, and M. Hawn. 2003. Duplicate publications in the otolaryngology literature. *Laryngoscope* 113(5):772–774.

Ross, J. S., G. K. Mulvey, E. M. Hines, S. E. Nissen, and H. M. Krumholz. 2009. Trial publication after registration in clinicaltrials.gov: A cross-sectional analysis. *PLoS Medicine* 6(9):e1000144.

Rothwell, P. M. 1995. Can overall results of clinical trials be applied to all patients? *Lancet* 345(8965):1616–1619.

Rothwell, P. M. 2005. External validity of randomised controlled trials: To whom do the results of this trial apply? *Lancet* 365(9453):82–93.

Rothwell, P. M. 2006. Factors that can affect the external validity of randomised controlled trials. *PLOS Clinical Trials* 1(1):e9.

Roundtree, A. K., M. A. Kallen, M. A. Lopez-Olivo, B. Kimmel, B. Skidmore, Z. Ortiz, V. Cox, and M. E. Suarez-Almazor. 2008. Poor reporting of search strategy and conflict of interest in over 250 narrative and systematic reviews of two biologic agents in arthritis: A systematic review. *Journal of Clinical Epidemiology* 62(2):128–137.

Royle, P., and R. Milne. 2003. Literature searching for randomized controlled trials used in Cochrane reviews: Rapid versus exhaustive searches. *International Journal of Technology Assessment in Health Care* 19(4):591–603.

Royle, P., and N. Waugh. 2003. Literature searching for clinical and cost-effectiveness studies used in health technology assessment reports carried out for the National Institute for Clinical Excellence appraisal system. *Health Technology Assessment* 7(34):1–51.

Royle, P., L. Bain, and N. Waugh. 2005. Systematic reviews of epidemiology in diabetes: Finding the evidence. *BMC Medical Research Methodology* 5(1):2.

Sampson, M., and J. McGowan. 2006. Errors in search strategies were identified by type and frequency. *Journal of Clinical Epidemiology* 59(10):1057.e1–1057.e9.

Sampson, M., K. G. Shojania, C. Garritty, T. Horsley, M. Ocampo, and D. Moher. 2008. Systematic reviews can be produced and published faster. *Journal of Clinical Epidemiology* 61(6):531–536.

Sampson, M., J. McGowan, E. Cogo, J. Grimshaw, D. Moher, and C. Lefebvre. 2009. An evidence-based practice guideline for the peer review of electronic search strategies. *Journal of Clinical Epidemiology* 62(9):944–952.

Sanderson, S., I. D. Tatt, and J. P. Higgins. 2007. Tools for assessing quality and susceptibility to bias in observational studies in epidemiology: A systematic review and annotated bibliography. *International Journal of Epidemiology* 36(3):666–676.

Savoie, I., D. Helmer, C. J. Green, and A. Kazanjian. 2003. Beyond MEDLINE: Reducing bias through extended systematic review search. *International Journal of Technology Assessment in Health Care* 19(1):168–178.

Schein, M., and R. Paladugu. 2001. Redundant surgical publications: Tip of the iceberg? *Surgery* 129(6):655–661.

Scherer, R. W., P. Langenberg, and E. Von Elm. 2007. Full publication of results initially presented in abstracts. *Cochrane Database of Systematic Reviews* 2:MR000005.

Schmidt, L. M., and P. C. Gøtzsche. 2005. Of mites and men: Reference bias in narrative review articles: A systematic review. *Journal of Family Practice* 54(4):334–338.

Schulz, K. F., L. Chalmers, R. J. Hayes, and D. G. Altman. 1995. Empirical evidence of bias: Dimensions of methodological quality associated with estimates of treatment effects in controlled trials. *JAMA* 273(5):408–412.

Scopus. 2010. *Scopus in detail*. http://info.scopus.com/scopus-in-detail/content-coverage-guide/ (accessed May 28, 2010).

Shikata, S., T. Nakayama, Y. Noguchi, Y. Taji, and H. Yamagishi. 2006. Comparison of effects in randomized controlled trials with observational studies in digestive surgery. *Annals of Surgery* 244(5):668–676.

Shojania, K. G., M. Sampson, M. T. Ansari, J. Ji, S. Doucette, and D. Moher. 2007. How quickly do systematic reviews go out of date? A survival analysis. *Annals of Internal Medicine* 147(4):224–233.

Silagy, C. A., P. Middleton, and S. Hopewell. 2002. Publishing protocols of systematic reviews: Comparing what was done to what was planned. *JAMA* 287(21):2831–2834.

Sismondo, S. 2008. Pharmaceutical company funding and its consequences: A qualitative systematic review. *Contemporary Clinical Trials* 29(2):109–113.

Song, F., S. Parekh-Bhurke, L. Hooper, Y. K. Loke, J. J. Ryder, A. J. Sutton, C. B. Hing, and I. Harvey. 2009. Extent of publication bias in different categories of research cohorts: A meta-analysis of empirical studies. *BMC Medical Research Methodology* 9(1):79–93.

Song, F., S. Parekh, L. Hooper, Y. K. Loke, J. Ryder, A. J. Sutton, C. Hing, C. S. Kwok, C. Pang, and I. Harvey. 2010. Dissemination and publication of research findings: An updated review of related biases. *Health Technology Assessment* 14(8):1–193.

Sterne, J., M. Egger, and D. Moher, eds. 2008. *Chapter 10: Addressing reporting biases*. In *Cochrane handbook for systematic reviews of interventions*, edited by J. P. T. Higgins and S. Green. Chichester, U.K.: The Cochrane Collaboration.

Sutton, A. J., S. Donegan, Y. Takwoingi, P. Garner, C. Gamble, and A. Donald. 2009. An encouraging assessment of methods to inform priorities for updating systematic reviews. *Journal of Clinical Epidemiology* 62(3):241–251.

Thompson, R. L., E. V. Bandera, V. J. Burley, J. E. Cade, D. Forman, J. L. Freudenheim, D. Greenwood, D. R. Jacobs, Jr., R. V. Kalliecharan, L. H. Kushi, M. L. McCullough, L. M. Miles, D. F. Moore, J. A. Moreton, T. Rastogi, and M. J. Wiseman. 2008. Reproducibility of systematic literature reviews on food, nutrition, physical activity and endometrial cancer. *Public Health Nutrition* 11(10):1006–1014.

Thomson Reuters. 2010. *EndNote web information*. http://endnote.com/enwebinfo. asp (accessed July 2, 2010).

Tramer, M. R., D. J. Reynolds, R. A. Moore, and H. J. McQuay. 1997. Impact of covert duplicate publication on meta-analysis: A case study. *BMJ* 315(7109):635–640.

Tricco, A. C., J. Tetzlaff, M. Sampson, D. Fergusson, E. Cogo, T. Horsley, and D. Moher. 2008. Few systematic reviews exist documenting the extent of bias: A systematic review. *Journal of Clinical Epidemiology* 61(5):422–434.

Turner, E. H., A. M. Matthews, E. Linardatos, R. A. Tell, and R. Rosenthal. 2008. Selective publication of antidepressant trials and its influence on apparent efficacy. *New England Journal of Medicine* 358(3):252–260.

Van de Voorde, C., and C. Leonard. 2007. *Search for evidence and critical appraisal*. Brussels, Belgium: Belgian Health Care Knowledge Centre.

van Tulder, M. W., M. Suttorp, S. Morton, L. M. Bouter, and P. Shekelle. 2009. Empirical evidence of an association between internal validity and effect size in randomized controlled trials of low-back pain. *Spine (Phila PA 1976)* 34(16):1685–1692.

Vandenbroucke, J. P. 2004. Benefits and harms of drug treatments: Observational studies and randomised trials should learn from each other. *BMJ* 329(7456):2–3.

Vedula, S. S., L. Bero, R. W. Scherer, and K. Dickersin. 2009. Outcome reporting in industry-sponsored trials of gabapentin for off-label use. *New England Journal of Medicine* 361(20):1963–1971.

Voisin, C. E., C. de la Varre, L. Whitener, and G. Gartlehner. 2008. Strategies in assessing the need for updating evidence-based guidelines for six clinical topics: An exploration of two search methodologies. *Health Information and Libraries Journal* 25(3):198–207.

von Elm, E., G. Poglia, B. Walder, and M. R. Tramer. 2004. Different patterns of duplicate publication: An analysis of articles used in systematic reviews. *JAMA* 291(8):974–980.

Walker, C. F., K. Kordas, R. J. Stoltzfus, and R. E. Black. 2005. Interactive effects of iron and zinc on biochemical and functional outcomes in supplementation trials. *American Journal of Clinical Nutrition* 82(1):5–12.

WAME (World Association of Medical Editors). 2010. *Publication ethics policies for medical journals.* http://www.wame.org/resources/publication-ethics-policies-for-medical-journals (accessed November 10, 2010).

Wennberg, D. E., F. L. Lucas, J. D. Birkmeyer, C. E. Bredenberg, and E. S. Fisher. 1998. Variation in carotid endarterectomy mortality in the Medicare population: Trial hospitals, volume, and patient characteristics. *JAMA* 279(16):1278–1281.

Whitlock, E. P., E. A. O'Connor, S. B. Williams, T. L. Beil, and K. W. Lutz. 2008. *Effectiveness of weight management programs in children and adolescents.* Rockville, MD: AHRQ.

WHO (World Health Organization). 2006. *African Index Medicus.* http://indexmedicus.afro.who.int/ (accessed June 2, 2010).

WHO. 2010. *International Clinical Trials Registry Platform.* http://www.who.int/ictrp/en/ (accessed June 17, 2010).

Wieland, S., and K. Dickersin. 2005. Selective exposure reporting and Medline indexing limited the search sensitivity for observational studies of the adverse effects of oral contraceptives. *Journal of Clinical Epidemiology* 58(6):560–567.

Wilczynski, N. L., R. B. Haynes, A. Eady, B. Haynes, S. Marks, A. McKibbon, D. Morgan, C. Walker-Dilks, S. Walter, S. Werre, N. Wilczynski, and S. Wong. 2004. Developing optimal search strategies for detecting clinically sound prognostic studies in MEDLINE: An analytic survey. *BMC Medicine* 2:23.

Wilt, T. J. 2006. *Comparison of endovascular and open surgical repairs for abdominal aortic aneurysm.* Rockville, MD: AHRQ.

Wood, A. J. J. 2009. Progress and deficiencies in the registration of clinical trials. *New England Journal of Medicine* 360(8):824–830.

Wood, A. M., I. R. White, and S. G. Thompson. 2004. Are missing outcome data adequately handled? A review of published randomized controlled trials in major medical journals. *Clinical Trials* 1(4):368–376.

Wood, L., M. Egger, L. L. Gluud, K. F. Schulz, P. Jüni, D. G. Altman, C. Gluud, R. M. Martin, A. J. Wood, and J. A. Sterne. 2008. Empirical evidence of bias in treatment effect estimates in controlled trials with different interventions and outcomes: Meta-epidemiological study. *BMJ* 336(7644):601–605.

Wortman, P. M., and W. H. Yeaton. 1983. Synthesis of results in controlled trials of coronary bypass graft surgery. In *Evaluation studies review annual*, edited by R. L. Light. Beverly Hills, CA: Sage.

Yoshii, A., D. A. Plaut, K. A. McGraw, M. J. Anderson, and K. E. Wellik. 2009. Analysis of the reporting of search strategies in Cochrane systematic reviews. *Journal of the Medical Library Association* 97(1):21–29.

Zarin, D. A. 2005. Clinical trial registration. *New England Journal of Medicine* 352(15):1611.

Zarin, D. A., T. Tse, and N. C. Ide. 2005. Trial registration at ClinicalTrials.gov between May and October 2005. *New England Journal of Medicine* 353(26):2779–2787.

4

Standards for Synthesizing the Body of Evidence

Abstract: *This chapter addresses the qualitative and quantitative synthesis (meta-analysis) of the body of evidence. The committee recommends four related standards. The systematic review (SR) should use prespecified methods; include a qualitative synthesis based on essential characteristics of study quality (risk of bias, consistency, precision, directness, reporting bias, and for observational studies, dose–response association, plausible confounding that would change an observed effect, and strength of association); and make an explicit judgment of whether a meta-analysis is appropriate. If conducting meta-analyses, expert methodologists should develop, execute, and peer review the meta-analyses. The meta-analyses should address heterogeneity among study effects, accompany all estimates with measures of statistical uncertainty, and assess the sensitivity of conclusions to changes in the protocol, assumptions, and study selection (sensitivity analysis). An SR that uses rigorous and transparent methods will enable patients, clinicians, and other decision makers to discern what is known and not known about an intervention's effectiveness and how the evidence applies to particular population groups and clinical situations.*

More than a century ago, Nobel prize-winning physicist J. W. Strutt Lord Rayleigh observed that "the work which deserves . . .

the most credit is that in which discovery and explanation go hand in hand, in which not only are new facts presented, but their relation to old ones is pointed out" (Rayleigh, 1884). In other words, the contribution of any singular piece of research draws not only from its own unique discoveries, but also from its relationship to previous research (Glasziou et al., 2004; Mulrow and Lohr, 2001). Thus, the synthesis and assessment of a body of evidence is at the heart of a systematic review (SR) of comparative effectiveness research (CER).

The previous chapter described the considerable challenges involved in assembling all the individual studies that comprise current knowledge on the effectiveness of a healthcare intervention: the "body of evidence." This chapter begins with the assumption that the body of evidence was identified in an optimal manner and that the risk of bias in each individual study was assessed appropriately—both according to the committee's standards. This chapter addresses the synthesis and assessment of the collected evidence, focusing on those aspects that are most salient to setting standards. The science of SR is rapidly evolving; much has yet to be learned. The purpose of standards for evidence synthesis and assessment—as in other SR methods—is to set performance expectations and to promote accountability for meeting those expectations without stifling innovation in methods. Thus, the emphasis is not on specifying preferred technical methods, but rather the building blocks that help ensure objectivity, transparency, and scientific rigor.

As it did elsewhere in this report, the committee developed this chapter's standards and elements of performance based on available evidence and expert guidance from the Agency for Healthcare Research and Quality (AHRQ) Effective Health Care Program, the Centre for Reviews and Dissemination (CRD, part of University of York, UK), and the Cochrane Collaboration (Chou et al., 2010; CRD, 2009; Deeks et al., 2008; Fu et al., 2010; Lefebvre et al., 2008; Owens et al., 2010). Guidance on assessing quality of evidence from the Grading of Recommendations Assessment, Development, and Evaluation (GRADE) Working Group was another key source of information (Guyatt et al. 2010; Schünemann et al., 2009). See Appendix F for a detailed summary of AHRQ, CRD, and Cochrane guidance for the assessment and synthesis of a body of evidence.

The committee had several opportunities for learning the perspectives of stakeholders on issues related to this chapter. SR experts and representatives from medical specialty associations, payers, and consumer groups provided both written responses to the committee's questions and oral testimony in a public workshop (see Appendix C). In addition, staff conducted informal, structured interviews with other key stakeholders.

The committee recommends four standards for the assessment and qualitative and quantitative synthesis of an SR's body of evidence. Each standard consists of two parts: first, a brief statement describing the related SR step and, second, one or more elements of performance that are fundamental to carrying out the step. Box 4-1 lists all of the chapter's recommended standards. This chapter provides the background and rationale for the recommended standards and elements of performance, first outlining the key considerations in assessing a body of evidence, and followed by sections on the fundamental components of qualitative and quantitative synthesis. The order of the chapter's standards and the presentation of the discussion do not necessarily indicate the sequence in which the various steps should be conducted. Although an SR synthesis should always include a qualitative component, the feasibility of a quantitative synthesis (meta-analysis) depends on the available data. If a meta-analysis is conducted, its interpretation should be included in the qualitative synthesis. Moreover, the overall assessment of the body of evidence cannot be done until the syntheses are complete.

In the context of CER, SRs are produced to help consumers, clinicians, developers of clinical practice guidelines, purchasers, and policy makers to make informed healthcare decisions (Federal Coordinating Council for Comparative Effectiveness Research, 2009; IOM, 2009). Thus, the assessment and synthesis of a body of evidence in the SR should be approached with the decision makers in mind. An SR using rigorous and transparent methods allows decision makers to discern what is known and not known about an intervention's effectiveness and how the evidence applies to particular population groups and clinical situations (Helfand, 2005). Making evidence-based decisions—such as when a guideline developer recommends what should and should not be done in specific clinical circumstances—is a distinct and separate process from the SR and is outside the scope of this report. It is the focus of a companion IOM study on developing standards for trustworthy clinical practice guidelines.[1]

A NOTE ON TERMINOLOGY

The SR field lacks an agreed-on lexicon for some of its most fundamental terms and concepts, including what actually constitutes

---

[1] The IOM report, *Clinical Practice Guidelines We Can Trust*, is available at the National Academies Press website: http://www.nap.edu/.

BOX 4-1
Recommended Standards for Synthesizing
the Body of Evidence

Standard 4.1 Use a prespecified method to evaluate the body of evidence
Required elements:
    4.1.1 For each outcome, systematically assess the following characteristics of the body of evidence:
- Risk of bias
- Consistency
- Precision
- Directness
- Reporting bias

    4.1.2 For bodies of evidence that include observational research, also systematically assess the following characteristics for each outcome:
- Dose–response association
- Plausible confounding that would change the observed effect
- Strength of association

    4.1.3 For each outcome specified in the protocol, use consistent language to characterize the level of confidence in the estimates of the effect of an intervention

Standard 4.2 Conduct a qualitative synthesis
Required elements:
    4.2.1 Describe the clinical and methodological characteristics of the included studies, including their size, inclusion or exclusion of important subgroups, timeliness, and other relevant factors

---

the quality of a body of evidence. This leads to considerable confusion. Because this report focuses on SRs for the purposes of CER and clinical decision making, the committee uses the term "quality of the body of evidence" to describe the extent to which one can be confident that the estimate of an intervention's effectiveness is correct. This terminology is designed to support clinical decision making and is similar to that used by GRADE and adopted by the Cochrane Collaboration and other organizations for the same purpose (Guyatt et al., 2010; Schünemann et al., 2008, 2009).

Quality encompasses summary assessments of a number of characteristics of a body of evidence, such as within-study bias (methodological quality), consistency, precision, directness or applicability of the evidence, and others (Schünemann et al., 2009). Syn-

4.2.2 Describe the strengths and limitations of individual studies and patterns across studies

4.2.3 Describe, in plain terms, how flaws in the design or execution of the study (or groups of studies) could bias the results, explaining the reasoning behind these judgments

4.2.4 Describe the relationships between the characteristics of the individual studies and their reported findings and patterns across studies

4.2.5 Discuss the relevance of individual studies to the populations, comparisons, cointerventions, settings, and outcomes or measures of interest

Standard 4.3 Decide if, in addition to a qualitative analysis, the systematic review will include a quantitative analysis (meta-analysis)

Required element:

4.3.1 Explain why a pooled estimate might be useful to decision makers

Standard 4.4 If conducting a meta-analysis, then do the following:

Required elements:

4.2.1 Use expert methodologists to develop, execute, and peer review the meta-analyses

4.2.2 Address the heterogeneity among study effects

4.2.3 Accompany all estimates with measures of statistical uncertainty

4.2.4 Assess the sensitivity of conclusions to changes in the protocol, assumptions, and study selection (sensitivity analysis)

NOTE: The order of the standards does not indicate the sequence in which they are carried out.

thesis is the collation, combination, and summary of the findings of a body of evidence (CRD, 2009). In an SR, the synthesis of the body of evidence should always include a qualitative component and, if the data permit, a quantitative synthesis (meta-analysis).

The following section presents the background and rationale for the committee's recommended standard and performance elements for prespecifying the assessment methods.

A Need for Clarity and Consistency

Neither empirical evidence nor agreement among experts is available to support the committee's endorsement of a specific approach for assessing and describing the quality of a body of evi-

dence. Medical specialty societies, U.S. and other national government agencies, private research groups, and others have created a
multitude of systems for assessing and characterizing the quality
of a body of evidence (AAN, 2004; ACCF/AHA, 2009; ACCP, 2009;
CEBM, 2009; Chalmers et al., 1990; Ebell et al., 2004; Faraday et
al., 2009; Guirguis-Blake et al., 2007; Guyatt et al., 2004; ICSI, 2003;
NCCN, 2008; NZGG, 2007; Owens et al., 2010; Schünemann et al.,
2009; SIGN, 2009; USPSTF, 2008). The various systems share common
features, but employ conflicting evidence hierarchies; emphasize
different factors in assessing the quality of research; and use a con-
fusing array of letters, codes, and symbols to convey investigators'
conclusions about the overall quality of a body of evidence (Atkins
et al., 2004a, 2004b; Schünemann et al., 2003; West et al., 2002). The
reader cannot make sense of the differences (Table 4-1). Through
public testimony and interviews, the committee heard that numerous producers and users of SRs were frustrated by the number,
variation, complexity, and lack of transparency in existing systems.

One comprehensive review documented 40 different systems
for grading the strength of a body of evidence (West et al., 2002).
Another review, conducted several years later, found that more than
50 evidence-grading systems and 230 quality assessment instruments were in use (COMPUS, 2005).

Early systems for evaluating the quality of a body of evidence
used simple hierarchies of study design to judge the internal validity (risk of bias) of a body of evidence (Guyatt et al., 1995). For
example, a body of evidence that included two or more randomized
controlled trials (RCTs) was assumed to be "high-quality," "level
1," or "grade A" evidence whether or not the trials met scientific
standards. Quasi-experimental research, observational studies, case
series, and other qualitative research designs were automatically
considered lower quality evidence. As research documented the
variable quality of trials and widespread reporting bias in the publication of trial findings, it became clear that such hierarchies are too
simplistic because they do not assess the extent to which the design
and implementation of RCTs (or other study designs) avoid biases
that may reduce confidence in the measures of effectiveness (Atkins
et al., 2004b; Coleman et al., 2009; Harris et al., 2001).

The early hierarchies produced conflicting conclusions about
effectiveness. A study by Ferreira and colleagues analyzed the effect
of applying different "levels of evidence" systems to the conclusions
of six Cochrane SRs of interventions for low back pain (Ferreira
et al., 2002). They found that the conclusions of the reviews were
highly dependent on the system used to evaluate the evidence

TABLE 4-1 Examples of Approaches to Assessing the Body of Evidence for Therapeutic Interventions*

System	System for Assessing the Body of Evidence	
Agency for Healthcare Research and Quality	**High**	High confidence that the evidence reflects the true effect. Further research is very unlikely to change our confidence of the estimate of effect.
	Moderate	Moderate confidence that the evidence reflects the true effect. Further research may change our confidence in the estimate of effect and may change the estimate.
	Low	Low confidence that the evidence reflects the true effect. Further research is likely to change the confidence in the estimate of effect and is likely to change the estimate.
	Insufficient	Evidence either is unavailable or does not permit a conclusion.
American College of Chest Physicians	**High**	Randomized controlled trials (RCTs) without important limitations or overwhelming evidence from observational studies.
	Moderate	RCTs with important limitations (inconsistent results, methodological flaws, indirect, or imprecise) or exceptionally strong evidence from observational studies.
	Low	Observational studies or case series.
American Heart Association/ American College of Cardiology	**A**	Multiple RCTs or meta-analyses.
	B	Single RCT, or nonrandomized studies.
	C	Consensus opinion of experts, case studies, or standard of care.
Grading of Recommendations Assessment, Development and Evaluation (GRADE)		*Starting points for evaluating quality level:* • RCTs start high. • Observational studies start low. *Factors that may decrease or increase the quality level of a body of evidence:* • *Decrease:* Study limitations, inconsistency of results, indirectness of evidence, imprecision of results, and high risk of publication bias. • *Increase:* Large magnitude of effect, dose-response gradient, all plausible biases would reduce the observed effect.

continued

TABLE 4-1 Continued

System	System for Assessing the Body of Evidence	
	High	Further research is very unlikely to change our confidence in the estimate of effect.
	Moderate	Further research is likely to have an important impact on our confidence in the estimate of effect and may change the estimate.
	Low	Further research is very likely to have an important impact on our confidence in the estimate of effect and is likely to change the estimate.
	Very low	Any estimate of effect is very uncertain.
National Comprehensive Cancer Network	**High**	High-powered RCTs or meta-analysis.
	Lower	Ranges from Phase II Trials to large cohort studies to case series to individual practitioner experience.
Oxford Centre for Evidence-Based Medicine		Varies with type of question. Level may be graded down on the basis of study quality, imprecision, indirectness, inconsistency between studies, or because the absolute effect size is very small. Level may be graded up if there is a large or very large effect size.
	Level 1	Systematic review (SR) of randomized trials or n-of-1 trial. *For rare harms*: SR of case-control studies, or studies revealing dramatic effects.
	Level 2	SR of nested case-control or dramatic effect. *For rare harms*: Randomized trial or (exceptionally) observational study with dramatic effect.
	Level 3	Nonrandomized controlled cohort/follow-up study.
	Level 4	Case-control studies, historically controlled studies.
	Level 5	Opinion without explicit critical appraisal, based on limited/undocumented experience, or based on mechanisms.

Scottish Intercollegiate Guidelines Network	1++	High-quality meta-analyses, SRs of RCTs, or RCTs with a very low risk of bias.
	1+	Well-conducted meta-analyses, SRs, or RCTs with a low risk of bias.
	1−	Meta-analyses, SRs, or RCTs with a high risk of bias.
	2++	High-quality SRs of case control or cohort studies. High-quality case control or cohort studies with a very low risk of confounding or bias and a high probability that the relationship is causal.
	2−	Case control or cohort studies with a high risk of confounding or bias and a significant risk that the relationship is not causal.
	3	Nonanalytic studies, e.g., case reports, case series.
	4	Expert opinion.

* Some systems use different grading schemes depending on the type of intervention (e.g., preventive service, diagnostic tests, and therapies). This table includes systems for therapeutic interventions.

SOURCES: ACCF/AHA (2009); ACCP (2009); CEBM (2009); NCCN (2008); Owens et al. (2010); Schünemann et al. (2009); SIGN (2009).

primarily because of differences in the number and quality of trials required for a particular level of evidence. In many cases, the differences in the conclusions were so substantial that they could lead to contradictory clinical advice. For example, for one intervention, "back school,"[2] the conclusions ranged from "strong evidence that back schools are effective" to "no evidence" on the effectiveness of back schools.

One reason for these discrepancies was failure to distinguish between the quality of the evidence and the magnitude of net benefit. For example, an SR and meta-analysis might highlight a dramatic effect size regardless of the risk of bias in the body of evidence. Conversely, use of a rigid hierarchy gave the impression that any effect based on randomized trial evidence was clinically important, regardless of the size of the effect. In 2001, the U.S. Preventive Services Task Force broke new ground when it updated its review methods, separating its assessment of the quality of evidence from its assessment of the magnitude of effect (Harris et al., 2001).

What Are the Characteristics of Quality for a Body of Evidence?

Experts in SR methodology agree on the conceptual underpinnings for the systematic assessment of a body of evidence. The committee identified eight basic characteristics of quality, described below, that are integral to assessing and characterizing the quality of a body of evidence. These characteristics—risk of bias, consistency, precision, directness, and reporting bias, and for observational studies, dose–response association, plausible confounding that would change an observed effect, and strength of association—are used by GRADE; the Cochrane Collaboration, which has adopted the GRADE approach; and the AHRQ Effective Health Care Program, which adopted a modified version of the GRADE approach (Owens et al., 2010; Balshem et al., 2011; Falck-Ytter et al., 2010; Schünemann et al., 2008). Although their terminology varies somewhat, Falck-Ytter and his GRADE colleagues describe any differences between the GRADE and AHRQ quality characteristics as essentially semantic (Falck-Ytter et al., 2010). Owens and his AHRQ colleagues appear

---

[2] Back schools are educational programs designed to teach patients how to manage chronic low back pain to prevent future episodes. The curriculums typically include the natural history, anatomy, and physiology of back pain as well as a home exercise program (Hsieh et al., 2002).

BOX 4-2
Key Concepts Used in the GRADE Approach to
Assessing the Quality of a Body of Evidence

The Grading of Recommendations Assessment, Development, and Evaluation (GRADE) Working Group uses a point system to upgrade or downgrade the ratings for each quality characteristic. A grade of high, moderate, low, or very low is assigned to the body of evidence for each outcome. Eight characteristics of the quality of evidence are assessed for each outcome.

Five characteristics can lower the quality rating for the body of evidence:

- Limitations in study design and conduct
- Inconsistent results across studies
- Indirectness of evidence with respect to the study design, populations, interventions, comparisons, or outcomes
- Imprecision of the estimates of effect
- Publication bias

Three factors can increase the quality rating for the body of evidence because they raise confidence in the certainty of estimates (particularly for observational studies):

- Large magnitude of effect
- Plausible confounding that would reduce the demonstrated effect
- Dose–response gradient

SOURCES: Atkins et al. (2004a); Balshem et al. (2011); Falck-Ytter et al. (2010); Schünemann et al. (2009).

---

to agree (Owens et al., 2010). As Boxes 4-2 and 4-3 indicate, the two approaches are quite similar.[3]

Risk of Bias

In the context of a body of evidence, risk of bias refers to the extent to which flaws in the design and execution of a collection of studies could bias the estimate of effect for each outcome under study.

---

[3] For detailed descriptions of the AHRQ and GRADE methods, see the *GRADE Handbook for Grading Quality of Evidence and Strength of Recommendations* (Schünemann et al., 2009) and "Grading the Strength of a Body of Evidence When Comparing Medical Interventions—AHRQ and the Effective Health Care Program" (Owens et al., 2010).

BOX 4-3
Key Concepts Used in the AHRQ Approach to
Assessing the Quality of a Body of Evidence

The Agency for Healthcare Research and Quality (AHRQ) Effective Health Care Program refers to the evidence evaluation process as grading the "strength" of a body of evidence. It requires that the body of evidence for each major outcome and comparison of interest be assessed according to the concepts listed below. After a global assessment of the concepts, AHRQ systematic review teams assign a grade of high, moderate, low, or insufficient to the body of evidence for each outcome.

Evaluation components in all systematic reviews:

- Risk of bias in the design and conduct of studies
- Consistency in the estimates of effect across studies
- Directness of the evidence in linking interventions to health outcomes
- Precision or degree of certainty about an estimate of effect for an outcome
- Applicability of the evidence to specific contexts and populations

Other considerations (particularly with respect to observational studies):

- Dose–response association
- Publication bias
- Presence of confounders that would diminish an observed effect
- Strength of association (magnitude of effect)

SOURCE: Owens et al. (2010).

Chapter 3 describes the factors related to the design and conduct of randomized trials and observational studies that may influence the magnitude and direction of bias for a particular outcome (e.g., sequence generation, allocation concealment, blinding, incomplete data, selective reporting of outcomes, confounding, etc.),[4] as well as

---

[4] Sequence generation refers to the method used to generate the random assignment of study participants in a trial. A trial is "blind" if participants are not told to which arm of the trial they have been assigned. Allocation concealment is a method used to prevent selection bias in clinical trials by concealing the allocation sequence from those assigning participants to intervention groups. Allocation concealment prevents researchers from (unconsciously or otherwise) influencing the intervention group to which each participant is assigned.

available tools for assessing risk of bias in individual studies. Assessing risk of bias for a body of evidence requires a cumulative assessment of the risk of bias across all individual studies for each specific outcome of interest. Study biases are outcome dependent in that potential sources of bias impact different outcomes in different ways; for example, blinding of outcome assessment to a treatment group might be less important for a study of the effect of an intervention on mortality than for a study measuring pain relief. The degree of confidence in the summary estimate of effect will depend on the extent to which specific biases in the included studies affect a specific outcome.

Consistency

For the appraisal of a body of evidence, consistency refers to the degree of similarity in the direction and estimated size of an intervention's effect on specific outcomes.[5] SRs and meta-analyses can provide clear and convincing evidence of a treatment's effect when the individual studies in the body of evidence show consistent, clinically important effects of similar magnitude (Higgins et al., 2003). Often, however, the results differ in the included studies. Large and unexplained differences (inconsistency) are of concern especially when some studies suggest substantial benefit, but other studies indicate no effect or possible harm (Guyatt et al., 2010).

However, inconsistency across studies may be due to true differences in a treatment's effect related to variability in the included studies' populations (e.g., differences in health status), interventions (e.g., differences in drug doses, cointerventions, or comparison interventions), and health outcomes (e.g., diminishing treatment effect with time). Examples of inconsistency in a body of evidence include statistically significant effects in opposite directions, confidence intervals that are wide or fail to overlap, and clinical or statistical heterogeneity that cannot be explained. When differences in estimates across studies reflect true differences in a treatment's effect, then inconsistency provides the opportunity to understand and characterize those differences, which may have important implications for clinical practice. If the inconsistency results from biases in study design or improper study execution, then a thorough assessment of these differences may inform future study design.

---

[5] In analyses involving indirect comparisons, network meta-analyses, or mixed-treatment comparisons, the term consistency refers to the degree to which the direct comparisons (head-to-head comparisons) and the indirect comparisons agree with each other with respect to the magnitude of the treatment effect of interest.

Precision

A measure of the likelihood of random errors in the estimates of effect, precision refers to the degree of certainty about the estimates for specific outcomes. Confidence intervals about the estimate of effect from each study are one way of expressing precision, with a narrower confidence interval meaning more precision.

Directness

The concept of directness has two dimensions, depending on the context:

- When interventions are compared, directness refers to the extent to which the individual studies were designed to address the link between the healthcare intervention and a specific health outcome. A body of evidence is considered indirect if the included studies only address surrogate or biological outcomes or if head-to-head (direct) comparisons of interventions are not available (e.g., intervention A is compared to intervention C, and intervention B is compared to C, when comparisons of A vs. B studies are of primary interest, but not available).
- The other dimension of "directness" is applicability (also referred to as generalizability or external validity).[6] A body of evidence is applicable if it focuses on the specific condition, patient population, intervention, comparators, and health outcomes that are the focus of the SR's research protocol. SRs should assess the applicability of the evidence to patients seen in everyday clinical settings. This is especially important because numerous clinically relevant factors distinguish clinical trial participants from most patients, such as health status and comorbidities as well as age, gender, race, and ethnicity (Pham et al., 2007; Slone Survey, 2006; Vogeli et al., 2007).

---

[6] As noted in Chapter 1, applicability is one of seven criteria that the committee used to guide its selection of SR standards. In that context, applicability relates to the aim of CER, that is, to help consumers, clinicians, purchasers, and policy makers to make informed decisions that will improve health care at both the individual and population levels. The other criteria are acceptability/credibility, efficiency of conducting the review, patient-centeredness, scientific rigor, timeliness, and transparency.

Reporting Bias

Chapter 3 describes the extent of reporting bias in the biomedical literature. Depending on the nature and direction of a study's results, research findings or findings for specific outcomes are often selectively published (publication bias and outcome reporting bias), published in a particular language (language bias), or released in journals with different ease of access (location bias) (Dickersin, 1990; Dwan et al., 2008; Gluud, 2006; Hopewell et al., 2008, 2009; Kirkham et al., 2010; Song et al., 2009, 2010; Turner et al., 2008). Thus, for each outcome, the SR should assess the probability of a biased subset of studies comprising the collected body of evidence.

Dose–Response Association

When findings from similar studies suggest a dose–response relationship across studies, it may increase confidence in the overall body of evidence. "Dose–response association" is defined as a consistent association across similar studies of a larger effect with greater exposure to the intervention. For a drug, a dose–response relationship might be observed with the treatment dosage, intensity, or duration. The concept of dose–response also applies to non-drug exposures. For example, in an SR of nutritional counseling to encourage a healthy diet, dose was measured as "the number and length of counseling contacts, the magnitude and complexity of educational materials provided, and the use of supplemental intervention elements, such as support groups sessions or cooking classes" (Ammerman et al., 2002, p. 6). Care needs to be exercised in the interpretation of dose–response relationships that are defined across, rather than within, studies. Cross-study comparisons of different "doses" may reflect other differences among studies, in addition to dose, that is, dose may be confounded with other study characteristics, populations included, or other aspects of the intervention.

The absence of a dose–response effect, in the observed range of doses, does not rule out a true causal relationship. For example, drugs are not always available in a wide range of doses. In some instances, any dose above a particular threshold may be sufficient for effectiveness.

Plausible Confounding That Would Change an Observed Effect

Although controlled trials generally minimize confounding by randomizing subjects to intervention and control groups, observational studies are particularly prone to selection bias, especially when there is little or no adjustment for potential confounding factors among comparison groups (Norris et al., 2010). This characteristic of quality refers to the extent to which systematic differences in baseline characteristics, prognostic factors, or co-occurring interventions among comparison groups may reduce or increase an observed effect. Generally, confounding results in effect sizes that are overestimated. However, sometimes, particularly in observational studies, confounding factors may lead to an underestimation of the effect of an intervention. If the confounding variables were not present, the measured effect would have been even larger. The AHRQ and GRADE systems use the term "plausible confounding that would decrease observed effect" to describe such situations. The GRADE Handbook provides the following examples (Schünemann et al., 2009, p. 125):

- A rigorous systematic review of observational studies including a total of 38 million patients demonstrated higher death rates in private for-profit versus private not-for-profit hospitals (Devereaux et al., 2004). One possible bias relates to different disease severity in patients in the two hospital types. It is likely, however, that patients in the not-for-profit hospitals were sicker than those in the for-profit hospitals. Thus, to the extent that residual confounding existed, it would bias results against the not-for-profit hospitals. The second likely bias was the possibility that higher numbers of patients with excellent private insurance coverage could lead to a hospital having more resources and a spill-over effect that would benefit those without such coverage. Since for-profit hospitals are [more] likely to admit a larger proportion of such well-insured patients than not-for-profit hospitals, the bias is once again against the not-for-profit hospitals. Because the plausible biases would all diminish the demonstrated intervention effect, one might consider the evidence from these observational studies as moderate rather than low quality.
- A parallel situation exists when observational studies have failed to demonstrate an association but all plausible biases would have increased an intervention effect. This situation will usually arise in the exploration of apparent harmful effects. For example, because the hypoglycemic drug phenformin causes lactic acidosis, the related agent metformin is under suspicion for the same toxicity. Nevertheless, very large observational studies have failed to demonstrate an association (Salpeter et al., 2004). Given the likelihood that

clinicians would be more alert to lactic acidosis in the presence of the agent and overreport its occurrence, one might consider this moderate, or even high-quality evidence refuting a causal relationship between typical therapeutic doses of metformin and lactic acidosis.

Strength of Association

Because observational studies are subject to many confounding factors (e.g., patients' health status, demographic characteristics) and greater risk of bias compared to controlled trials, the design, execution, and statistical analyses in each study should be assessed carefully to determine the influence of potential confounding factors on the observed effect. Strength of association refers to the likelihood that a large observed effect in an observational study is *not* due to bias from potential confounding factors.

Evidence on Assessment Methods Is Elusive

Applying the above concepts in a systematic way across multiple interventions and numerous outcomes is clearly challenging. Although many SR experts agree on the concepts that should underpin the assessment of the quality of body of evidence, the committee did not find any research to support existing methods for using these basic concepts in a systematic method such as the GRADE and AHRQ approaches. The GRADE Working Group reports that 50 organizations have either endorsed or are using an adapted version of their system (GRADE Working Group, 2010). However, the reliability and validity of the GRADE and AHRQ methods have not been evaluated, and not much literature assesses other approaches. Furthermore, many GRADE users are apparently selecting aspects of the system to suit their needs rather than adopting the entire method. The AHRQ method is one adaptation.

The committee heard considerable anecdotal evidence suggesting that many SR producers and users had difficulty using GRADE. Some organizations seem reluctant to adopt a new, more complex system that has not been sufficiently evaluated. Others are concerned that GRADE is too time consuming and difficult to implement. There are also complaints about the method's subjectivity. GRADE advocates acknowledge that the system does not eliminate subjectivity, but argue that a strength of the system is that, unlike other approaches, it makes transparent any judgments or disagreements about evidence (Brozek et al., 2009).

RECOMMENDED STANDARD FOR ASSESSING AND DESCRIBING THE QUALITY OF A BODY OF EVIDENCE

The committee recommends the following standard for assessing and describing the quality of a body of evidence. As noted earlier, this overall assessment should be done once the qualitative and quantitative syntheses are completed (see Standards 4.2–4.4 below). The order of this chapter's standards does not indicate the sequence in which the various steps should be conducted. Standard 4.1 is presented first to reflect the committee's recommendation that the SR specifies its methods *a priori* in the research protocol.[7]

Standard 4.1—Use a prespecified method to evaluate the body of evidence
> Required elements:
>> 4.1.1   For each outcome, systematically assess the following characteristics of the body of evidence:
>> • Risk of bias
>> • Consistency
>> • Precision
>> • Directness
>> • Reporting bias
>>
>> 4.1.2   For bodies of evidence that include observational research, also systematically assess the following characteristics for each outcome:
>> • Dose–response association
>> • Plausible confounding that would change the observed effect
>> • Strength of association
>>
>> 4.1.3   For each outcome specified in the protocol, use consistent language to characterize the level of confidence in the estimates of the effect of an intervention

Rationale

If an SR is to be objective, it should use prespecified, analytic methods. If the SR's assessment of the quality of a body of evidence is to be credible and true to scientific principles, it should be based on agreed-on concepts of study quality. If the SR is to be comprehensible, it should use unambiguous language, free from jar-

---

[7] See Chapter 2 for the committee's recommended standards for developing the SR research protocol.

gon, to describe the quality of evidence for each outcome. Decision makers—whether clinicians, patients, or others—should not have to decipher undefined and possibly conflicting terms and symbols in order to understand the methods and findings of SRs.

Clearly, the assessment of the quality of a body of evidence—for each outcome in the SR—must incorporate multiple dimensions of study quality. Without a sound conceptual framework for scrutinizing the body of evidence, the SR can lead to the wrong conclusions about an intervention's effectiveness, with potentially serious implications for clinical practice.

The lack of an evidence-based system for assessing and characterizing the quality of a body of evidence is clearly problematic. A plethora of systems are in use, none have been evaluated, and all have their proponents and critics. The committee's recommended quality characteristics are well-established concepts for evaluating quality; however, the SR field needs unambiguous, jargon-free language for systematically applying these concepts. GRADE merits consideration, but should be rigorously evaluated before it becomes a required component of SRs in the United States. Until a well-validated standard language is developed, SR authors should use their chosen lexicon and provide clear definitions of their terms.

QUALITATIVE SYNTHESIS OF THE BODY OF EVIDENCE

As noted earlier, the term "synthesis" refers to the collation, combination, and summary of the results of an SR. The committee uses the term "qualitative synthesis" to refer to an assessment of the body of evidence that goes beyond factual descriptions or tables that, for example, simply detail how many studies were assessed, the reasons for excluding other studies, the range of study sizes and treatments compared, or quality scores of each study as measured by a risk of bias tool. While an accurate description of the body of evidence is essential, it is not sufficient (Atkins, 2007; Mulrow and Lohr, 2001).

The primary focus of the qualitative synthesis should be to develop and to convey a deeper understanding of how an intervention works, for whom, and under what circumstances. The committee identified nine key purposes of the qualitative synthesis (Table 4-2).

If crafted to inform clinicians, patients, and other decision makers, the qualitative synthesis would enable the reader to judge the relevance and validity of the body of evidence for specific clinical

TABLE 4-2 Key Purposes of the Qualitative Synthesis

Purpose	Relevant Content in the Systematic Review (SR)
To orient the reader to the clinical landscape	A description of the clinical environment in which the research was conducted. It should enable the reader to grasp the relevance of the body of evidence to specific patients and clinical circumstances. It should describe the settings in which care was provided, how the intervention was delivered, by whom, and to whom.
To describe what actually happened to subjects during the course of the studies	A description of the actual care and experience of the study participants (in contrast with the original study protocol).
To critique the strengths and weaknesses of the body of evidence	A description of the strengths and weaknesses of the individual studies' design and execution, including their common features and differences. It should highlight well-designed and executed studies, contrasting them with others, and include an assessment of the extent to which the risk of bias affects summary estimates of the intervention's effect. It should also include a succinct summary of the issues that lead to the use of particular adjectives (e.g., "poor," "fair," "low quality," "high risk of bias," etc.) in describing the quality of the evidence.
To identify differences in the design and execution of the individual studies that explain why their results differ	An examination of how heterogeneity in the treatment's effects may be due to clinical differences in the study population (e.g., demographics, coexisting conditions, or treatments) as well as methodological differences in the studies' designs.

To describe how the design and execution of the individual studies affect their relevance to real-world clinical settings	A description of the applicability of the studies' health conditions, patient population, intervention, comparators, and health outcomes to the SR research question. It should also address how adherence of patients and providers may limit the applicability of the results. For example, the use of prescribed medications, as directed, may differ substantially between patients in the community compared with study participants.
To integrate the general summary of the evidence and the subgroup analyses based on setting and patient populations	For each important outcome, an overview of the nested subgroup analyses, as well as a presentation of the overall summary and assessment of the evidence.
To call attention to patient populations that have been inadequately studied or for whom results differ	A description of important patient subgroups (e.g., by comorbidity, age, gender, race, or ethnicity) that are unaddressed in the body of evidence.
To interpret and assess the robustness of the meta-analysis results	A clear synthesis of the evidence that goes beyond presentation of summary statistics. The summary statistics should not dominate the discussion; instead, the synthesis of the evidence should be carefully articulated, using the summary statistics to support the key conclusions.
To describe how the SR findings contrast with conventional wisdom	Sometimes commonly held notions about an intervention or a type of study design are not supported by the body of evidence. If this occurs, the qualitative synthesis should clearly explain how the SR findings differ from the conventional wisdom.

decisions and circumstances. Guidance from the Editors of *Annals of Internal Medicine* is noteworthy:

> We are disappointed when a systematic review simply lists the characteristics and findings of a series of single studies without attempting, in a sophisticated and clinically meaningful manner, to discover the pattern in a body of evidence. Although we greatly value meta-analyses, we look askance if they seem to be mechanistically produced without careful consideration of the appropriateness of pooling results or little attempt to integrate the finds into the contextual background. We want all reviews, including meta-analyses to include rich qualitative synthesis. (Editors, 2005, p. 1019)

Judgments and Transparency Are Key

Although the qualitative synthesis of CER studies should be based in systematic and scientifically rigorous methods, it nonetheless involves numerous judgments—judgments about the relevance, legitimacy, and relative uncertainty of some aspects of the evidence; the implications of missing evidence (a commonplace occurrence); the soundness of technical methods; and the appropriateness of conducting a meta-analysis (Mulrow et al., 1997). Such judgments may be inherently subjective, but they are always valuable and essential to the SR process. If the SR team approaches the literature from an open-minded perspective, team members are uniquely positioned to discover and describe patterns in a body of evidence that can yield a deeper understanding of the underlying science and help readers to interpret the findings of the quantitative synthesis (if conducted). However, the SR team should exercise extreme care to keep such discussions appropriately balanced and, whenever possible, driven by the underlying data.

RECOMMENDED STANDARDS FOR QUALITATIVE SYNTHESIS

The committee recommends the following standard and elements of performance for conducting the qualitative synthesis.

Standard 4.2—Conduct a qualitative synthesis
Required elements:
    4.2.1   Describe the clinical and methodological characteristics of the included studies, including their size, inclusion or exclusion of important subgroups, timeliness, and other relevant factors

4.2.2   Describe the strengths and limitations of individual studies and patterns across studies

4.2.3   Describe, in plain terms, how flaws in the design
or execution of the study (or groups of studies)
could bias the results, explaining the reasoning
behind these judgments

4.2.4   Describe the relationships between the characteristics of the individual studies and their reported
findings and patterns across studies

4.2.5   Discuss the relevance of individual studies to the
populations, comparisons, cointerventions, settings, and outcomes or measures of interest

Rationale

The qualitative synthesis is an often undervalued component of
an SR. Many SRs lack a qualitative synthesis altogether or simply
provide a nonanalytic recitation of the facts (Atkins, 2007). Patients,
clinicians, and others should feel confident that SRs accurately
reflect what is known and not known about the effects of a healthcare intervention. To give readers a clear understanding of how the
evidence applies to real-world clinical circumstances and specific
patient populations, SRs should describe—in easy-to-understand
language—the clinical and methodological characteristics of the
individual studies, including their strengths and weaknesses and
their relevance to particular populations and clinical settings.

META-ANALYSIS

This section of the chapter presents the background and rationale for the committee's recommended standards for conducting a
meta-analysis: first, considering the issues that determine whether
a meta-analysis is appropriate, and second, exploring the fundamental considerations in undertaking a meta-analysis. A detailed
description of meta-analysis methodology is beyond the scope of this
report; however, excellent reference texts are available (Borenstein,
2009; Cooper et al., 2009; Egger et al., 2001; Rothstein et al., 2005;
Sutton et al., 2000). This discussion draws from these sources as well
as guidance from the AHRQ Effective Health Care Program, CRD,
and the Cochrane Collaboration (CRD, 2009; Deeks et al., 2008; Fu
et al., 2010).

Meta-analysis is the statistical combination of results from
multiple individual studies. Meta-analytic techniques have been

used for more than a century for a variety of purposes (Sutton and Higgins, 2008). The nomenclature for SRs and meta-analysis has evolved over time. Although often used as a synonym for SR in the past, meta-analysis has come to mean the quantitative analysis of data in an SR. As noted earlier, the committee views "meta-analysis" as a broad term that encompasses a wide variety of methodological approaches whose goal is to quantitatively synthesize and summarize data across a set of studies. In the context of CER, meta-analyses are undertaken to combine and summarize existing evidence comparing the effectiveness of multiple healthcare interventions (Fu et al., 2010). Typically, the objective of the analysis is to increase the precision and power of the overall estimated effect of an intervention by producing a single pooled estimate, such as an odds ratio. In CER, large numbers are often required to detect what may be modest or even small treatment effects. Many studies are themselves too small to yield conclusive results. By combining the results of multiple studies in a meta-analysis, the increased number of study participants can reduce random error, improve precision, and increase the likelihood of detecting a real effect (CRD, 2009).

Fundamentally, a meta-analysis provides a weighted average of treatment effects from the studies in the SR. While varying in details, the weights are set up so that the most informative studies have the greatest impact on the average. While the term "most informative" is vague, it is usually expressed in terms of the sample size and precision of the study. The largest and most precisely estimated studies receive the greatest weights. In addition to an estimate of the average effect, a measure of the uncertainty of this estimate that reflects random variation is necessary for a proper summary.

In many circumstances, CER meta-analyses focus on the average effect of the difference between two treatments across all studies, reflecting the common practice in RCTs of providing a single number summary. While a meta-analysis is itself a nonrandomized study, even if the individual studies in the SR are themselves randomized, it can fill a confirmatory or an exploratory role (Anello and Fleiss, 1995). Although it has been underused for this purpose, meta-analysis is a valuable tool for assessing the pattern of results across studies and for identifying the need for primary research (CRD, 2009; Sutton and Higgins, 2008).

In other circumstances, individual studies in SRs of more than two treatments evaluate different subsets of treatments so that direct, head-to-head comparisons between two treatments of interest, for example, are limited. Treatment networks allow indirect comparisons in which the two treatments are each compared to a common third treatment (e.g., a placebo). The indirect treatment estimate then consists of the difference between the two comparisons with the common treatment. The network is said to be consistent if the indirect estimates are the same as the direct estimates (Lu and Ades, 2004). Consistency is most easily tested when some studies test all three treatments. Finding consistency increases confidence that the estimated effects are valid. Inconsistency suggests a bias in either or both of the indirect or direct estimates. While the direct estimate is often preferred, bias in the design of the direct comparison studies may suggest that the indirect estimate is better (Salanti et al., 2010). Proper consideration of indirect evidence requires that the full network be considered. This facilitates determining which treatments work best for which reported outcomes.

Many clinical readers view meta-analyses as confirmatory summaries that resolve conflicting evidence from previous studies. In this role, all the potential decision-making errors in clinical trials (e.g., Type 1 and Type 2 errors or excessive subgroup analyses)[8] apply to meta-analyses as well. However, in an exploratory role, meta-analysis may be more useful as a means to explore heterogeneity among study findings, recognize types of patients who might differentially benefit from (or be harmed by) treatment or treatment protocols that may work more effectively, identify gaps in knowledge, and suggest new avenues for research (Lau et al., 1998). Many of the methodological developments in meta-analysis in recent years have been motivated by the desire to use the information available from a meta-analysis for multiple purposes.

When Is Meta-Analysis Appropriate?

Meta-analysis has the potential to inform and explain, but it also has the potential to mislead if, for example, the individual studies are not similar, are biased, or publication or reporting biases are large (Deeks et al., 2008). A meta-analysis should not be assumed to always be an appropriate step in an SR. The decision to conduct a meta-analysis is neither purely analytical nor statistical in nature. It will depend on a number of factors, such as the availability of suitable data and the likelihood that the analysis could inform clinical decision making. Ultimately, it is a subjective judgment that should be made in consultation with the entire SR team, including both clinical and methodological perspectives. For purposes of transpar-

---

[8] A Type 1 error is a false-positive result. A Type 2 error is a false-negative result.

ency, the review team should clearly explain the rationale for each subjective determination (Fu et al., 2010).

Data Considerations

Conceptually a meta-analysis may make sense, and the studies may appear sufficiently similar, but without unbiased data that are in (or may be transformed into) similar metrics, the meta-analysis simply may not be feasible. There is no agreed-on definition of "similarity" with respect to CER data. Experts agree that similarity should be judged across three dimensions (Deeks et al., 2008; Fu et al., 2010): First, are the studies clinically similar, with comparable study population characteristics, interventions, and outcome measures? Second, are the studies alike methodologically in study design, conduct, and quality? Third, are the observed treatment effects statistically similar? All three of these questions should be considered before deciding a meta-analysis is appropriate.

Many meta-analyses use aggregate summary data for the comparison groups in each trial. Meta-analysis can be much more powerful when outcome, treatment, and patient data—individual patient data (IPD)—are available from individual patients. IPD, the raw data for each study participant, permit data cleaning and harmonization of variable definitions across studies as well as reanalysis of primary studies so that they are more readily combined (e.g., clinical measurement reported at a common time). IPD also allow valid analyses for effect modification by factors that change at the patient level, such as age and gender, for which use of aggregate data are susceptible to ecological bias (Berlin et al., 2002; Schmid et al., 2004). By permitting individual modeling in each study, IPD also focus attention on study-level differences that may contribute to heterogeneity of treatment effects across studies. When IPD are not available from each study in the meta-analysis, they can be analyzed together with summary data from the other studies (Riley and Steyerberg, 2010). The IPD inform the individual-level effects and both types of data inform the study-level effects. The increasing availability of data repositories and registries may make this hybrid modeling the norm in the future.

Advances in health information technology, such as electronic health records (EHRs) and disease registries, promise new sources of evidence on the effectiveness of health interventions. As these data sources become more readily accessible to investigators, they are likely to supplement or even replace clinical trials data in SRs of

CER. Furthermore, as with other data sources, the potential for bias and confounding will need to be addressed.

The Food and Drug Administration Sentinel Initiative and related activities (e.g., Observational Medical Outcomes Partnership) may be an important new data source for future SRs. When operational, the Sentinel Initiative will be a national, integrated, electronic database built on EHRs and claims records databases for as many as 100 million individuals (HHS, 2010; Platt et al., 2009). Although the principal objective of the system is to detect adverse effects of drugs and other medical products, it may also be useful for SRs of CER questions. A "Mini-Sentinel" pilot is currently under development at Harvard Pilgrim Health Care (Platt, 2010). The system will be a distributed network, meaning that separate data holders will contribute to the network, but the data will never be put into one common repository. Instead, all database holders will convert their data into a common data model and retain control over their own data. This allows a single "program" to be run (e.g., a statistical analysis in SAS) on all the disparate datasets, generating an estimated relative risk (or other measure) from each database. These then can be viewed as a type of meta-analysis.

Will the Findings Be Useful?

The fact that available data are conducive to pooling is not in itself sufficient reason to conduct a meta-analysis (Fu et al., 2010). The meta-analysis should not be undertaken unless the anticipated results are likely to produce meaningful answers that are useful to patients, clinicians, or other decision makers. For example, if the same outcomes are measured differently in the individual studies and the measures cannot be converted to a common scale, doing a meta-analysis may not be appropriate (Cummings, 2004). This situation may occur in studies comparing the effect of an intervention on a variety of important patient outcomes such as pain, mental health status, or pulmonary function.

Conducting the Meta-Analysis

Addressing Heterogeneity

Good statistical analyses quantify the amount of variability in the data in order to obtain estimates of the precision with which estimates may be made. Large amounts of variability reduce our confidence that effects are accurately measured. In meta-analysis, variability arises from three sources—clinical diversity, methodological diversity, and statistical heterogeneity—which should be separately considered in presentation and discussion (Fu et al., 2010). Clinical diversity describes variability in study population characteristics, interventions, and outcome ascertainments. Methodological diversity encompasses variability in study design, conduct, and quality, such as blinding and concealment of allocation. Statistical heterogeneity, relating to the variability in observed treatment effects across studies, may occur because of random chance, but may also arise from real clinical and methodological diversity and bias.

Assessing the amount of variability is fundamental to determining the relevance of the individual studies to the SR's research questions. It is also key to choosing which statistical model to use in the quantitative synthesis. Large amounts of variability may suggest a poorly formulated question or many sources of uncertainty that can influence effects. As noted above, if the individual studies are so diverse in terms of populations, interventions, comparators, outcomes, time lines, and/or settings, summary data will not yield clinically meaningful conclusions about the effect of an intervention for important subgroups of the population (West et al., 2010).

In general, quantifying heterogeneity helps determine whether and how the data may be combined, but specific tests of the presence of heterogeneity can be misleading and should not be used because of their poor statistical properties and because an assumption of complete homogeneity is nearly always unrealistic (Higgins et al., 2003). Graphical representations of among-study variation such as forest plots can be informative (Figure 4-1) (Anzures-Cabrera and Higgins, 2010).

When pooling is feasible, investigators typically use one of two statistical techniques—fixed-effects or random-effects models—to analyze and integrate the data, depending on the extent of heterogeneity. Each model has strengths and limitations. A fixed-effects model assumes that the treatment effect is the same for each study. A random-effects model assumes that some heterogeneity is present and acceptable, and the data can be pooled. Exploring the potential sources of heterogeneity may be more important than a decision about the use of fixed- or random-effects models. Although the committee does not believe that any single statistical technique should be a methodological standard, it is essential that the SR team clearly explain and justify the reasons why it chose the technique actually used.

183

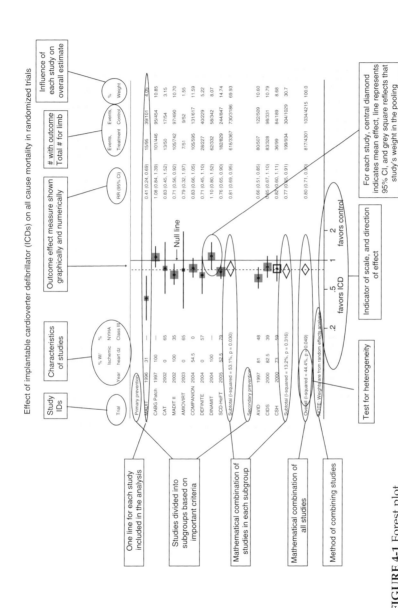

FIGURE 4-1 Forest plot.
SOURCE: Schriger et al. (2010).

Statistical Uncertainty

In meta-analyses, the amount of within- and between-study variation determines how precisely study and aggregate treatment effects are estimated. Estimates of effects without accompanying measures of their uncertainty, such as confidence intervals, cannot be correctly interpreted. A forest plot can provide a succinct representation of the size and precision of individual study effects and aggregated effects. When effects are heterogeneous, more than one summary effect may be necessary to fully describe the data. Measures of uncertainty should also be presented for estimates of heterogeneity and for statistics that quantify relationships between treatment effects and sources of heterogeneity.

Between-study heterogeneity is common in meta-analysis because studies differ in their protocols, target populations, settings, and ages of included subjects. This type of heterogeneity provides evidence about potential variability in treatment effects. Therefore, heterogeneity is not a nuisance or an undesirable feature, but rather an important source of information to be carefully analyzed (Lau et al., 1998). Instead of eliminating heterogeneity by restricting study inclusion criteria or scope, which can limit the utility of the review, heterogeneity of effect sizes can be quantified, and related to aspects of study populations or design features through statistical techniques such as meta-regression, which associates the size of treatment effects with effect modifiers. Meta-regression is most useful in explaining variation that occurs from sources that have no effect within studies, but big effects among studies (e.g., use of randomization or dose employed). Except in rare cases, meta-regression analyses are exploratory, motivated by the need to explain heterogeneity, and not by prespecification in the protocol. Meta-regression is observational in nature, and if the results of meta-regression are to be considered valid, they should be clinically plausible and supported by other external evidence. Because the number of studies in a meta-regression is often small, the technique has low power. The technique is subject to spurious findings because many potential covariates may be available, and adjustments to levels of significance may be necessary (Higgins and Thompson, 2004). Users should also be careful of relationships driven by anomalies in one or two studies. Such influential data do not provide solid evidence of strong relationships.

Research Trends in Meta-Analysis

As mentioned previously, a detailed discussion of meta-analysis methodology is beyond the scope of this report. There are many unresolved questions regarding meta-analysis methods. Fortunately, meta-analysis methodological research is vibrant and ongoing. Box 4-4 describes some of the research trends in meta-analysis and provides relevant references for the interested reader.

Sensitivity of Conclusions

Meta-analysis entails combining information from different studies; thus, the data may come from very different study designs. A small number of studies in conjunction with a variety of study designs contribute to heterogeneity in results. Consequently, verifying that conclusions are robust to small changes in the data and to changes in modeling assumptions solidifies the belief that they are robust to new information that could appear. Without a sensitivity analysis, the credibility of the meta-analysis is reduced.

Results are considered robust if small changes in the meta-analytic protocol, in modeling assumptions, and in study selection do not affect the conclusions. Robust estimates increase confidence in the SR's findings. Sensitivity analyses subject conclusions to such tests by perturbing these characteristics in various ways.

The sensitivity analysis could, for example, assess whether the results change when the meta-analysis is rerun leaving one study out at a time. One statistical test for stability is to check that the predictive distribution of a new study from a meta-analysis with one of the studies omitted would include the results of the omitted study (Deeks et al., 2008). Failure to meet this criterion implies that the result of the omitted study is unexpected given the remaining studies. Another common criterion is to determine whether the estimated average treatment effect changes substantially upon omission of one of the studies. A common definition of substantial involves change in the determination of statistical significance of the summary effect, although this definition is problematic because a significance threshold may be crossed with an unimportant change in the magnitude or precision of the effect (i.e., loss of statistical significance may result from omission of a large study that reduces the precision, but not the magnitude, of the effect).

In addition to checking sensitivity to inclusion of single studies, it is important to evaluate the effect of changes in the protocol that may alter the composition of the studies in the meta-analysis. Changes to the inclusion and exclusion criteria—such as the inclusion of non-English literature or the exclusion of studies that enroll some participants not in the target population or the focus on studies with low risk of bias—may all modify results sufficiently to question robustness of inferences.

BOX 4-4
Research Trends in Meta-Analysis

Meta-analytic research is a dynamic and rapidly changing field. The following describes key areas of research with recommended citations for additional reading:

Prospective meta-analysis—In this approach, studies are identified and evaluated prior to the results of any individual studies being known. Prospective meta-analysis (PMA) allows selection criteria and hypotheses to be defined a priori to the trials being concluded. PMA can implement standardization across studies so that heterogeneity is decreased. In addition, small studies that lack statistical power individually can be conducted if large studies are not feasible. See for example: Berlin and Ghersi, 2004, 2005; Ghersi et al., 2008; The Cochrane Collaboration, 2010.

Meta-regression—In this method, potential sources of heterogeneity are represented as predictors in a regression model, thereby enabling estimation of their relationship with treatment effects. Such analyses are exploratory in the majority of cases, motivated by the need to explain heterogeneity. See for example: Schmid et al., 2004; Smith et al., 1997; Sterne et al., 2002; Thompson and Higgins, 2002.

Bayesian methods in meta-analysis—In these approaches, as in Bayesian approaches in other settings, both the data and parameters in the meta-analytic model are considered random variables. This approach allows the incorporation of prior information into subsequent analyses, and may be more flexible in complex situations than standard methodologies. See for example: Berry et al., 2010; O'Rourke and Altman, 2005; Schmid, 2001; Smith et al., 1995; Sutton and Abrams, 2001; Warn et al., 2002.

Meta-analysis of multiple treatments—In this setting, direct treatment comparisons are not available, but an indirect comparison through a common comparator is. Multiple treatment models, also called mixed comparison models or network meta-analysis, may be used to more efficiently model treatment comparisons of interest. See for example: Cooper et al., 2009; Dias et al., 2010; Salanti et al., 2009.

Individual participant data meta-analysis—In some cases, study data may include outcomes, treatments, and characteristics of individual participants. Meta-analysis with such individual participant data (IPD) offers many advantages over meta-analysis of aggregate study-level data. See for example: Berlin et al., 2002; Simmonds et al., 2005; Smith et al., 1997; Sterne et al., 2002; Stewart, 1995; Thompson and Higgins, 2002; Tierney et al., 2000.

Another good practice is to evaluate sensitivity to choices about outcome metrics and statistical models. While one metric and one model may in the end be chosen as best for scientific reasons, results that are highly model dependent require more trust in the modeler and may be more prone to being overturned with new data. In any case, support for the metrics and models chosen should be provided.

Meta-analyses are also frequently sensitive to assumptions about missing data. In meta-analysis, missing data include not only missing outcomes or predictors, but also missing variances and correlations needed when constructing weights based on study precision. As with any statistical analysis, missing data pose two threats: reduced power and bias. Because the number of studies is often small, loss of even a single study's data can seriously affect the ability to draw conclusive inferences from a meta-analysis. Bias poses an even more dangerous problem. Seemingly conclusive analyses may give the wrong answer if studies that were excluded—because of missing data—differ from the studies that supplied the data. The conclusion that the treatment improved one outcome, but not another, may result solely from the different studies used. Interpreting such results requires care and caution.

RECOMMENDED STANDARDS FOR META-ANALYSIS

The committee recommends the following standards and elements of performance for conducting the quantitative synthesis.

Standard 4.3—Decide if, in addition to a qualitative analysis, the systematic review will include a quantitative analysis (meta-analysis)
Required element:
    4.3.1 Explain why a pooled estimate might be useful to decision makers

Standard 4.4—If conducting a meta-analysis, then do the following:
Required elements:
    4.4.1 Use expert methodologists to develop, execute, and peer review the meta-analyses
    4.4.2 Address heterogeneity among study effects
    4.4.3 Accompany all estimates with measures of statistical uncertainty
    4.4.4 Assess the sensitivity of conclusions to changes in the protocol, assumptions, and study selection (sensitivity analysis)

Rationale

A meta-analysis is usually desirable in an SR because it provides reproducible summaries of the individual study results and has potential to offer valuable insights into the patterns of results across studies. However, many published analyses have important methodological shortcomings and lack scientific rigor (Bailar, 1997; Gerber et al., 2007; Mullen and Ramirez, 2006). One must always look beyond the simple fact that an SR contains a meta-analysis to examine the details of how it was planned and conducted. A strong meta-analysis emanates from a well-conducted SR and features and clearly describes its subjective components, scrutinizes the individual studies for sources of heterogeneity, and tests the sensitivity of the findings to changes in the assumptions and set of studies (Greenland, 1994; Walker et al., 2008).

REFERENCES

AAN (American Academy of Neurology). 2004. *Clinical practice guidelines process manual.* http://www.aan.com/globals/axon/assets/3749.pdf (accessed February 1, 2011).

ACCF/AHA. 2009. *Methodology manual for ACCF/AHA guideline writing committees.* http://www.americanheart.org/downloadable/heart/12378388766452009Methodology ManualACCF_AHAGuidelineWritingCommittees.pdf (accessed July 29, 2009).

ACCP (American College of Chest Physicians). 2009. *The ACCP grading system for guideline recommendations.* http://www.chestnet.org/education/hsp/gradingSystem.php (accessed February 1, 2011).

Ammerman, A., M. Pignone, L. Fernandez, K. Lohr, A. D. Jacobs, C. Nester, T. Orleans, N. Pender, S. Woolf, S. F. Sutton, L. J. Lux, and L. Whitener. 2002. *Counseling to promote a healthy diet.* http://www.ahrq.gov/downloads/pub/prevent/pdfser/dietser.pdf (accessed September 26, 2010).

Anello, C., and J. L. Fleiss. 1995. Exploratory or analytic meta-analysis: Should we distinguish between them? *Journal of Clinical Epidemiology* 48(1):109–116.

Anzures-Cabrera, J., and J. P. T. Higgins. 2010. Graphical displays for meta-analysis: An overview with suggestions for practice. *Research Synthesis Methods* 1(1):66–89.

Atkins, D. 2007. Creating and synthesizing evidence with decision makers in mind: Integrating evidence from clinical trials and other study designs. *Medical Care* 45(10 Suppl 2):S16–S22.

Atkins, D., D. Best, P. A. Briss, M. Eccles, Y. Falck-Ytter, S. Flottorp, and GRADE Working Group. 2004a. Grading quality of evidence and strength of recommendations. *BMJ* 328(7454):1490–1497.

Atkins, D., M. Eccles, S. Flottorp, G. Guyatt, D. Henry, S. Hill, A. Liberati, D. O'Connell, A. D. Oxman, B. Phillips, H. Schünemann, T. T. Edejer, G. Vist, J. Williams, and the GRADE Working Group. 2004b. Systems for grading the quality of evidence and the strength of recommendations I: Critical appraisal of existing approaches. *BMC Health Services Research* 4(1):38.

Bailar, J. C., III. 1997. The promise and problems of meta-analysis. *New England Journal of Medicine* 337(8):559–561.

Balshem, H., M. Helfand, H. J. Schünemann, A. D. Oxman, R. Kunz, J. Brozek, G. E. Vist, Y. Falck-Ytter, J. Meerpohl, S. Norris, and G. H. Guyatt. 2011. GRADE guidelines: 3. Rating the quality of evidence. *Journal of Clinical Epidemiology* (In press).

Berlin, J. A., J. Santanna, C. H. Schmid, L. A. Szczech, H. I. Feldman, and the Antilymphocyte Antibody Induction Therapy Study Group. 2002. Individual patient versus group-level data meta-regressions for the investigation of treatment effect modifiers: Ecological bias rears its ugly head. *Statistics in Medicine* 21(3):371–387.

Berlin, J., and D. Ghersi. 2004. Prospective meta-analysis in dentistry. *The Journal of Evidence-Based Dental Practice* 4(1):59–64.

———. 2005. Preventing publication bias: Registries and prospective meta-analysis. *Publication bias in meta-analysis: Prevention, assessment and adjustments*, edited by H. R. Rothstein, A. J. Sutton, and M. Borenstein, pp. 35–48.

Berry, S., K. Ishak, B. Luce, and D. Berry. 2010. Bayesian meta-analyses for comparative effectiveness and informing coverage decisions. *Medical Care* 48(6):S137.

Borenstein, M. 2009. *Introduction to meta-analysis*. West Sussex, U.K.: John Wiley & Sons.

Brozek, J. L., E. A. Aki, P. Alonso-Coello, D. Lang, R. Jaeschke, J. W. Williams, B. Phillips, M. Lelgemann, A. Lethaby, J. Bousquet, G. Guyatt, H. J. Schünemann, and the GRADE Working Group. 2009. Grading quality of evidence and strength of recommendations in clinical practice guidelines: Part 1 of 3. An overview of the GRADE approach and grading quality of evidence about interventions. *Allergy* 64(5):669–677.

CEBM (Centre for Evidence-based Medicine). 2009. *Oxford Centre for Evidence-based Medicine—Levels of evidence (March 2009)*. http://www.cebm.net/index.aspx?o=1025 (accessed February 1, 2011).

Chalmers, I., M. Adams, K. Dickersin, J. Hetherington, W. Tarnow-Mordi, C. Meinert, S. Tonascia, and T. C. Chalmers. 1990. A cohort study of summary reports of controlled trials. *JAMA* 263(10):1401–1405.

Chou, R., N. Aronson, D. Atkins, A. S. Ismaila, P. Santaguida, D. H. Smith, E. Whitlock, T. J. Wilt, and D. Moher. 2010. AHRQ series paper 4: Assessing harms when comparing medical interventions: AHRQ and the Effective Health Care Program. *Journal of Clinical Epidemiology* 63(5):502–512.

Cochrane Collaboration. 2010. *Cochrane prospective meta-analysis methods group*. http://pma.cochrane.org/ (accessed January 27, 2011).

Coleman, C. I., R. Talati, and C. M. White. 2009. A clinician's perspective on rating the strength of evidence in a systematic review. *Pharmacotherapy* 29(9):1017–1029.

COMPUS (Canadian Optimal Medication Prescribing and Utilization Service). 2005. *Evaluation tools for Canadian Optimal Medication Prescribing and Utilization Service.* http://www.cadth.ca/media/compus/pdf/COMPUS_Evaluation_Methodology_final_e.pdf (accessed September 6, 2010).

Cooper, H. M., L. V. Hedges, and J. C. Valentine. 2009. *The handbook of research synthesis and meta-analysis*, 2nd ed. New York: Russell Sage Foundation.

Cooper, N., A. Sutton, D. Morris, A. Ades, and N. Welton. 2009. Addressing between-study heterogeneity and inconsistency in mixed treatment comparisons: Application to stroke prevention treatments in individuals with non-rheumatic atrial fibrillation. *Statistics in Medicine* 28(14):1861–1881.

CRD (Centre for Reviews and Dissemination). 2009. *Systematic reviews: CRD's guidance for undertaking reviews in health care*. York, U.K.: York Publishing Services, Ltd.

Cummings, P. 2004. Meta-analysis based on standardized effects is unreliable. *Archives of Pediatrics & Adolescent Medicine* 158(6):595–597.

Deeks, J., J. Higgins, and D. Altman, eds. 2008. Chapter 9: Analysing data and undertaking meta-anayses. In *Cochrane handbook for systematic reviews of interventions*, edited by J. P. T. Higgins and S. Green. Chichester, UK: John Wiley & Sons.

Devereaux, P. J., D. Heels-Ansdell, C. Lacchetti, T. Haines, K. E. Burns, D. J. Cook, N. Ravindran, S. D. Walter, H. McDonald, S. B. Stone, R. Patel, M. Bhandari, H. J. Schünemann, P. T. Choi, A. M. Bayoumi, J. N. Lavis, T. Sullivan, G. Stoddart, and G. H. Guyatt. 2004. Payments for care at private for-profit and private not-for-profit hospitals: A systematic review and meta-analysis. *Canadian Medical Association Journal* 170(12):1817–1824.

Dias, S., N. Welton, D. Caldwell, and A. Ades. 2010. Checking consistency in mixed treatment comparison meta analysis. *Statistics in Medicine* 29(7 8):932–944.

Dickersin, K. 1990. The existence of publication bias and risk factors for its occurrence. *JAMA* 263(10):1385–1389.

Dwan, K., D. G. Altman, J. A. Arnaiz, J. Bloom, A.-W. Chan, E. Cronin, E. Decullier, P. J. Easterbrook, E. Von Elm, C. Gamble, D. Ghersi, J. P. A. Ioannidis, J. Simes, and P. R. Williamson. 2008. Systematic review of the empirical evidence of study publication bias and outcome reporting bias. *PLoS ONE* 3(8):e3081.

Ebell, M. H., J. Siwek, B. D. Weiss, S. H. Woolf, J. Susman, B. Ewigman, and M. Bowman. 2004. Strength of recommendation taxonomy (SORT): A patient-centered approach to grading evidence in medical literature. *American Family Physician* 69(3):548–556.

Editors. 2005. Reviews: Making sense of an often tangled skein of evidence. *Annals of Internal Medicine* 142(12 Pt 1):1019–1020.

Egger, M., G. D. Smith, and D. G. Altman. 2001. *Systematic reviews in health care: Meta-analysis in context*. London, U.K.: BMJ Publishing Group.

Falck-Ytter, Y., H. Schünemann, and G. Guyatt. 2010. AHRQ series commentary 1: Rating the evidence in comparative effectiveness reviews. *Journal of Clinical Epidemiology* 63(5):474–475.

Faraday, M., H. Hubbard, B. Kosiak, and R. Dmochowski. 2009. Staying at the cutting edge: A review and analysis of evidence reporting and grading; The recommendations of the American Urological Association. *BJU International* 104(3): 294–297.

Federal Coordinating Council for Comparative Effectiveness Research. 2009. *Report to the President and the Congress*. Available from http://www.hhs.gov/recovery/programs/cer/cerannualrpt.pdf.

Ferreira, P. H., M. L. Ferreira, C. G. Maher, K. Refshauge, R. D. Herbert, and J. Latimer. 2002. Effect of applying different "levels of evidence" criteria on conclusions of Cochrane reviews of interventions for low back pain. *Journal of Clinical Epidemiology* 55(11):1126–1129.

Fu, R., G. Gartlehner, M. Grant, T. Shamliyan, A. Sedrakyan, T. J. Wilt, L. Griffith, M. Oremus, P. Raina, A. Ismaila, P. Santaguida, J. Lau, and T. A. Trikalinos. 2010. Conducting quantitative synthesis when comparing medical interventions: AHRQ and the Effective Health Care Program. In *Methods guide for comparative effectiveness reviews*, edited by Agency for Healthcare Research and Quality. http://www.effectivehealthcare.ahrq.gov/index.cfm/search-for-guides-reviews-and-reports/?pageaction=displayProduct&productID=554 (accessed January 19, 2011).

Gerber, S., D. Tallon, S. Trelle, M. Schneider, P. Jüni, and M. Egger. 2007. Bibliographic study showed improving methodology of meta-analyses published in leading journals: 1993–2002. *Journal of Clinical Epidemiology* 60(8):773–780.

Ghersi, D., J. Berlin, and L. Askie, eds. 2008. *Chapter 19: Prospective meta-analysis.* Edited by J. Higgins and S. Green, *Cochrane handbook for systematic reviews of interventions.* Chichester, UK: John Wiley & Sons.

Glasziou, P., J. Vandenbroucke, and I. Chalmers. 2004. Assessing the quality of research. *BMJ* 328(7430):39–41.

Gluud, L. L. 2006. Bias in clinical intervention research. *American Journal of Epidemiology* 163(6):493–501.

GRADE Working Group. 2010. *Organizations that have endorsed or that are using GRADE.* http://www.gradeworkinggroup.org/society/index.htm (accessed September 20, 2010).

Greenland, S. 1994. Invited commentary: A critical look at some popular meta-analytic methods. *American Journal of Epidemiology* 140(3):290–296.

Guirguis-Blake, J., N. Calonge, T. Miller, A. Siu, S. Teutsch, E. Whitlock, and for the U.S. Preventive Services Task Force. 2007. Current processes of the U.S. Preventive Services Task Force: Refining evidence-based recommendation development. *Annals of Internal Medicine* 147:117–122.

Guyatt, G. H., D. L. Sackett, J. C. Sinclair, R. Hayward, D. J. Cook, and R. J. Cook. 1995. Users' guides to the medical literature: A method for grading health care recommendations. *JAMA* 274(22):1800–1804.

Guyatt, G., H. J. Schünemann, D. Cook, R. Jaeschke, and S. Pauker. 2004. Applying the grades of recommendation for antithrombotic and thrombolytic therapy: The seventh ACCP conference on antithrombotic and thrombolytic therapy. *Chest* 126(3 Suppl):179S–187S.

Guyatt, G., A. D. Oxman, E.A. Akl, R. Kunz, G. Vist, J. Brozek, S. Norris, Y. Falck-Ytter, P. Glasziou, H. deBeer, R. Jaeschke, D. Rind, J. Meerpohl, P. Dahm, and H. J. Schünemann. 2010. GRADE guidelines 1. Introduction—GRADE evidence profiles and summary of findings tables. *Journal of Clinical Epidemiology* (In press).

Harris, R. P., M. Helfand, S. H. Woolf, K. N. Lohr, C. D. Mulrow, S. M. Teutsch, D. Atkins, and the Methods Work Group Third U. S. Preventive Services Task Force. 2001. Current methods of the U.S. Preventive Services Task Force: A review of the process. *American Journal of Preventive Medicine* 20(3 Suppl):21–35.

Helfand, M. 2005. Using evidence reports: Progress and challenges in evidence-based decision making. *Health Affairs* 24(1):123–127.

HHS (U.S. Department of Health and Human Services). 2010. *The Sentinel Initiative: A national strategy for monitoring medical product safety.* Available from http://www.fda.gov/Safety/FDAsSentinelInitiative/ucm089474.htm.

Higgins, J. P. T., and S. G. Thompson. 2004. Controlling the risk of spurious findings from meta-regression. *Statistics in Medicine* 23(11):1663–1682.

Higgins, J. P. T., S. G. Thompson, J. J. Deeks, and D. G. Altman. 2003. Measuring inconsistency in meta-analyses. *BMJ* 327(7414):557–560.

Hopewell, S., K. Loudon, M. J. Clarke, A. D. Oxman, and K. Dickersin. 2009. Publication bias in clinical trials due to statistical significance or direction of trial results (Review). *Cochrane Database of Systematic Reviews* 1:MR000006.

Hopewell, S., J. Clarke Mike, L. Stewart, and J. Tierney. 2008. Time to publication for results of clinical trials (Review). *Cochrane Database of Systematic Reviews* (2).

Hsieh, C., A. H. Adams, J. Tobis, C. Hong, C. Danielson, K. Platt, F. Hoehler, S. Reinsch, and A. Rubel. 2002. Effectiveness of four conservative treatments for subacute low back pain: A randomized clinical trial. *Spine* 27(11):1142–1148.

ICSI (Institute for Clinical Systems Improvement). 2003. *Evidence grading system.* http://www.icsi.org/evidence_grading_system_6/evidence_grading_system_pdf_.html (accessed September 8, 2009).

IOM (Institute of Medicine). 2009. *Initial national priorities for comparative effectiveness research*. Washington, DC: The National Academies Press.

Kirkham, J. J., K. M. Dwan, D. G. Altman, C. Gamble, S. Dodd, R. Smyth, and P. R. Williamson. 2010. The impact of outcome reporting bias in randomised controlled trials on a cohort of systematic reviews. *BMJ* 340:c365.

Lau, J., J. P. A. Ioannidis, and C. H. Schmid. 1998. Summing up evidence: One answer is not always enough. *Lancet* 351(9096):123–127.

Lefebvre, C., E. Manheimer, and J. Glanville. 2008. Chapter 6: Searching for studies. In *Cochrane handbook for systematic reviews of interventions*, edited by J. P. T. Higgins and S. Green. Chichester, UK: John Wiley & Sons.

Lu, G., and A. E. Ades. 2004. Combination of direct and indirect evidence in mixed treatment comparisons. *Statistics in Medicine* 23(20):3105–3124.

Mullen, P. D., and G. Ramirez. 2006. The promise and pitfalls of systematic reviews. *Annual Review of Public Health* 27:81–102.

Mulrow, C. D., and K. N. Lohr. 2001. Proof and policy from medical research evidence. *Journal of Health Politics Policy and Law* 26(2):249–266.

Mulrow, C., P. Langhorne, and J. Grimshaw. 1997. Integrating heterogeneous pieces of evidence in systematic reviews. *Annals of Internal Medicine* 127(11):989–995.

NCCN (National Comprehensive Cancer Network). 2008. *About the NCCN clinical practice guidelines in oncology*. http://www.nccn.org/professionals/physician_gls/about.asp (accessed September 8, 2009).

Norris, S., D. Atkins, W. Bruening, S. Fox, E. Johnson, R. Kane, S. C. Morton, M. Oremus, M. Ospina, G. Randhawa, K. Schoelles, P. Shekelle, and M. Viswanathan. 2010. Selecting observational studies for comparing medical interventions. In *Methods guide for comparative effectiveness reviews*, edited by Agency for Healthcare Research and Quality. http://www.effectivehealthcare.ahrq.gov/index.cfm/search-for-guides-reviews-and-reports/?pageaction=displayProduct&productID=454 (accessed January 19, 2011).

NZGG (New Zealand Guidelines Group). 2007. *Handbook for the preparation of explicit evidence-based clinical practice guidelines*. http://www.nzgg.org.nz/download/files/nzgg_guideline_handbook.pdf (accessed February 1, 2011).

O'Rourke, K., and D. Altman. 2005. Bayesian random effects meta-analysis of trials with binary outcomes: Methods for the absolute risk difference and relative risk scales *Statistics in Medicine* 24(17):2733–2742.

Owens, D. K., K. N. Lohr, D. Atkins, J. R. Treadwell, J. T. Reston, E. B. Bass, S. Chang, and M. Helfand. 2010. Grading the strength of a body of evidence when comparing medical interventions: AHRQ and the Effective Health Care Program. *Journal of Clinical Epidemiology* 63(5):513–523.

Pham, H. H., D. Schrag, A. S. O'Malley, B. Wu, and P. B. Bach. 2007. Care patterns in Medicare and their implications for pay for performance. *New England Journal of Medicine* 356(11):1130–1139.

Platt, R. 2010. *FDA's Mini-Sentinel program*. http://www.brookings.edu/~/media/Files/events/2010/0111_sentinel_workshop/06%20Sentinel%20Initiative%20Platt%20Brookings%2020100111%20v05%20distribution.pdf (accessed October 25, 2010).

Platt, R., M. Wilson, K. A. Chan, J. S. Benner, J. Marchibroda, and M. McClellan. 2009. The new Sentinel Network: Improving the evidence of medical-product safety. *New England Journal of Medicine* 361(7):645–647.

Rayleigh, J. W. 1884. Address by the Rt. Hon. Lord Rayleigh. In *Report of the fifty-fourth meeting of the British Association for the Advancement of Science*, edited by Murray J. Montreal.

Riley, R. D., and E. W. Steyerberg. 2010. Meta-analysis of a binary outcome using individual participant data and aggregate data. *Research Synthesis Methods* 1(1):2–19.

Rothstein, H. R., A. J. Sutton, and M. Borenstein, editors. 2005. *Publication bias in meta-analysis: Prevention, assessment and adjustments*. Chichester, U.K.: Wiley.

Salanti, G., V. Marinho, and J. Higgins. 2009. A case study of multiple-treatments meta-analysis demonstrates that covariates should be considered. *Journal of Clinical Epidemiology* 62(8):857–864.

Salanti, G., S. Dias, N. J. Welton, A. Ades, V. Golfinopoulos, M. Kyrgiou, D. Mauri, and J. P. A. Ioannidis. 2010. Evaluating novel agent effects in multiple-treatments meta-regression. *Statistics in Medicine* 29(23):2369–2383.

Salpeter, S., E. Greyber, G. Pasternak, and E. Salpeter. 2004. Risk of fatal and nonfatal lactic association with metformin use in type 2 diabetes mellitus. *Cochrane Database of Systematic Reviews* 4:CD002967.

Schmid, C. 2001. Using bayesian inference to perform meta-analysis. *Evaluation & the Health Professions* 24(2):165.

Schmid, C. H., P. C. Stark, J. A. Berlin, P. Landais, and J. Lau. 2004. Meta-regression detected associations between heterogeneous treatment effects and study-level, but not patient-level, factors. *Journal of Clinical Epidemiology* 57(7):683–697.

Schriger, D. L., D. G. Altman, J. A. Vetter, T. Heafner, and D. Moher. 2010. Forest plots in reports of systematic reviews: A cross-sectional study reviewing current practice. *International Journal of Epidemiology* 39(2):421–429.

Schünemann, H., D. Best, G. Vist, and A. D. Oxman. 2003. Letters, numbers, symbols and words: How to communicate grades of evidence and recommendations. *Canadian Medical Association Journal* 169(7):677–680.

Schünemann, H., A. D. Oxman, G. Vist, J. Higgins, J. Deeks, P. Glasziou, and G. Guyatt. 2008. Chapter 12: Interpreting results and drawing conclusions. In *Cochrane handbook for systematic reviews of interventions*, edited by J. P. T. Higgins and S. Green. Chichester, UK: John Wiley & Sons.

Schünemann, H. J., J. Brożek, and A. D. Oxman. 2009. *GRADE handbook for grading quality of evidence and strength of recommendations*. Version 3.2 [updated March 2009]. http://www.cc-ims.net/gradepro (accessed November 10, 2010).

SIGN (Scottish Intercollegiate Guidelines Network). 2009. *SIGN 50: A guideline developer's handbook*. http://www.sign.ac.uk/guidelines/fulltext/50/index.html (accessed Februray 1, 2011).

Silagy, C.A., P. Middelton, and S. Hopewell. 2002. Publishing protocols of systematic reviews: Comparing what was done to what was planned. *JAMA* 287:2831–2834.

Simmonds, M., J. Higginsa, L. Stewartb, J. Tierneyb, M. Clarke, and S. Thompson. 2005. Meta-analysis of individual patient data from randomized trials: A review of methods used in practice. *Clinical Trials* 2(3):209.

Slone Survey. 2006. *Patterns of medication use in the United States, 2006: A report from the Slone Survey*. http://www.bu.edu/slone/SloneSurvey/AnnualRpt/SloneSurveyWebReport2006.pdf (accessed February 1, 2011).

Smith, G., M. Egger, and A. Phillips. 1997. Meta-analysis: Beyond the grand mean? *BMJ* 315(7122):1610.

Smith, T., D. Spiegelhalter, and A. Thomas. 1995. Bayesian approaches to random-effects meta-analysis: A comparative study. *Statistics in Medicine* 14(24):2685–2699.

Song, F., S. Parekh-Bhurke, L. Hooper, Y. Loke, J. Ryder, A.J. Sutton, C.B. Hing, and I. Harvey. 2009. Extent of publication bias in different categories of research cohorts: a meta-analysis of empirical studies. *BMC Medical Research Methodology* 9:79.

Song, F., S. Parekh, L. Hooper, Y. K. Loke, J. Ryder, A. J. Sutton, C. Hing, C. S. Kwok, C. Pang, and I. Harvey. 2010. Dissemination and publication of research findings: an updated review of related biases. *Health Technology Assessment* 14(8).

Sterne, J., P. Jüni, K. Schulz, D. Altman, C. Bartlett, and M. Egger. 2002. Statistical methods for assessing the influence of study characteristics on treatment effects in 'meta epidemiological' research. *Statistics in Medicine* 21(11):1513–1524.

Stewart, L. 1995. Practical methodology of meta-analyses (overviews) using updated individual patient data. *Statistics in Medicine* 14(19):2057–2079.

Sutton, A., and K. Abrams. 2001. Bayesian methods in meta-analysis and evidence synthesis. *Statistical Methods in Medical Research* 10(4):277.

Sutton, A. J., and J. P. Higgins. 2008. Recent developments in meta-analysis. *Statistics in Medicine* 27(5):625–650.

Sutton, A. J., K. R. Abams (Q: Abrams?), D. R. Jones, T. A. Sheldon, and F. Song. 2000. *Methods for meta-analysis in medical research, Wiley series in probability and statistics.* Chichester, U.K.: John Wiley & Sons.

Thompson, S., and J. Higgins. 2002. How should meta-regression analyses be undertaken and interpreted? *Statistics in Medicine* 21(11):1559–1573.

Tierney, J., M. Clarke, and L. Stewart. 2000. Is there bias in the publication of individual patient data meta-analyses? *International Journal of Technology Assessment in Health Care* 16(02):657–667.

Turner, E. H., A. M. Matthews, E. Linardatos, R. A. Tell, and R. Rosenthal. 2008. Selective publication of antidepressant trials and its influence on apparent efficacy. *New England Journal of Medicine* 358(3):252–260

USPSTF (U.S. Preventive Services Task Force). 2008. *Grade definitions.* http://www.ahrq.gov/clinic/uspstf/grades.htm (accessed January 6, 2010).

Vogeli, C., A. Shields, T. Lee, T. Gibson, W. Marder, K. Weiss, and D. Blumenthal. 2007. Multiple chronic conditions: Prevalence, health consequences, and implications for quality, care management, and costs. *Journal of General Internal Medicine* 22(Suppl. 3):391–395.

Walker, E., A. V. Hernandez, and M. W. Kattan. 2008. Meta-analysis: Its strengths and limitations. *Cleveland Clinic Journal of Medicine* 75(6):431–439.

Warn, D., S. Thompson, and D. Spiegelhalter. 2002. Bayesian random effects meta-analysis of trials with binary outcomes: Methods for the absolute risk difference and relative risk scales. *Statistics in Medicine* 21(11):1601–1623.

West, S., V. King, T. S. Carey, K. N. Lohr, N. McKoy, S. F. Sutton, and L. Lux. 2002. Systems to rate the strength of scientific evidence. Evidence Report/Technology Assessment No. 47 (prepared by the Research Triangle Institute–University of North Carolina Evidence-based Practice Center under Contract No. 290-97-0011). *AHRQ Publication No. 02-E016*:64–88.

West, S. L., G. Gartlehner, A. J. Mansfield, C. Poole, E. Tant, N. Lenfestey, L. J. Lux, J. Amoozegar, S. C. Morton, T. C. Carey, M. Viswanathan, and K. N. Lohr. 2010. *Comparative effectiveness review methods: Clinical heterogeneity.* http://www.effectivehealthcare.ahrq.gov/ehc/products/93/533/Clinical_Heteogeneity_Revised_Report_FINAL%209-24-10.pdf (accessed September 28, 2010).

5

Standards for Reporting Systematic Reviews

Abstract: *Authors of publicly sponsored systematic reviews (SRs) should produce a detailed, comprehensive final report. The committee recommends three related standards for documenting the SR process, responding to input from peer reviewers and other users and stakeholders, and making the final report publicly available. The standards draw extensively from the Preferred Reporting Items for Systematic Reviews and Meta-Analyses (PRISMA) checklist. The committee recommends several reporting items in addition to the PRISMA requirements to ensure that the final report (1) describes all of the steps and judgments required by the standards in the previous chapters and (2) focuses on informing patient and clinical decision making.*

High-quality systematic review (SR) reports should accurately document all of the steps and judgments in the SR process using clear language that is understandable to users and stakeholders. A report should provide enough detail that a knowledgeable reader could reproduce the SR. The quality of a final report has profound implications for patients and clinicians. Too often the information that researchers report in published SRs does not adequately reflect their study methods (Devereaux et al., 2004).[1] If SRs are poorly reported, patients and clinicians have difficulty determining whether an SR is trustworthy enough to be used to guide decision making or the development of clinical practice guidelines (Moher et al., 2007). High-quality SR reports summarize the methodological strengths and weaknesses of the SR and include language designed to help nonexperts interpret and judge the value of the SR (AHRQ, 2010b; CRD, 2010a; Higgins and Green, 2008; Liberati et al. 2009; Moher et al. 2009). However, according to an extensive literature, many published SRs inadequately document important aspects of the SR process (Delaney et al., 2005, 2007; Golder et al., 2008; McAlister et al., 1999; Moher et al., 2007; Mulrow, 1987; Roundtree et al., 2008; Sacks et al., 1987). A seminal study conducted by Mulrow, for example, assessed 50 review articles published in four leading medical journals and found that many reviews failed to report the methods of identifying, selecting, and validating information, and choosing areas for future research (Mulrow, 1987). More recently, Moher and colleagues (2007) evaluated 300 SRs indexed in MEDLINE during November 2004. They concluded that information continues to be poorly reported, with many SRs failing to report key components of SRs, such as assessing for publication bias, aspects of the searching and screening process, and funding sources. Other studies have found that SRs published in journals often inadequately report search strategies, validity assessments of included studies, and authors' conflicts of interest (Delaney et al., 2005; Golder et al., 2008; Roundtree et al., 2008).

Authors of all publicly sponsored SRs must produce a detailed final report, which is typically longer and more detailed than the version submitted for journal publication. The sponsor typically publishes the final report on its website, where it stands as the definitive documentation of the review. The standards recommended by the committee apply to this definitive comprehensive final report. The committee recommends three standards for producing a comprehensive SR final report (Box 5-1), including standards for documenting the SR process, responding to input from peer reviewers and other users and stakeholders, and making the final reports publicly available. Each standard includes elements of performance that the committee deems essential. The evidence base for developing standards for the final report is sparse. In addition, most evaluations of the quality of published SRs have focused on

---

[1] See Chapter 3 for a review of the literature on reporting bias and dearth of adequate documentation in most SRs of comparative effectiveness.

BOX 5-1
Recommended Standards for
Reporting Systematic Reviews

Standard 5.1 Prepare the final report using a structured format
Required elements:

5.1.1   Include a report title*
5.1.2   Include an abstract*
5.1.3   Include an executive summary
5.1.4   Include a summary written for the lay public
5.1.5   Include an introduction (rationale and objectives)*
5.1.6   Include a methods section. Describe the following:
- Research protocol*
- Eligibility criteria (criteria for including and excluding studies in the sysematic review)*
- Analytic framework and key questions
- Databases and other information sources used to identify relevant studies*
- Search strategy*
- Study selection process*
- Data extraction process*
- Methods for handling missing information*
- Information to be extracted from included studies*
- Methods to appraise the quality of individual studies*
- Summary measures of effect size (e.g., risk ratio, difference in means)*
- Rationale for pooling (or not pooling) results of included studies
- Methods of synthesizing the evidence (qualitative and meta-analysis*)
- Additional analyses, if done, indicating which were prespecified*

5.1.7   Include a results section. Organize the presentation of results around key questions. Describe the following (repeat for each key question):
- Study selection process*
- List of excluded studies and reasons for their exclusion*
- Appraisal of individual studies' quality*
- Qualitative synthesis
- Meta-analysis of results, if performed (explain rationale for doing one)*
- Additional analyses, if done, indicating which were prespecified*
- Tables and figures

5.1.8   Include a discussion section. Include the following:
- Summary of the evidence*

continued

BOX 5-1 Continued

- Strengths and limitations of the systematic review*
- Conclusions for each key questions*
- Gaps in evidence
- Future research needs

5.1.9   Include a section describing funding sources* and COI

Standard 5.2 Peer review the draft report
Required elements:
    5.2.1   Use a third party to manage the peer review process
    5.2.2   Provide a public comment period for the report and publicly report on disposition of comments

Standard 5.3 Publish the final report in a manner that ensures free public access

---

* Indicates items from the PRISMA checklist. (The committee endorses all of the PRISMA checklist items.)

journal articles rather than SR reports. The committee developed the standards by first reviewing existing expert guidance, particularly the Preferred Reporting Items for Systematic Reviews and Meta-Analyses (PRISMA) checklist (Liberati et al., 2009). However, PRISMA is focused on journal articles, not comprehensive final reports to public sponsors. The committee recommended including items that were not on the PRISMA checklist because it believed that the report of an SR should describe all the steps and judgments required by the committee's standards in Chapters 2 through 4 to improve the transparency of the SR process and to inform patient and clinical decision making. The committee also took into account the legislatively mandated reporting requirements for the Patient-Centered Outcomes Research Institute (PCORI), as specified by the 2010 *Patient Protection and Affordable Care Act* (ACA). Box 5-2 describes the ACA reporting requirements for research funded by PCORI. See Appendix G for the Agency for Healthcare Research and Quality (AHRQ), Centre for Reviews and Dissemination (CRD), and Cochrane Collaboration guidance on writing an SR final report. Appendix H contains the PRISMA checklist.

BOX 5-2
Requirements for Research Funded by the
Patient-Centered Outcomes Research Institute

The 2010 *Patient Protection and Affordable Care Act* created the Patient-Centered Outcomes Research Institute (PCORI), a nonprofit corporation intended to advance comparative effectiveness research. The act stipulates that research funded by PCORI, including systematic reviews, adhere to the following reporting and publication requirements:

- For each research study, the following information should be posted on PCORI's website:
    o A research protocol, including measures taken, methods of research and analysis, research results, and other information the institute determines appropriate.
    o The research findings conveyed in a manner that is comprehensible and useful to patients and providers in making healthcare decisions.
    o Considerations specific to certain subpopulations, risk factors, and comorbidities, as appropriate.
    o The limitations of the research and what further research may be needed as appropriate.
    o The identity of the entity and the investigators conducting the research.
    o Conflicts of interest, including the type, nature, and magnitude of the interests.
- PCORI is required to:
    o Provide a public comment period for systematic reviews to increase public awareness, and to obtain and incorporate public input and feedback on research findings.
    o Ensure there is a process for peer review to assess a study's scientific integrity and adherence to methodological standards.
    o Disseminate research to physicians, healthcare providers, patients, payers, and policy makers.

SOURCE: *The Patient Protection and Affordable Care Act*, Public Law 111-148, 111th Cong., Subtitle D, § 6301 (March 23, 2010).

REPORTING GUIDELINES

Over the past decade, several international, multidisciplinary groups have collaborated to develop guidelines for reporting the methods and results of clinical research (reporting guidelines). Reporting guidelines exist for many types of health research (Ioannidis et al., 2004; Liberati et al., 2009; Moher et al., 1999, 2001a,b,

2009; Stroup et al., 2000). These guideline initiatives were undertaken out of concern that reports on health research were poorly documenting the methods and results of the research studies (IOM, 2008). Detailed reporting requirements are also seen as a line of defense against reporting bias.[2] For SRs to be trustworthy enough to inform healthcare decisions, accurate, thorough, and transparent reporting are essential. The adoption of reporting guidelines furthers this goal. Examples of reporting guidelines include the Consolidated Standards of Reporting Trials (CONSORT) statement for reporting randomized clinical trials (Ioannidis et al., 2004; Moher et al., 2001b), and the Strengthening the Reporting of Observational Studies in Epidemiology (STROBE) statement for reporting observational studies in epidemiology (von Elm et al., 2007). The major reporting guideline for SRs and meta-analyses is PRISMA (Liberati et al., 2009; Moher et al., 2009), an update to the 1999 Quality of Reporting of Meta-analyses (QUOROM) statement (Moher et al., 1999). In 2006, the Enhancing Quality and Transparency of Health Research (EQUATOR) Network was launched to coordinate initiatives to promote transparent and accurate reporting of health research and to assist in the development of reporting guidelines (EQUATOR Network, 2010). See Box 5-3 for a historical overview of reporting guidelines.

The methodological quality of SRs (i.e., how well the SR is conducted) is distinct from reporting quality (i.e., how well reviewers report their methodology and results) (Shea et al., 2007). Whether reporting guidelines improve the underlying methodological quality of research studies is unknown. However, incomplete documentation of the SR process makes it impossible to evaluate its methodological quality, so that it is impossible to tell whether a step in the SR process was performed correctly but not reported (poor reporting quality), completed inadequately, or not completed at all and therefore not reported (poor methodological quality).

At present, the evidence that reporting guidelines improve the quality of reports of SRs and meta-analyses is weak. The few observational studies that have addressed the issue have serious flaws. For example, Delaney and colleagues (2005) compared the quality of reports of meta-analyses addressing critical care, including topics related to shock, resuscitation, inotropes, and mechanical ventilation, published before and after the release of the QUOROM statement (the precursor to PRISMA). They found that reports of meta-analyses published after QUOROM were of higher quality

---

[2] See Chapter 3 for a discussion on reporting bias.

BOX 5-3
A History of Reporting Guidelines for
Comparative Effectiveness Research

In 1993 the Standards for Reporting Trials (SORT) group met to address inadequate reporting of randomized controlled trials (RCTs). This group developed the concept of a structured reporting guideline, and proposed a checklist of essential items for reporting RCTs. Five months later the Asilomar Working group met independently to discuss challenges in reporting RCTs and developed a reporting checklist. The Consolidated Standards of Reporting Trials (CONSORT) statement was developed in 1996 and consolidated the recommendation from both groups. The CONSORT statement consists of a checklist of reporting items, such as the background, methods, results, discussion, and conclusion sections, as well as a flow diagram for documenting participants through the trial. Many journals have adopted the CONSORT statement. It has been extended to address a number of specific issues in the reporting of RCTs (e.g., reporting of harms, noninferiority and equivalence RCTs, cluster RCTs).

Following the success of the CONSORT statement, two international groups of review authors, methodologists, clinicians, medical editors, and consumers developed standard formats for reporting systematic reviews (SRs) and meta-analyses: Quality of Reporting of Meta-analyses (QUOROM) and Meta-analysis of Observational Studies in Epidemiology (MOOSE). The statements consist of checklists of items to include in reports and flow diagrams for documenting the search process. However, unlike CONSORT, reporting guidelines for SRs and meta-analyses have not been widely adopted by prominent journals.

In 2009, the Preferred Reporting Items for Systematic Reviews and Meta-analyses (PRISMA) statement was published to update the QUOROM statement. According to its developers, PRISMA reflects the conceptual and practical advances made in the science of SRs since the development of QUOROM. These conceptual advances include the following: completing an SR is an iterative process; the conduct and reporting of research are distinct processes; the assessment of risk of bias requires both a study-level assessment (e.g., adequacy of allocation concealment) and outcome-level assessment (i.e., reliability and validity of the data for each outcome); and the importance of addressing reporting bias. PRISMA decouples several checklist items that were a single item on the QUOROM checklist and links other items to improve the consistency across the SR report. PRISMA was funded by the Canadian Institutes of Health Research; Universita di Modena e Reggio Emilia, Italy; Cancer Research U.K.; Clinical Evidence BMJ Knowledge; The Cochrane Collaboration; and GlaxoSmithKline, Canada.[a] It has been endorsed by a number of organizations and journals, including the Centre for Reviews and Dissemination, Cochrane Collaboration, *British Medical Journal*, and *Lancet*.[b]

---

[a] The following Institute of Medicine committee members were involved in the development of PRISMA: Jesse Berlin, Kay Dickersin, and Jeremy Grimshaw.

[b] See the following website for a full list of organizations endorsing PRISMA: http://www.prisma-statement.org/endorsers.htm (accessed July 14, 2010).

SOURCES: Begg et al. (1996); Ioannidis et al. (2004); IOM (2008); Liberati et al. (2009); Moher et al. (1999, 2001a, 2001b, 2007, 2009); Stroup et al. (2000).

than reports published before and were more likely to describe whether a comprehensive literature search was conducted; the criteria for screening the studies; and the methods used to combine the findings of relevant studies (Delaney et al., 2005). Mrkobrada and colleagues (2008) evaluated 90 SRs published in 2005 in the field of nephrology. They found that only a minority of journals (4 out of 48) recommended adherence to SR reporting guidelines. The four journals that endorsed or adopted reporting guidelines published SRs of significantly higher methodological quality than the other journals, and were more likely to report assessing methodological quality of included studies and taking precautions to avoid bias in study selection. Neither of these studies, however, assessed whether the journals endorsing QUOROM published higher quality reviews than the other journals prior to the adoption of QUOROM. In addition, journals that endorse reporting guidelines, such as QUOROM, may merely recommend that authors comply with the reporting items, but may not require authors to show compliance by submitting a checklist stating whether or not they adhered to each item as a condition of accepting the SR for review. As a result, whether the reporting improvements were due to QUOROM or other developments in the field is unclear. No controlled trials have evaluated the effectiveness of PRISMA on improving the reporting of SRs (Liberati et al., 2009).

In light of this history of reporting guidelines for medical journals, the committee decided to develop reporting guidelines specifically for the final report to the sponsor of an SR. The committee intends for its reporting requirements to improve the documentation of SR final report study methodology and results, and to increase the likelihood that SR final reports will provide enough information for patients and clinicians to determine whether an SR is trustworthy enough to be used to guide decision making.

SYSTEMATIC REVIEWS PUBLISHED IN JOURNALS

The committee recognizes that a journal publishing SRs will choose the level of documentation that is most appropriate for its readers. It also recognizes that its reporting requirements for final reports to public sponsors of SRs are quite detailed and comprehensive, and will produce manuscripts that are too long and too detailed for most journals to publish in full. Ideally, all published SRs (both final reports to sponsors and journal publications) should follow one reporting standard. With the advent of electronic-only appendixes to journal articles, journals can now require authors to meet the committee's full reporting guidelines (i.e., journals can post any reporting items not included in the actual journal publication in an online appendix). Alternatively, journals can publish a link to the website of the full SR report to the public sponsor, explaining what information readers would find only at the sponsor's website.

RECOMMENDED STANDARD FOR PREPARING THE FINAL REPORT

The committee recommends the following standard for preparing the final report:

Standard 5.1—Prepare the final report using a structured format
> Required elements:
> 5.1.1   Include a report title
> 5.1.2   Include an abstract
> 5.1.3   Include an executive summary
> 5.1.4   Include a summary written for the lay public
> 5.1.5   Include an introduction (rationale and objectives)
> 5.1.6   Include a methods section
> 5.1.7   Include a results section. Organize the presentation of results around key questions
> 5.1.8   Include a discussion section
> 5.1.9   Include a section describing funding sources and COI

Rationale

All SR reports to public sponsors should use a structured format to help guide the readers to relevant information, to improve the documentation of the SR process, and to promote consistency in reporting. More than 150 journals have adopted the PRISMA requirements (PRISMA, 2010). Because of this support, the committee used the PRISMA checklist as its starting point for developing its reporting standards. However, PRISMA is focused on journal articles, which are usually subject to length restrictions in the print version of the article, and the committee's reporting standards are directed at comprehensive, final reports to public sponsors (e.g., AHRQ, PCORI), which typically do not have word limits. Most of the committee's additions and revisions to PRISMA were necessary to make the standards for the final report consistent with *all* of the steps and judgments in the SR process required by the standards for performing an SR, as recommended in Chapters 2 through 4 of this report. In addition, the committee added several items to PRISMA because of the committee's focus on setting standards for public agencies that sponsor SRs of comparative effectiveness research (CER), which place a strong emphasis on generating evidence to inform patient and clinical decision making.

Therefore, the committee's reporting recommendations build on PRISMA, but incorporate the following revisions: greater specificity in reporting the data collection and study selection process, and eight new checklist items. The checklist items are as follows: (1) an executive summary, (2) a summary written for the lay public, (3) an analytic framework and description of the chain of logic for how the intervention may improve a health outcome, (4) rationale for pooling (or not pooling) results across studies, (5) results of the qualitative synthesis, including findings of differences in responses to the intervention for key subgroups (this requirement reflects a specific characteristic of CER: the search for evidence to help patients and clinicians tailor the decisions to the characteristics and needs of the individual patient), (6) tables and figures summarizing the results, (7) gaps in evidence, and (8) future research needs.

The following sections present the committee's recommendations for the key components of a final SR report: title, abstract and summaries, introduction, methods, results, discussion, and funding and conflict-of-interest (COI) sections of SR reports (see Box 5-1 for a complete list of all required reporting elements).

Report Title

The title should identify the report as an SR, a meta-analysis, or both (if appropriate). This may improve the indexing and identification of SRs in bibliographic databases (Liberati et al., 2009). The title should also reflect the research questions addressed in the review in order to help the reader understand the scope of the SR. PRISMA provides the following example of a clear title: "Recurrence Rates of Video-assisted Thoracoscopic versus Open Surgery in the Prevention of Recurrent Pneumothoraces: A Systematic Review of Randomized and Nonrandomized Trials" (Barker et al., 2007; Liberati et al., 2009).

Abstract, Executive Summary, and Plain-Language Summary

The SR final report should include a structured abstract organized under a series of headings corresponding to the background, methods, results, and conclusions (Haynes et al., 1990; Mulrow et al., 1988). A structured abstract helps readers to quickly determine the scope, processes, and findings of a review without reading the entire report. Structured abstracts also give the reader more complete information than unstructured abstracts (Froom and Froom, 1993; Hartley, 2000; Hartley et al., 1996; Pocock et al., 1987). In SR final reports, the abstract should address, as applicable: background; objectives; data sources; study eligibility criteria (inclusion/exclusion criteria), participants, and interventions; study appraisal and synthesis methods; results; appraisal of the body of evidence; limitations; conclusions and implications of key findings; and SR registration number[3] (Liberati et al., 2009). See Box 5-4 for an example of a structured abstract.

The final report should also include an executive summary. Many users and stakeholders find concise summaries that highlight the main findings and allow for rapid scanning of results very useful (Lavis et al., 2005; Oxman et al., 2006). Because the length of abstracts is often limited they may not provide enough information to satisfy decision makers. The committee's recommendation to include an executive summary and abstract in final reports is consistent with guidance from AHRQ and CRD (AHRQ, 2009a; CRD, 2009).

SR reports, including their abstracts and executive summaries, are often written in language that is too technical for consumers and patients to use in decision making. This is especially problematic for SRs of CER studies because one of the major goals of CER is to help patients and consumers make healthcare decisions (IOM, 2009). To improve the usability of SRs for patients and consumers, the committee recommends that final reports include summaries written in nontechnical language (the plain-language summary) (see Box 5-5 for an example). The plain-language summary should include background information about the healthcare condition, population, intervention, and main findings. The committee believes the plain-language summary should explain the shortcomings of the body of evidence, so the public can form a realistic appreciation of the limitations of the science. Developing plain-language summaries requires specialized knowledge and skills. An important resource in this area is the John M. Eisenberg Clinical Decisions and Communications Science Center at Baylor College of Medicine in Houston, Texas. The Center, with AHRQ funding, translates SRs of CER conducted by the

---

[3] An SR registration number is the unique identification number assigned to a protocol in an electronic registry. See Chapter 2 for a discussion on protocol publication.

BOX 5-4
Example of a Structured Abstract:
Clinical Utility of Cancer Family History
Collection in Primary Care

Objectives: This systematic review aimed to evaluate, within unselected populations, the:

1. Performance of family history (FHx)-based models in predicting cancer risk.
2, Overall benefits and harms associated with established cancer prevention interventions.
3. Impact of FHx-based risk information on the uptake of preventive interventions.
4. Potential for harms associated with collecting cancer FHx.

Data sources: MEDLINE, EMBASE, CINAHL Cochrane Central, Cochrane Database of Systematic Reviews, and PsycINFO were searched from 1990 to June 2008. Cancer guidelines and recommendations were searched from 2002 forward and systematic reviews from 2003 to June 2008.

Review methods: Standard systematic review methodology was employed. Eligibility criteria included English studies evaluating breast, colorectal, ovarian, or prostate cancers. Study designs were restricted to systematic review, experimental and diagnostic types. Populations were limited to those unselected for cancer risk. Interventions were limited to collection of cancer FHx; primary and/or secondary prevention interventions for breast, colorectal, ovarian, and prostate cancers.

Results:
- *Accuracy of models:* Seven eligible studies evaluated systems based on the Gail model, and on the Harvard Cancer Risk Index. No evaluations demonstrated more than modest discriminatory

---

EPCs into short, easy-to-read guides and tools that can be used by consumers, clinicians, and policy makers (AHRQ, 2010b).

Advice about the best method of presenting the research results for a consumer audience has a substantial body of evidence to support it (Akl et al., in press; Glenton, 2002; Glenton et al., 2006a; Glenton et al., 2006b; Lipkus, 2007; Santesso et al., 2006; Schünemann et al., 2004; Schwartz et al., 2009; Trevena et al., 2006; Wills and Holmes-Rovner, 2003). For example, Glenton (2010) conducted a series of semi-structured interviews with members of the public and

accuracy at an individual level. No evaluations were identified relevant to ovarian or prostate cancer risk.

- *Efficacy of preventive interventions:* From 29 eligible systematic reviews, 7 found no experimental studies evaluating interventions of interest. Of the remaining 22, none addressed ovarian cancer prevention. The reviews were generally based on limited numbers of randomized or controlled clinical trials. There was no evidence either to support or refute the use of selected chemoprevention interventions, there was some evidence of effectiveness for mammography and fecal occult blood testing.

- *Uptake of intervention:* Three studies evaluated the impact of FHx-based risk information on uptake of clinical preventive interventions for breast cancer. The evidence is insufficient to draw conclusions on the effect of FHx-based risk information on change in preventive behavior.

- *Potential harms of FHx taking:* One uncontrolled trial evaluated the impact of FHx-based breast cancer risk information on psychological outcomes and found no evidence of significant harm.

Conclusions: Our review indicates a very limited evidence base with which to address all four of the research questions:

1. The few evaluations of cancer risk prediction models do not suggest useful individual predictive accuracy.
2. The experimental evidence base for primary and secondary cancer prevention is very limited.
3. There is insufficient evidence to assess the effect of FHx-based risk assessment on preventive behaviors.
4. There is insufficient evidence to assess whether FHx-based personalized risk assessment directly causes adverse outcomes.

SOURCE: AHRQ (2009b).

---

found that summarizing SR results using both qualitative statements and numbers in tables improves consumer comprehension (Glenton, 2010). Other research has found that consumer comprehension is improved if authors use frequencies (e.g., 1 out of 100) rather than percentages or probabilities; use a consistent numeric format to summarize research results; and use absolute risk rather than relative risk (Akl et al., in press; Lipkus, 2007; Wills and Holmes-Rovner, 2003). The recommendation to include a plain-language summary follows guidance from AHRQ and Cochrane (AHRQ, 2010a; Higgins

BOX 5-5
Example of a Plain-Language Summary:
Antenatal Corticosteroids for Accelerating
Fetal Lung Maturation for Women at Risk of Preterm Birth

Corticosteroids given to women in early labor help the babies' lungs to mature and so reduce the number of babies who die or suffer breathing problems at birth.

Babies born very early are at risk of breathing difficulties (respiratory distress syndrome) and other complications at birth. Some babies have developmental delay and some do not survive the initial complications. In animal studies, corticosteroids are shown to help the lungs to mature and so it was suggested these drugs may help babies in preterm labor too. This review of 21 trials shows that a single course of corticosteroid, given to the mother in preterm labor and before the baby is born, helps to develop the baby's lungs and reduces complications like respiratory distress syndrome. Furthermore, this treatment results in fewer babies dying and fewer common serious neurological and abdominal problems, e.g. cerebroventricular haemorrhage and necrotising enterocolitis, that affect babies born very early. There does not appear to be any negative effects of the corticosteroid on the mother. Long-term outcomes on both baby and mother are also good.

SOURCE: Roberts and Dalziel (2006).

and Green, 2008). Also consistent with the requirement is that PCORI convey the research findings so patients can understand and apply them to their personal circumstances.[4]

Introduction to the Final Report

The introduction section of an SR final report should describe the research questions as well as the rationale for undertaking the review. The description should address the perspectives of both patients and clinicians, the current state of knowledge, and what the SR aims to add to the body of knowledge. It should indicate whether the review is new or an update of an existing one. If it is an update, the authors should state why the update is needed and describe in general terms how the evidence base has changed since the previous

---

[4] *The Patient Protection and Affordable Care Act*, Public Law 111-148, 111th Cong., Subtitle D, § 6301(d)(8)(A)(i).

review (e.g., three new, large randomized controlled trials have been published in the past 2 years).

Methods Section

Detailed reporting of methods is important because it allows the reader to assess the reliability and validity of the review. Table 5-1 lists and describes the topics that should be included in the methods section.

Results Section

The results section should logically lay out the key findings from the SR and include all the topics described in Table 5-2.

Discussion Section

The discussion should include a summary of the main findings; the strength of evidence; a general interpretation of the results for each key question; the strengths and limitations of the study; and gaps in evidence, including future research needs. The discussion should draw conclusions only if they are clearly supported by the evidence (Docherty and Smith, 1999; Higgins and Green, 2008). At the same time, the discussion should provide an interpretation of the data that are useful to users and stakeholders. The peer review process often improves the quality of discussion sections and can provide an evaluation of whether the authors went beyond the evidence in their interpretation of the results (Goodman et al., 1994).

Future research is particularly important for authors to discuss because most SRs identify significant gaps in the body of evidence (Clarke et al., 2007). The ACA language specifies that reports funded by PCORI should "include limitations of the research and what further research may be needed as appropriate."[5] Policy makers and research funders rely on well-written discussions of future research needs to set research agendas and funding priorities. When information gaps are reported clearly, SRs can bring attention to future research needs. Odierna and Bero, for example, used Drug Effectiveness Review Project SRs to identify the need for better drug studies in non-white and economically disadvantaged populations (Odierna and Bero, 2009).

---

[5] *The Patient Protection and Affordable Care Act*, Public Law 111-148, 111th Cong., Subtitle D, § 6301(d)(8)(A)(iii) (March 23, 2010).

TABLE 5-1 Topics to Include in the Methods Section

Methods Topic	Include
Research protocol	• Rationale for deviations from the protocol in the conduct of the systematic review (SR) • Registration number (if applicable)
Eligibility criteria (for including and excluding studies in the SR)	• Research designs (trials, observational studies), patients, interventions, comparators, outcomes, length of follow-up • Report characteristics (e.g., publication period, language) • Rationale for each criterion
Analytic framework and key questions	• A diagram illustrating the chain of logic describing the mechanism by which the intervention could improve a health outcome • Key questions written in a structured format (e.g., PICO[TS])
Databases and other information sources	• All sources of information about potentially eligible articles (including contact with study authors) • Date of last search
Search strategy	• Electronic search strategy for at least one database, including any limits used and the date of searches (include all search strategies in an electronic appendix)
Study selection	• Process for screening studies, including the number of individual screeners and their qualifications • Process for resolving differences among screeners
Data extraction	• Process for extracting data from included studies, including the data collection form, number of individual data extractors and their qualifications, and whether more than one person independently extracted data from the same study • Process for resolving differences among extractors
Missing information	• Researchers contacted, information requested, and success of requests
Information to be extracted	• All variables for which data were sought (e.g., PICO[TS]) • Any assumptions made about missing and unclear data
Appraisal of individual studies	• Description of how risk of bias was assessed • Description of how the relevance of the studies to the populations, interventions, and outcome measures was assessed • Description of how the fidelity of the implementation of interventions was assessed
Summary measures	• Principal summary measures (e.g., risk ratio, difference in means)
Data pooling across studies	• Rationale for pooling decision

TABLE 5-1 Continued

Methods Topic	Include
Synthesizing the results	• Summary of qualitative and quantitative synthesis methods, including how heterogeneity, sensitivity, and statistical uncertainty were addressed • Description of the methods for assessing the characteristics of the body of evidence
Additional analyses	• Description of analyses (e.g., subgroup analyses, meta-regression) not prespecified in the protocol

NOTE: PICO(TS) = population, intervention, comparator, outcome, timing, and setting.

Unfortunately, many SRs are not explicit when recommending future research and not specific enough about recommending types of participants, interventions, or outcomes that need additional examination (Clarke et al., 2007). The EPICOT acronym is a helpful guide for organizing the discussion of future research needs: Evidence, Population, Intervention, Comparison, Outcomes, and Time Stamp (see Table 5-3 for an example recommending that further evidence be collected on the efficacy and adverse effects of intensive blood-pressure lowering in representative populations) (Brown et al., 2006). This tool indicates that recommendations on future research needs should be specific on all of the PICO elements that are required in SR topic formulation (see Chapter 2). The discussion should also report the strength of existing evidence on the topic, using consistent language when discussing different studies (see Chapter 4) and the date of the most recent literature search or recommendation.

Funding and Conflict-of-Interest Section

The final report should describe the sources of funding for the SR; the role of the funder in carrying out the review (including approval of the content); the review authors', contributing users', and stakeholders' biases and COIs; and how any potential conflicts were managed (See Box 5-6 for examples of how to report funding and COI statements).[6] The sponsor of an SR can have a significant impact on the SR process and resulting conclusions. SRs funded by industry, for example, are more likely to favor the sponsor's product

---

[6] See Chapter 2 for an overview of COI and bias in the review team, and a discussion of the role of the sponsor in the SR process.

TABLE 5-2 Topics to Include in the Results Section (repeat for each key question)

Results Topic	Include
Study selection	• Numbers of studies that were screened, assessed for eligibility, and included in the review • A flow chart that shows the number of studies that remain after each stage of the selection process • Provide a citation for each included study
Excluded studies	• Excluded studies that experts might expect to see included and reason for their exclusion
Appraisal of individual studies	• Summarize the threats to validity in each study and, if available, any outcome-level assessment of the effects of bias • Summarize the relevance of the studies to the populations, interventions, and outcome measures • Summarize the fidelity of the implementation of interventions

Qualitative synthesis	• Summarize clinical and methodological characteristics of the included studies, such as:
	  o Number and characteristics of study participants, including factors that may impact generalizability of results to real-world settings (e.g., comorbidities in studies of older patients or race/ethnicity in conditions where disparities exist)
	  o Clinical settings
	  o Interventions
	  o Primary and secondary outcome measures
	  o Follow-up period
	• Observed patterns of threats to validity across studies, strengths, and weaknesses of the evidence, and confidence in the results
	• Description of the overall body of evidence across the following domains:
	  o Risk of bias
	  o Consistency
	  o Precision
	  o Directness
	  o Reporting bias
	  o Dose–response association
	  o Plausible confounding that would change the observed effect
	  o Strength of association
	• Findings of differences in responses to the intervention for key subgroups (e.g., by age, race, gender, socioeconomic status, and/or clinical findings)

TABLE 5-2 Continued

Results Topic	Include
Meta-analysis (if performed)	• Justification for why a pooled estimate might be more useful to decision makers than the results of each study individually • Examination of how heterogeneity in the treatment's effects may be due to clinical differences in the study population or methodological differences in the studies' design • Results of each meta-analysis, including a measure of statistical uncertainty and the sensitivity of the conclusions to changes in the protocol, assumptions, and study selection
Additional analyses	• If done, results of additional analyses (e.g., subgroup analyses, meta-regression), indicating whether the analysis was prespecified or exploratory
Tables and figures	• An evidence table summarizing the characteristics of included studies • Graphic displays of results (e.g., forest plots to summarize quantitative findings, GRADE summary tables)

NOTE: GRADE = Grading of Recommendations Assessment, Development and Evaluation.

than SRs funded through other sources (Lexchin et al., 2003; Yank et al., 2007). Identifying the sources of funding and the role of the sponsor (including whether the sponsor reserved the right to approve the content of the report) in the final report improves the transparency and is critical for the credibility of the report (Liberati et al., 2009).

Currently, many peer-reviewed publications fail to provide complete or consistent information regarding the authors' biases and COI (Chimonas et al., 2011; McPartland, 2009; Roundtree et al., 2008). A recent study of payments received by physicians from orthopedic device companies identified 41 individuals who each received $1 million or more in 2007. In 2008 and 2009, these individuals published a total of 95 articles relating to orthopedics. Fewer than half the articles disclosed the authors' relationships with the orthopedic device manufacturers, and an even smaller number provided information on the amount of the physicians' payments (Chimonas et al., 2011). Requiring authors to disclose *any* potential outside influences on their judgment, not just industry relationships, improves the

TABLE 5-3 EPICOT Format for Formulating Future Research Recommendations

EPICOT Component	Issues to Consider	Example
E Evidence	What is the current evidence?	One systematic review dominated by a large randomized controlled study conducted in hospital setting
P Population	Diagnosis, disease stage, comorbidity, risk factor, sex, age, ethnic group, specific inclusion or exclusion criteria, clinical setting	Primary care patients with confirmed stroke or transient ischemic attack (mean age $\geq$ 75 years, female–male ratio 1:1, time since last cerebrovascular event $\geq$ 1 year)
I Intervention	Type, frequency, dose, duration, prognostic factor	Intensive blood pressure lowering
C Comparison	Placebo, routine care, alternative treatment/management	No active treatment or placebo
O Outcomes	Which clinical or patient-related outcomes will the researcher need to measure, improve, influence, or accomplish? Which methods of measurement should be used?	Major vascular events (stroke, myocardial infarction, vascular death); adverse events, risk of discontinuation of treatment because of adverse events
T Time stamp	Date of literature search or recommendation	February 2006

SOURCE: Brown et al. (2006).

transparency and trustworthiness of the review. The ACA contains a similar requirement for authors of research funded by PCORI.[7]

RECOMMENDED STANDARD FOR REPORT REVIEW

The committee recommends one overarching standard for review by scientific peers, other users and stakeholders, and the public:

Standard 5.2—Peer review the draft report
    Required elements:
        5.2.1   Use a third party to manage the peer review process

---

[7] *The Patient Protection and Affordable Care Act* at § 6301(h)(3)(B).

BOX 5-6
Reporting Funding and Conflict of Interest:
Selected Examples

Source of Funding
"PRISMA was funded by the Canadian Institutes of Health Research; Universita' di Modena e Reggio Emilia, Italy; Cancer Research UK; Clinical Evidence BMJ Knowledge; the Cochrane Collaboration; and GlaxoSmith-Kline, Canada. AL is funded, in part, through grants of the Italian Ministry of University (COFIN–PRIN 2002 prot. 2002061749 and COFIN–PRIN 2006 prot. 2006062298). DGA is funded by Cancer Research UK. DM is funded by a University of Ottawa Research Chair."

Role of Funders
"None of the sponsors had any involvement in the planning, execution, or write-up of the PRISMA documents. Additionally, no funder played a role in drafting the manuscript."

Potential Conflicts of Interest
"The authors have declared that no competing interests exist."

SOURCE: Moher et al. (2009).

5.2.2   Provide a public comment period for the report and publicly report on disposition of comments

Rationale

SR final reports should be critically reviewed by peer reviewers to ensure accuracy and clarity and to identify any potential methodological flaws (e.g., overlooked studies, methodological errors). The original protocol for the SR (including any amendments) should be made available to the peer reviewers. A small body of empirical evidence suggests that the peer review process improves the quality of published research by making the manuscripts more readable and improving the comprehensiveness of reporting (Goodman et al., 1994; Jefferson et al., 2002; Weller, 2002). In addition, the critical assessment of manuscripts by peer reviewers is an essential part of the scientific process (ICMJE, 2010). Journals rely on the peer review process to establish when a study is suitable for publication and to improve the quality of reporting and compliance with reporting guidelines (ICMJE, 2010). Some version of peer review is recommended in the guidance from all the major producers of SRs (CRD, 2009; Higgins and Green, 2008; Slutsky et al., 2010). Peer review of research funded through PCORI will be required, either directly through a process established by PCORI or by an appropriate medical journal or other entity.[8]

The evidence is unclear on how to select peer reviewers, the qualifications that are important for peer reviewers to possess, and what type of training and instructions improve the peer review process (Callaham and Tercier, 2007; Jefferson et al., 2002; Schroter et al., 2004, 2006). In the context of publicly funded SRs, the committee recommends that peer reviewers include a range of relevant users and stakeholders, such as practicing clinicians, statisticians and other methodologists, and consumers. This process can be used to gather input from perspectives that were not represented on the review team (e.g., individuals with diverse clinical specialties).

The committee also recommends that the public be given an opportunity to comment on SR reports as part of the peer review process. Allowing public comments encourages publicly funded research that is responsive to the public's interests and concerns and is written in language that is understandable and usable for patient and clinical decision making. Requiring a public comment period is also consistent with the ACA, which directs PCORI to obtain public input on research findings,[9] as well as guidance from AHRQ and Cochrane (Higgins and Green, 2008; Whitlock et al., 2010).

The review team should be responsive to the feedback provided by the peer reviewers and the public, and publicly report how it revised the SR in response to the comments. The authors should document the major comments and input received; how the final report was or was not modified accordingly; and the rationale for the course of action. The authors' response to this feedback can be organized into general topic areas of response, rather than responding to each individual comment. Requiring authors to report on the disposition of comments holds the review authors accountable for responding to the peer reviewers' comments and improves the public's confidence in the scientific integrity and credibility of the SR (Whitlock et al., 2010).

A neutral third party should manage and oversee the entire peer review process. The main role of the third party should be to provide an independent judgment about the adequacy of the authors' responses (Helfand and Balshem, 2010). This recommendation is

---

[8] *The Patient Protection and Affordable Care Act* at § 6301(d)(7).
[9] *The Patient Protection and Affordable Care Act* at § 6301(h).

consistent with the rules governing PCORI that allow, but do not require, the peer review process to be overseen by a medical journal or outside entity.[10] It also furthers SR authors' accountability for responding to reviewers' feedback and it is consistent with AHRQ guidance (Helfand and Balshem, 2010; Whitlock et al., 2010). The National Academies has an office that manages the review of all Academies studies. A monitor and coordinator, chosen by the report review office from the membership of the Academies, oversee the response to external review. They must approve the response to review before release of the report.

RECOMMENDED STANDARD FOR PUBLISHING THE FINAL REPORT

The committee recommends one standard for publishing the final report:

Standard 5.3—Publish the final report in a manner that ensures free public access

Rationale

The final report should be publicly available. PCORI will be required to post research findings on a website accessible to clinicians, patients, and the general public no later than 90 days after receipt of the research findings and completion of the peer review process.[11] This requirement should be extended to all publicly funded SRs of effectiveness research. Publishing final reports is consistent with leading guidance (AHRQ, 2010c; CRD, 2009; Higgins and Green, 2008) and this committee's criteria of transparency and credibility. Public sponsors should not prevent the SR team from publishing the SR in a peer-reviewed journal and should not interfere with the journal's peer review process. Ideally, the public sponsor will cooperate with the journal to ensure timely, thorough peer review, so that journal publication and posting on the sponsor's website can take place simultaneously. In any case, posting an SR final report on a government website should not qualify as a previous publication, in the same way that journals have agreed that publication of an abstract describing clinical trial results in clinicaltrials.gov (which is required by federal law) does not count as prior publication (ICMJE,

---

[10] *The Patient Protection and Affordable Care Act* at § 6301(d)(7).
[11] *The Patient Protection and Affordable Care Act* at § 6301(d)(8)(A).

2009). In addition, public sponsors should encourage the review team to post the research results in international SR registries, such as the one being developed by the CRD (CRD, 2010b).

REFERENCES

AHRQ (Agency for Healthcare Research and Quality). 2009a. *AHRQ Evidence-based Practice Centers partners guide*. Gaithersburg, MD: AHRQ.

AHRQ. 2009b. *Cancer, clinical utility of family history*. http://www.ahrq.gov/clinic/tp/famhist2tp.htm (accessed September 20, 2010).

AHRQ. 2010a. *Consumers and patients*. http://www.ahrq.gov/consumer/compare.html (accessed September 10, 2010).

AHRQ. 2010b. *About the Eisenberg Center*. http://www.effectivehealthcare.ahrq.gov/index.cfm/who-is-involved-in-the-effective-health-care-program1/about-the-eisenberg-center/ (accessed December 27, 2010).AHRQ. 2010c. *Search for guides, reviews, and reports*. http://www.effectivehealthcare.ahrq.gov/index.cfm/search-for-guides-reviews-and-reports/ (accessed July 2, 2010).

AHRQ. 2010c. *Search for guides, reviews, and reports*. http://www.effectivehealthcare.ahrq.gov/index.cfm/search-for-guides-reviews-and-reports/ (accessed July 2, 2010).

Akl, E., A. D. Oxman, J. Herrin, G. E. Vist, I. Terrenato, F. Sperati, C. Costiniuk, D. Blank, and H. Schunemann. In press. Using alternative statistical formats for presenting risks and risk reduction. *Cochrane Database of Systematic Reviews*.

Barker, A., E. C. Maratos, L. Edmonds, and M. Lim. 2007. Recurrence rates of video-assisted thoracoscopic versus open surgery in the prevention of recurrent pneumothoraces: A systematic review of randomised and non-randomised trials. *Lancet* 370(9584):329–335.

Begg, C., M. Cho, S. Eastwood, R. Horton, D. Moher, I. Olkin, R. Pitkin, D. Rennie, K. F. Schulz, D. Simel, and D. F. Stroup. 1996. Improving the quality of reporting of randomized controlled trials: The CONSORT statement. *JAMA* 276(8):637–639.

Brown, P., K. Brunnhuber, K. Chalkidou, I. Chalmers, M. Clarke, M. Fenton, C. Forbes, J. Glanville, N. J. Hicks, J. Moody, S. Twaddle, H. Timimi, and P. Young. 2006. How to formulate research recommendations. *BMJ* 333(7572):804–806.

Callaham, M. L., and J. Tercier. 2007. The relationship of previous training and experience of journal peer reviewers to subsequent review quality. *PLoS Medicine* 4(1):e40.

Chimonas, S., Z. Frosch, and D. J. Rothman. 2011. From disclosure to transparency: The use of company payment data. *Archives of Internal Medicine*.171(1):81–86.

Clarke, L., M. Clarke, and T. Clarke. 2007. How useful are Cochrane reviews in identifying health needs? *Journal of Health Services & Research Policy* 12(2):101–103.

CRD (Centre for Reviews and Dissemination). 2009. *Systematic reviews: CRD's guidance for undertaking reviews in health care*. York, UK: York Publishing Services, Ltd.

CRD. 2010a. *Database of Abstracts of Reviews of Effects (DARE)*. http://www.crd.york.ac.uk/crdweb/Home.aspx?DB=DARE (accessed December 27, 2010).

CRD. 2010b. *Register of ongoing systematic reviews*. http://www.york.ac.uk/inst/crd/projects/register.htm (accessed June 17, 2010).

Delaney, A., S. Bagshaw, A. Ferland, B. Manns, K. Laupland, and C. Doig. 2005. A systematic evaluation of the quality of meta-analyses in the critical care literature. *Critical Care* 9(5):R575–R582.

Delaney, A., S. M. Bagshaw, A. Ferland, K. Laupland, B. Manns, and C. Doig. 2007. The quality of reports of critical care meta-analyses in the Cochrane Database of Systematic Reviews: An independent appraisal. *Critical Care Medicine* 35(2): 589–594.

Devereaux, P. J., P. Choi, S. El-Dika, M. Bhandari, V. M. Montori, H. J. Schünemann, A. X. Garg, J. W. Busse, D. Heels-Ansdell, W. A. Ghali, B. J. Manns, and G. H. Guyatt. 2004. An observational study found that authors of randomized controlled trials frequently use concealment of randomization and blinding, despite the failure to report these methods. *Journal of Clinical Epidemiology* 57(12):1232–1236.

Docherty, M., and R. Smith. 1999. The case for structuring the discussion of scientific papers. *BMJ* 318(7193):1224–1225.

EQUATOR Network. 2010. *Welcome to the EQUATOR Network website: The resource centre for good reporting of health research studies.* http://www.equator-network.org/home/ (accessed June 29, 2010).

Froom, P., and J. Froom. 1993. Deficiencies in structured medical abstracts. *Journal of Clinical Epidemiology* 46(7):591–594.

Glenton, C. 2002. Developing patient-centered information for back pain patients. *Health Expectations* 5(4):319–329.

Glenton, C. 2010. Presenting the results of Cochrane systematic reviews to a consumer audience: A qualitative study. *Medical Decision Making* 30(5):566–577.

Glenton, C., E. Nilsen, and B. Carlsen. 2006a. Lay perceptions of evidence-based information: A qualitative evaluation of a website for back pain sufferers. *BMC Health Services Research* 6(1):34.

Glenton, C., V. Underland, M. Kho, V. Pennick, and A. D. Oxman. 2006b. Summaries of findings, descriptions of interventions and information about adverse effects would make reviews more informative. *Journal of Clinical Epidemiology* 59(8):770–778.

Golder, S., Y. Loke, and H. M. McIntosh. 2008. Poor reporting and inadequate searches were apparent in systematic reviews of adverse effects. *Journal of Clinical Epidemiology* 61(5):440–448.

Goodman, S. N., J. Berlin, S. W. Fletcher, and R. H. Fletcher. 1994. Manuscript quality before and after peer review and editing at *Annals of Internal Medicine*. *Annals of Internal Medicine* 121(1):11–21.

Hartley, J. 2000. Clarifying the abstracts of systematic literature reviews. *Bulletin of the Medical Library Association* 88(4):332–337.

Hartley, J., M. Sydes, and A. Blurton. 1996. Obtaining information accurately and quickly: Are structured abstracts more efficient? *Journal of Information Science* 22(5):349–356.

Haynes, R. B., C. D. Mulrow, E. J. Huth, D. G. Altman, and M. J. Gardner. 1990. More informative abstracts revisited. *Annals of Internal Medicine* 113(1):69–76.

Helfand, M., and H. Balshem. 2010. AHRQ Series Paper 2: Principles for developing guidance: AHRQ and the Effective Health-Care Program. *Journal of Clinical Epidemiology* 63(5):484–490.

Higgins, J. P. T., and S. Green, eds. 2008. *Cochrane handbook for systematic reviews of interventions.* Chichester, UK: John Wiley & Sons.

ICMJE (International Committee of Medical Journal Editors). 2009. *Obligation to register clinical trials.* http://www.icmje.org/publishing_10register.html (accessed September 9, 2010).

ICMJE. 2010. *Uniform requirements for manuscripts submitted to biomedical journals: Ethical considerations in the conduct and reporting of research: Peer review.* http://www.icmje.org/ethical_3peer.html (accessed July 12, 2010).

Ioannidis, J. P., J. W. Evans, P. C. Gøtzsche, R. T. O'Neill, D. Altman, K. Schulz, and D. Moher. 2004. Better reporting of harms in randomized trials: An extension of the CONSORT Statement. *Annals of Internal Medicine* 141(10):781–788.

IOM (Institute of Medicine). 2008. *Knowing what works in health care: A roadmap for the nation.* Edited by J. Eden, B. Wheatley, B. McNeil, and H. Sox. Washington, DC: The National Academies Press.

IOM. 2009. *Initial national priorities for comparative effectiveness research.* Washington, DC: The National Academies Press.

Jefferson, T., P. Alderson, E. Wager, and F. Davidoff. 2002. Effects of editorial peer review: A systematic review. *JAMA* 287(21):2784–2786.

Lavis, J., H. Davies, A. D. Oxman, J. L. Denis, K. Golden-Biddle, and E. Ferlie. 2005. Towards systematic reviews that inform health care management and policy-making. *Journal of Health Services & Research Policy* 10(Suppl 1):35–48.

Lexchin, J., L. A. Bero, B. Djubegovic, and O. Clark. 2003. Pharmaceutical industry sponsorship and research outcome and quality: Systematic review. *BMJ* 326(7400):1167–1170.

Liberati, A., D. G. Altman, J. Tetzlaff, C. Mulrow, P. Gotzsche, J. P. Ioannidis, M. Clarke, P. J. Devereaux, J. Kleijnen, and D. Moher. 2009. The PRISMA Statement for reporting systematic reviews and meta-analysis of studies that evaluate health care interventions: Explanation and elaboration. *Annals of Internal Medicine* 151(4):W11–W30.

Lipkus, I. M. 2007. Numeric, verbal, and visual formats of conveying health risks: Suggested best practices and future recommendations. *Medical Decision Making* 27(5):696–713.

McAlister, F. A., H. D. Clark, C. van Walraven, S. E. Straus, F. Lawson, D. Moher, and C. D. Mulrow. 1999. The medical review article revisited: Has the science improved? *Annals of Internal Medicine* 131(12):947–951.

McPartland, J. M. 2009. Obesity, the endocannabinoid system, and bias arising from pharmaceutical sponsorship. *PLoS One* 4(3):e5092.

Moher, D., D. J. Cook, S. Eastwood, I. Olkin, D. Rennie, and D. F. Stroup. 1999. Improving the quality of reports of meta-analyses of randomised controlled trials: The QUOROM statement. *Lancet* 354(9193):1896–1900.

Moher, D., A. Jones, and L. Lepage. 2001a. Use of the CONSORT statement and quality of reports of randomized trials: A comparative before-and-after evaluation. *JAMA* 285:1992–1995.

Moher, D., K. F. Schulz, D. Altman, and the CONSORT Group. 2001b. The CONSORT statement: Revised recommendations for improving the quality of reports of parallel-group randomized trials. *JAMA* 285(15):1987–1991.

Moher, D., J. Tetzlaff, A. C. Tricco, M. Sampson, and D. G. Altman. 2007. Epidemiology and reporting characteristics of systematic reviews. *PLoS Medicine* 4(3):447–455.

Moher, D., A. Liberati, J. Tetzlaff, and D. G. Altman. 2009. Preferred reporting items for systematic reviews and meta-analyses: The PRISMA statement. *PLoS Medicine* 6(7):1–6.

Mrkobrada, M., H. Thiessen-Philbrook, R. B. Haynes, A. V. Iansavichus, F. Rehman, and A. X. Garg. 2008. Need for quality improvement in renal systematic reviews. *Clinical Journal of the American Society of Nephrology* 3(4):1102–1114.

Mulrow, C. D. 1987. The medical review article: State of the science. *Annals of Internal Medicine* 106(3):485–488.

Mulrow, C. D., S. B. Thacker, and J. A. Pugh. 1988. A proposal for more informative abstracts of review articles. *Annals of Internal Medicine* 108(4):613–615.

Odierna, D. H., and L. A. Bero. 2009. Systematic reviews reveal unrepresentative evidence for the development of drug formularies for poor and nonwhite populations. *Journal of Clinical Epidemiology* 62(12):1268–1278.

Oxman, A. D., H. Schunemann, and A. Fretheim. 2006. Improving the use of research evidence in guideline development: Synthesis and presentation of evidence. *Health Research Policy and Systems* 4:20.

Pocock, S., M. D. Hughes, and R. J. Lee. 1987. Statistical problems in the reporting of clinical trials. A survey of three medical journals. *New England Journal of Medicine* 317(7):426–432.

PRISMA (Preferred Reporting Items for Systematic Reviews and Meta-Analyses). 2010. *PRISMA endorsers.* http://www.prisma-statement.org/endorsers.htm (accessed September 13, 2010).

Roberts, D., and S. Dalziel. 2006. Antenatal corticosteroids for accelerating fetal lung maturation for women at risk of preterm birth. In *Cochrane Database of Systematic Reviews.* http://www.cochrane.org/cochrane-reviews/sample-review#PLS (accessed October 6, 2010).

Roundtree, A. K., M. A. Kallen, M. A. Lopez-Olivo, B. Kimmel, B. Skidmore, Z. Ortiz, V. Cox, and M. E. Suarez-Almazor. 2008. Poor reporting of search strategy and conflict of interest in over 250 narrative and systematic reviews of two biologic agents in arthritis: A systematic review. *Journal of Clinical Epidemiology* 62(2):128–137

Sacks, H. S., D. Reitman, V. A. Ancona-Berk, and T. C. Chalmers. 1987. Meta–analysis of randomized controlled trials. *New England Journal of Medicine* 316(8):450–455.

Santesso, N., L. Maxwell, P. S. Tugwell, G. A. Wells, A. M. Connor, M. Judd, and R. Buchbinder. 2006. Knowledge transfer to clinicians and consumers by the Cochrane Musculoskeletal Group. *The Journal of Rheumatology* 33(11):2312–2318.

Schroter, S., N. Black, S. Evans, J. Carpenter, F. Godlee, and R. Smith. 2004. Effects of training on quality of peer review: Randomised controlled trial. *BMJ* 328(7441):657–658.

Schroter, S., L. Tite, A. Hutchings, and N. Black. 2006. Differences in review quality and recommendations for publication between peer reviewers suggested by authors or by editors. *JAMA* 295(3):314–317.

Schünemann, H. J., E. Ståhl, P. Austin, E. Akl, D. Armstrong, and G. H. Guyatt. 2004. A comparison of narrative and table formats for presenting hypothetical health states to patients with gastrointestinal or pulmonary disease. *Medical Decision Making* 24(1):53–60.

Schwartz, L. M., S. Woloshin, and H. G. Welch. 2009. Using a drug facts box to communicate drug benefits and harms. *Annals of Internal Medicine* 150(8):516–527.

Shea, B., L. M. Bouter, J. Peterson, M. Boers, N. Andersson, Z. Ortiz, T. Ramsay, A. Bai, V. K. Shukla, and J. M. Grimshaw. 2007. External validation of a measurement tool to assess systematic reviews (AMSTAR). *PLoS ONE* 2(12):e1350.

Slutsky, J., D. Atkins, S. Chang, and B. A. Collins Sharp. 2010. AHRQ Series Paper 1: Comparing medical interventions: AHRQ and the Effective Health-Care Program. *Journal of Clinical Epidemiology* 63(5):481–483.

Stroup, D. F., J. Berlin, S. Morton, I. Olkin, G. D. Williamson, D. Rennie, D. Moher, B. J. Becker, T. A. Sipe, S. B. Thacker, and the Meta-analysis of Observational Studies in Epidemiology Group. 2000. Meta-analysis of observational studies in epidemiology: A proposal for reporting. *JAMA* 283(15):2008–2012.

Trevena, L. J., A. Barratt, P. Butow, and P. Caldwell. 2006. A systematic review on communicating with patients about evidence. *Journal of Evaluation in Clinical Practice* 12(1):13–23.

von Elm, E., D. G. Altman, M. Egger, S. J. Pocock, P. C. Gotzsche, J. P. Vandenbroucke, and the Strobe Initiative. 2007. The Strengthening the Reporting of Observational Studies in Epidemiology (STROBE) statement: Guidelines for reporting observational studies. *Annals of Internal Medicine* 147(8):573–577.

Weller, A. C. 2002. *Editorial peer review: Its strengths and weaknesses.* Medford, NJ: American Society for Information Science and Technology. http://books.google. com/books?hl=en&lr=&id=lH3DVnkbTFsC&oi=fnd&pg=PR12&dq=ICMJE+P EER+REVIEW&ots=rpXA8rZOna&sig=nCltaFOsxGxyrVSoGCeWWhRNLIE# v=onepage&q=ICMJE%20PEER%20REVIEW&f=false (accessed July 12, 2010).

Whitlock, E. P., S. A. Lopez, S. Chang, M. Helfand, M. Eder, and N. Floyd. 2010. AHRQ Series Paper 3: Identifying, selecting, and refining topics for comparative effectiveness systematic reviews: AHRQ and the Effective Health-Care Program. *Journal of Clinical Epidemiology* 63(5):491–501.

Wills, C. E., and M. Holmes-Rovner. 2003. Patient comprehension of information for shared treatment decision making: State of the art and future directions. *Patient Education and Counseling* 50(3):285–290.

Yank, V., D. Rennie, and L. A. Bero. 2007. Financial ties and concordance between results and conclusions in meta-analyses: Retrospective cohort study. *BMJ* 335(7631):1202–1205.

6

Improving the Quality of
Systematic Reviews: Discussion,
Conclusions, and Recommendations[1]

Abstract: *The committee recommends that sponsors of systematic reviews (SRs) of comparative effectiveness research (CER) should adopt appropriate standards for the design, conduct, and reporting of SRs and require adherence to the standards as a condition for funding. The newly created Patient-Centered Outcomes Research Institute and agencies of the U.S. Department of Health and Human Services should collaborate to improve the science and environment for SRs of CER. Although the recommended SR standards presented in this report are based on the best available evidence and current practice of respected organizations, many of the standards should be considered provisional pending more methods research. This chapter presents a framework for improving the quality of the science underpinning SRs in several broad categories: involving the right people, methods for conducting reviews, methods for grading and synthesizing evidence, and methods for communicating and using results.*

Systematic reviews (SRs) should be at the center of programs developing a coordinated approach to comparative effectiveness

---

[1] This chapter does not include references. Citations for the findings presented appear in the preceding chapters.

research (CER), both for setting priorities among individual CER studies and for appropriately focusing studies during their design. The committee recognizes that fully implementing all of the SR standards proposed in this report will be costly, resource intensive, and time consuming. Further, as previous chapters make clear, the evidence base supporting many elements of SRs is incomplete and, for some steps, nonexistent. Finally, the committee is fully aware that there is little direct evidence linking high-quality SRs to clinical guidance that then leads to improved health. Nonetheless, designing and conducting new comparative effectiveness studies without first being fully informed about the state of the evidence from an SR risks even higher costs and waste by conducting studies that are poorly designed or redundant. Research organizations such as the Agency for Healthcare Research and Quality (AHRQ) Effective Health Care Program, Centre for Reviews and Dissemination (CRD) (University of York), and the Cochrane Collaboration have published standards, but none of these are generally accepted and consistently applied during planning, conducting, reporting, and peer reviewing of SRs. Furthermore, the environment supporting development of a robust SR enterprise in the United States lacks both adequate funding and coordination; many organizations conduct SRs, but do not typically work together. Thus the committee concludes that improving the quality of SRs will require advancing not only the science supporting the steps in the SR process and linking SRs to improved health, but also providing a more supportive environment for the conduct of SRs. In this chapter the committee outlines some of the principal issues that must be addressed in both of these domains.

Throughout the chapter and in its final recommendations, the committee refers to the newly established Patient-Centered Outcomes Research Institute (PCORI) and, in particular, its Methodology Committee, as a potentially appropriate organization to provide comprehensive oversight and coordination of the development of the science and to promote the environment for SRs in support of CER in the United States. The committee views PCORI as an unusually timely development—albeit untested—that should help advance the field of SRs as an essential component of its overall mission, building on the strengths of well-established programs in the United States (e.g., AHRQ, National Institutes of Health [NIH]) and internationally (e.g., Cochrane Collaboration, National Institute for Health and Clinical Excellence in the United Kingdom), that either produce or rely on SRs for policy purposes. Nonetheless, while the committee views PCORI as relevant and promising, PCORI is by no means the only way to achieve the stated aims. Other agencies, working individually, are able to contribute to advancing the field as well. However, the committee believes that collaborative relationships among agencies, both public and private, would be most effective at contributing to progress. Furthermore, the committee recognizes that U.S. developments are only part of a substantial international effort focused on how best to conduct SRs, an effort that in some countries is advanced and highly sophisticated. Given the potential for duplication of efforts, the need to ensure that gaps in the information base are appropriately addressed, and the need for efficient use of limited available resources, the coordination across multiple organizations within the United States and throughout the world will have clear benefits and should be viewed as essential.

IMPROVING THE SCIENCE OF SYSTEMATIC REVIEWS

Establishing a process for ongoing development of the research agenda in SRs must be an important part of the path forward. Although the committee believes the recommended standards and elements of performance presented in this report are founded on the best available evidence and current practice of respected organizations, all SR standards should be considered provisional pending additional experience and research on SR methods. The committee recognizes that each of its recommended standards could be examined in appropriately designed research, with the expectation that some items would be validated, some discarded, and some added. Future research to develop methods that promote efficiency and scientific rigor is especially important. A detailed description of research that might be conducted on each step, however, is outside the committee's scope of work and would require substantial time and resources. We also note that some of the needed work may be more appropriately categorized as program development and evaluation than research.

The committee promotes the goal of developing a coordinated approach to improving the science of SR, embedded in a program of innovation, implementation, and evaluation that improves the quality of SRs overall. PCORI is an appropriate organization to provide comprehensive oversight and coordination of the development of the science of SRs in support of CER, in cooperation with agencies of the U.S. Department of Health and Human Services (HHS). It could, also function as an important U.S. collaborator with international organizations similarly focused (e.g., Cochrane Collaboration, Campbell Collaboration, and CRD). Among other goals, such a coordinated program would support a description of methods currently employed, methodological research, and comparative studies of alternative approaches, working with international partners to efficiently advance the research agenda. By supporting innovation, the incorporation of a feedback loop into design and reporting of trials and observational studies, and the appropriate and intentional (not accidental or wasteful) replication of methodological research and SRs of methods, PCORI will contribute to ensuring that standards are evidence based. SR methods research will also help to identify gaps in the literature and, through the application of the findings of empirical, "meta-epidemiologic" approaches (i.e., investigations of how particular features of study design or study populations relate to the validity and applicability of primary studies), will provide information about how well standards are being applied.

In this section, the committee proposes a framework for improving the quality of the science underpinning SRs in several broad categories: strategies for involving the right people, methods for conducting the SR, methods for synthesizing and evaluating evidence, and methods for communicating and using results.

Strategies for Involving the Right People[2]

Successful execution and effective use of an SR is a collaborative activity requiring a wide range of experience and expertise among the contributors (the review team). The committee believes that involving people with sufficient experience in each step of the SR process has not received enough attention. While noting that a typical review will require people with certain expertise in specific steps, the committee resisted proposing a standard that a particular menu of experts and stakeholders must be a part of every SR, regardless of topic and purpose. On the other hand, the committee believes that current practice, particularly among groups with modest resources, probably underestimates and undervalues the need for certain kinds of expertise, with the result that SRs vary enormously in quality and credibility. In contrast to authors carrying out the traditional literature review, review teams need formal education and training, which should include hands-on experience and mentoring. There is also wide variability in the involvement of consumers and other users and stakeholders in SRs. Finally, the committee recognizes that

---

[2] See Chapter 2 for a discussion of the individuals who should be included on the review team and the importance of involving users and stakeholders in the SR process.

depth of experience in participating in SRs varies among individuals in a given field, so that the mere presence of an individual with general expertise in a relevant domain does not ensure that the issues will be covered adequately in the review. As an example, not all biostatisticians are fluent in methods of SRs, even though they may be experts in other areas. Similarly, generalist librarians and other information specialists may require special training or experience in conducting SRs, including special knowledge of bibliographic database-specific search terms, to design and execute the search strategy appropriately.

Little descriptive information is available about how the issues of personnel and expertise are handled in various SR enterprises, and the evidence base comparing different approaches is inadequate. For example, we believe comparative studies of models involving consumers and patients are needed. As another example, research on the effects of conflict of interest and bias is provocative, but the topic needs to be addressed more systematically using sophisticated research methods. The committee recognizes that performing such research will present challenges, beginning with defining appropriate outcome measures in these methodologic investigations.

Methods for Conducting the Systematic Review

Developing a review protocol, locating and screening studies, and collecting and appraising the data (the subject of Chapters 2 and 3) are many specific steps along the pathway to completing an SR. Some steps, such as the use of different databases and sensitive search filters to identify relevant literature, are supported with empirical data, but many other steps have not been examined in research. The committee believes an entity such as PCORI should systematically support research that examines key steps in the methods involved in conducting an SR. The committee's criteria (Table 1-2) might be a useful framework to identify topics for further research. For example, how do alternative approaches to some individual steps affect the scientific rigor and efficiency of SR? In addition, we have data on how particular steps in a review are potentially influenced by bias (e.g., reporting biases), but not on whether the bias is of concern in an individual review. The challenge will be not only to identify topics that can be researched, but also to set priorities among them. For example, those standards that have a substantial effect on cost (e.g., dual extraction) might be initially considered higher priority.

Methods for Synthesizing and Evaluating Evidence[3]

Quantitative synthesis of empirical data is a highly developed and active topic of research. Research ranges from the theoretical (with emphasis on the statistics) to comparisons of different modeling approaches. Despite ongoing research in the field, many outstanding questions remain, particularly related to the synthesis of complex multivariate data structures. The committee recommends a range of approaches to answering these questions, including theoretical, empirical, and simulation studies as appropriate.

Qualitative synthesis (i.e., a narrative description of available evidence without drawing conclusions based on statistical inference) has received less attention in research than quantitative synthesis, although the committee recommends that it be part of all SRs. Failing to perform a qualitative synthesis is problematic because the evidence available to answer specific SR questions often does not lend itself to quantitative methods. There is no empirical research to guide synthesis when a qualitative synthesis is the only approach possible. Even when a quantitative review is conducted, we need to understand what perspectives and judgments should be considered in undertaking qualitative synthesis that require authors to be reflective, critical, and as objective as possible in their presentation and interpretation of the data. Because an important goal of qualitative synthesis is communication to users and stakeholders, research in this area might also focus on effectiveness of communication, or perceived objectivity.

Furthermore, although a formal approach to assessing the quality of a body of evidence is recommended, there is little, if any, research testing the reliability and validity of existing approaches to evidence assessment (e.g., the Grading of Recommendations Assessment, Development, Evaluation, or GRADE model). Careful consideration of how to define validity for an SR (e.g., defining a reference standard) will be an important challenge in this research. Finally, the field clearly needs to develop a common lexicon and set of symbols for summarizing the quality of evidence, a process that will need to be coordinated among groups using SRs to develop clinical guidance where there is further variation in lexicon and symbols.

The committee believes that PCORI and its Methodology Committee should invest in research on quantitative and qualitative syntheses and grading of the body of evidence for SRs. This work

---

[3] See Chapter 4 for discussions on qualitative synthesis, quantitative synthesis, and evaluating the quality of a body of evidence.

should be done in close collaboration with other groups commissioning and doing SRs, including the U.S. Public Health Service (e.g., AHRQ, NIH, U.S. Preventive Services Task Force, and the Community Guide), professional organizations and associations, and existing international organizations (e.g., the Cochrane Collaboration).

Methods for Communicating and Using the Results[4]

The committee placed high value on public availability of, and transparency in reporting, SRs, but was not able to cite specific research supporting a particular format. Research on how to most effectively communicate the results of an SR to various users (e.g., clinicians, clinical guidelines panels, consumers, healthcare organizations, payers, both public and private, etc.) is limited, and more would be useful. The committee also notes that in current practice, the process of conducting some SRs is often formally separated from processes in which they are actually used. Although appropriate objectivity and freedom from undue influence need to be maintained, the committee believes that research examining the utility of connecting the SR with its intended users (e.g., clinical guidelines groups, practicing clinicians, and patients), as well as effectiveness and impact of current collaborative efforts, would be timely.

IMPROVING THE ENVIRONMENT FOR SUPPORTING SYSTEMATIC REVIEWS

Developing the science of SRs is not enough to address all the issues that the committee identified as important to improving the quality of SRs to inform CER. A number of environmental factors will critically influence whether the quality of SRs can be improved. Some are best described as infrastructure (e.g., training, registries), but others have to do with SRs as required elements for a culture aimed at improving CER overall.

The committee believes there is a need for greater collaboration among multiple stakeholder groups, including PCORI, government agencies (especially AHRQ and NIH), the Cochrane Collaboration, medical professional societies, researchers, healthcare delivery organizations, patient interest groups, and others. Such multidisciplinary and multiorganizational collaborations have the potential to improve the rigor, transparency, and efficiency of SRs; encourage standardization of methods and processes; set priorities

---

[4] See Chapter 5 for a discussion on preparing final reports of SRs.

for selection of clinical topics of interest to clinicians and patients; reduce unintentional duplication of efforts; provide a shared funding source for the generation of high-quality evidence reviews; more effectively manage conflicts of interest; and facilitate implementation of reviews. Developing effective collaborations, however, requires a transformation in current thinking and structural approaches to conducting SRs. The importance of including international collaborators in discussions of priorities for methodologic research, in particular, cannot be overstated; there is deep expertise and effective leadership in the SR field inside and outside U.S. borders.

The committee also underscores that its recommended standards and elements of performance for publicly funded SRs are provisional, subject to change as the science of SRs advances and lessons are learned from applying the standards in practice. A mechanism is needed to monitor the progress of the science and update the standards periodically to reflect current best practice.

As in the preceding section on developing the science, the committee found that dividing issues into four general categories was a useful way to organize our conclusions: (1) strategies for involving the right people; (2) methods for conducting SRs; (3) methods for synthesizing and evaluating evidence; and (4) methods for communicating and using results.

Strategies for Involving the Right People

The committee believes the environment must be improved to allow and encourage people with sufficient training and experience to be engaged in an SR. Training and professional development must be well established, supported, and recognized by the research community before aspiring researchers will feel secure in choosing careers in SR. Rewards and promotion systems for faculty and scientists in academic institutions need to recognize that the conduct of SRs and the research on SR methods are inherently collaborative efforts. Substantive intellectual contributions to such collaborative efforts need to be recognized in meaningful ways that will attract, not discourage, participation by top scientists. Training targeted to the specific skills needed for SRs needs to be addressed in any national program supporting CER. This research is often multidisciplinary, which training curriculums must take into account. This may require innovation as many disciplines narrowly focus their pre- and post-doctoral training.

Support for the training of users and stakeholders—such as consumers, patients, clinicians, payers, representatives from the insurance industry—in the design, conduct, and use of SRs will be essential if representatives from these groups are to contribute effectively to the choice of the clinical scenario for the review and otherwise fully participate in the conduct of a review and its dissemination. Finally, involving the right people requires providing an environment in which a transparent and robust approach to managing conflict of interest and bias is developed, implemented, and rigorously evaluated for all who participate in an SR. Key CER studies often involve proprietary interests, which involve confidentiality and legal issues. Promoting thorough, transparent analysis will require consideration of these interests, potentially including changes to rules and regulations.

Methods for Conducting Systematic Reviews and for Synthesizing and Evaluating Evidence

The science of conducting an SR, from design through review, synthesis, and evaluation, can only thrive in an environment in which all aspects are supported in a culture valuing the contribution of SRs to improvements in health care. The committee noted many specific ways in which the environment could provide such support. These include establishing a registry for SR protocols (under development by CRD at the University of York in the United Kingdom),[5] providing a repository for data extracted during the conduct of SRs (being explored by the Tufts Medical Center Evidence-based Practice Center),[6] publicly posting protocols and reviews, using public mechanisms to ensure timely updating of protocols and reviews, guaranteeing access to data from primary studies for use in SRs, and ensuring that SRs are a required part of planning, designing, and conducting future primary CER.

Establishing a collaborative methodologic research infrastructure will also be valuable to advancing the science of SRs. Some aspects of methodology might be amenable to rigorous study through the various organizations that fund SRs. For example, a study comparing

---

[5] CRD is developing a registry of SR protocols—focused initially on SRs of the effectiveness of health interventions—with the support of the UK National Institute of Health Research, the Canadian Institute of Health Research, and the International Network of Agencies for Health Technology Appraisal.

[6] The Tufts Medical Center Evidence-based Practice Center, Boston, Massachusetts, with support from AHRQ and the National Library of Medicine, is currently exploring methods for improving the efficiency and quality of SRs through the creation of an electronic SR data repository.

structures for presenting qualitative reviews might randomize SRs being performed by several organizations, measuring acceptability, efficiency, or transparency. The details of study designs are beyond the scope of this report, but the committee believes that a coordinated and collaborative approach to reviews that are already being conducted could offer rich opportunities for efficiently advancing research, particularly if this planning is done prospectively so that reviews are updated in a timely manner.

Methods for Communicating and Using the Results

The committee believes that developing an environment that supports the understanding and use of SRs is critical if the enterprise is to improve CER. Terminology should be consistent, and conventions and standards for publication uniform and well defined. When publicly funded SRs are intended to be used in support of clinical guidance, these reviews should be formally linked with guidelines committees that also meet rigorous standards. The use and usefulness of SRs commissioned as part of a guidelines process should be evaluated once the guideline is implemented, with a feedback loop into future reviews on similar topics and methods used to conduct the review.

CONCLUSIONS AND RECOMMENDATIONS

The committee explored a wide range of topics in its deliberations. The standards and elements of performance form the core of our conclusions, but the standards themselves do not indicate how the standards should be implemented, nor do the standards address issues of improving the science for SRs or improving the environment that supports the development and use of an SR enterprise. In consequence, the committee makes the following two recommendations.

Recommendation 1: Sponsors of SRs of CER should adopt standards for the design, conduct, and reporting of SRs and require adherence to the standards as a condition for funding.

SRs of CER in the United States are now commissioned and conducted by a vast array of private and public entities, some supported generously with adequate funding to meet the most exacting standards, others supported less generously with the result that compromises must be made at every step of the review. Regardless of the level of funding, all sponsors of SRs of CER should adopt standards for the planning, conducting, and reporting of SRs to ensure that a minimal level of quality is met, and should make the adopted standards publicly available. The committee recognizes that its recommended standards are provisional, subject to change as the science of SRs advances and lessons are learned from applying the standards in real-world situations. Also, its standards and elements of performance are at the "exacting" end of the continuum, some of which are within the control of the review team whereas others are contingent on the SR sponsor's compliance. However, high-quality reviews require adequate time and resources to reach reliable conclusions. The recommended standards are an appropriate starting point for publicly funded reviews in the United States (including PCORI, federal, state, and local funders) because of the heightened attention and potential clinical impact of major reviews sponsored by public agencies. The committee also recognizes that a range of SRs are supported by public funds derived from nonfederal sources (e.g., state public health agencies) and private sources where these standards will be seen as an aspiration rather than as a minimum bar. Application of the standards to reviews embedded within other programs that may be publicly funded (e.g., highly focused reviews conducted by individual investigators as part of research grants) also presents difficult operational issues. On the whole, however, the committee feels strongly that the standards (and their successor standards) should serve as a benchmark for all SRs of CER. They could even, for example, be used to inform other topic areas (e.g., risk assessment, epidemiologic research) where standards are also being developed. SRs that significantly deviate from the standards should clearly explain and justify the use of different methods.

> **Recommendation 2: PCORI and the Department of Health and Human Services (HHS) agencies (directed by the Secretary of HHS) should collaborate to improve the science and environment for SRs of CER. Primary goals of this collaboration should include**
>
> - **Developing training programs for researchers, users, consumers, and other stakeholders to encourage more effective and inclusive contributions to SRs of CER;**
> - **Systematically supporting research that advances the methods for designing and conducting SRs of CER;**
> - **Supporting research to improve the communication and use of SRs of CER in clinical decision making;**

- Developing effective coordination and collaboration between U.S. and international partners;
- Developing a process to ensure that standards for SRs of CER are regularly updated to reflect current best practice; and
- Using SRs to inform priorities and methods for primary CER.

This recommendation conveys the committee's view of how best to implement its recommendations to improve the science and support the environment for SRs of CER, which is clearly in the public's interest. PCORI is specifically named because of its statutory mandate to establish and carry out a CER research agenda. As noted above, it is charged with creating a methodology committee that will work to develop and improve the science and methods of SRs of CER and to update such standards regularly. PCORI is also required to assist the Comptroller General in reviewing and reporting on compliance with its research standards, the methods used to disseminate research findings, the types of training conducted and supported in CER, as well as the extent to which CER research findings are used by healthcare decision makers. The HHS agencies are specifically named because AHRQ, NIH, the Centers for Disease Control and Prevention, and other divisions of HHS are major funders and producers of SRs. In particular, the AHRQ Effective Health Care Program has been actively engaged in coordinating high-quality SRs and developing SR methodology. The committee assigns these groups with responsibility and accountability for coordinating and moving the agenda ahead.

The committee found compelling evidence that having high-quality SRs based on rigorous standards is a topic of international concern, and that individual colleagues, professional organizations, and publicly funded agencies in other countries make up a large proportion of the world's expertise on the topic. Nonetheless, the committee necessarily follows the U.S. law that facilitated this report, which suggests a management approach appropriate to the U.S. environment is useful. A successful implementation of our final recommendation should result in a U.S. enterprise that participates fully and harmonizes with the international development of SRs, serving in some cases in a primary role and in others as a facilitator or participant. The new enterprise should also fully understand that this cannot be entirely scripted and managed in advance—structures and processes must allow for innovation to arise naturally from among U.S. individuals and organizations already fully engaged in the topic.

A

Abbreviations and Acronyms

ACA	*Affordable Care Act*
ACCP	American College of Chest Physicians
AHRQ	Agency for Healthcare Research and Quality
AIM	African Index Medicus
ASD	autism spectrum disorder
C2-SPECTR	Campbell Collaboration Social, Psychological, Educational, & Criminological Trials Register
CDC	Centers for Disease Control and Prevention
CENTRAL	Cochrane Central Register of Controlled Trials
CER	comparative effectiveness research
CI	confidence interval
CINAHL	Cumulative Index to Nursing and Allied Health Literature
CMSG	Cochrane Musculoskeletal Group
COI	conflict of interest
CONSORT	Consolidated Standards of Reporting Trials
CPCG	Cochrane Pregnancy and Childbirth Group
CPG	clinical practice guideline
CPP	chronic pelvic pain
CRD	Centre for Reviews and Dissemination
DARE	Database of Abstracts of Reviews of Effectiveness
DERP	Drug Effectiveness Review Project

EHC	Effective Health Care Program
EPC	Evidence-based Practice Center
EPICOT	Evidence, Population, Intervention, Comparison, Outcomes, and Time
EQUATOR	Enhancing Quality and Transparency of Health Research
FDA	Food and Drug Administration
GRADE	Grading of Recommendations Assessment, Development, and Evaluation
HHS	Department of Health and Human Services
ICMJE	International Committee of Medical Journal Editors
IOM	Institute of Medicine
KDIGO	National Kidney Foundation's Kidney Disease: Improving Global Outcomes
LILACS	Latin American and Caribbean Health Sciences Literature
LOE	languages other than English
MOOSE	Meta-analysis of Observational Studies in Epidemiology
NDA	New Drug Application
NHS	National Health Service (UK)
NICE	National Institute for Health and Clinical Excellence (UK)
NIH	National Institutes of Health (U.S.)
NKF	National Kidney Foundation
NSAIDs	nonsteroidal anti-inflammatory drugs
OpenSIGLE	System for Information on Grey Literature in Europe
PCORI	Patient-Centered Outcomes Research Institute
PICO(TS)	population, intervention, comparator, and outcome (timing, and study design or setting)
PQDT	ProQuest Dissertations & Theses Database

PRISMA	Preferred Reporting Items for Systematic Reviews and Meta-Analyses
QUOROM	Quality of Reporting of Meta-analyses
RCT	randomized controlled trial
RR	risk ratio
SR	systematic review
TBI	traumatic brain injury
USPSTF	U.S. Preventive Services Task Force
WHO	World Health Organization

B

Glossary

Acceptability. Cultivates stakeholder understanding and acceptance of findings. Also referred to as credibility.

Applicability. Consistent with the aim of comparative effectiveness research, that is, to help consumers, clinicians, purchasers, and policy makers to make informed decisions that will improve health care at both the individual and population levels. Also referred to as external validity or generalizability.

Benefit. A positive or valued outcome of an action or event.

Bias (intellectual). Views stated or positions taken that are largely intellectually motivated or that arise from the close identification or association of an individual with a particular point of view or the positions or perspectives of a particular group.

Bias (study quality). The tendency for a study to produce results that depart systematically from the truth.

Clinical practice guidelines. Statements that include recommendations intended to optimize patient care that are informed by a systematic review (SR) of evidence and assessment of the benefits and harms of clinical interventions in particular circumstances.

Comparative effectiveness research (CER). The generation and synthesis of evidence that compares the benefits and harms of alternative methods to prevent, diagnose, treat, and monitor a clinical condition or to improve the delivery of care. The purpose of CER is to help consumers, clinicians, purchasers, and policy makers to make informed decisions that will improve health care at both the individual and population levels. Also referred to as clinical effectiveness research, evidence-based medicine, or health technology assessment.

Conflict of interest. A set of circumstances that creates a risk that professional judgment or actions regarding a primary interest will be unduly influenced by a secondary interest.

Consistency. The degree to which estimates of effect for specific outcomes are similar across included studies.

Directness. The extent to which studies in the body of evidence were designed to address the link between the healthcare intervention and a specific health outcome.

Dose–response association. A consistent association across similar studies of a larger effect with greater exposure to the intervention.

Efficiency of conducting review. Avoids unnecessary burden and cost of the process of conducting the review, and allows completion of the review in a timely manner.

Evidence. Information on which a decision or guidance is based. Evidence is obtained from a range of sources, including randomized controlled trials, observational studies, and expert opinion of clinical professionals and/or patients.

Harm. A hurtful or adverse outcome of an action or event, whether temporary or permanent.

Meta-analysis. The process of using statistical methods to combine quantitatively the results of similar studies in an attempt to allow inferences to be made from the sample of studies and be applied to the population of interest.

Patient-centeredness. Respect for and responsiveness to individual patient preferences, needs, and values; helps ensure that patient values and circumstances guide clinical decisions.

Precision. A measure of the likelihood of random errors in the estimates of effect; the degree of certainty about the estimates for specific outcomes.

Quality of evidence. The extent to which one can be confident that the estimate of an intervention's effectiveness is correct.

Reporting bias. A group of related biases that lead to overrepresentation of significant or positive studies in systematic reviews. Reporting bias includes publication bias, outcome reporting bias, time-lag bias, location bias, language bias, citation bias, and multiple- (duplicate-) publication bias.

Risk of bias. The extent to which flaws in the design and execution of a collection of studies could bias the estimate of effect for each outcome under study.

Scientific rigor. Improves objectivity, minimizes bias, provides reproducible results, and fosters more complete reporting.

Standard. A process, action, or procedure that is deemed essential to producing scientifically valid, transparent, and reproducible results. May be supported by scientific evidence, by a reasonable expectation that the standard helps achieve the anticipated level of quality, or by the broad acceptance of its practice.

Strength of association. The likelihood that a large observed effect in an observational study is not due to bias from potential confounding factors.

Study quality. For an individual study, study quality refers to all aspects of a study's design and execution and the extent to which bias is avoided or minimized. A related concept is internal validity, that is, the degree to which the results of a study are likely to be true and free of bias.

Systematic review. A scientific investigation that focuses on a specific question and that uses explicit, planned scientific methods to identify, select, assess, and summarize the findings of similar but separate studies. It may or may not include a quantitative synthesis of the results from separate studies (meta-analysis).

Timeliness. Currency of the review.

Transparency. Methods are explicitly defined, consistently applied, and available for public review so that observers can readily link judgments, decisions, or actions to the data on which they are based. Allows users to assess the strengths and weaknesses of the systematic review or clinical practice guideline.

Users and stakeholders. Refers to individuals who are likely to consult a specific SR to guide decision making or who have a particular interest in the outcome of an SR. This includes consumers, including patients, families, and informal (or unpaid) caregivers; clinicians, including physicians, nurses, and other healthcare professionals; payers; and policy makers, including guideline developers and other SR sponsors.

C

Workshop Agenda and Questions to Panelists

January 14, 2010

Keck Center of The National Academies
500 Fifth Street, N.W., Room 100
Washington, DC

Workshop Objective: To learn how various stakeholders use and develop systematic reviews (SRs), including expert developers of SRs, professional specialty societies, payers, and consumer advocates.

8:00   Breakfast served

8:30   **Welcome and Introductory Remarks**
          Alfred O. Berg, Chair, Institute of Medicine Committee

8:45   **Systematic Review Experts Panel**
          Kalipso Chalkidou, Director, NICE International,
              National Institute for Health and Clinical Excellence
          Naomi Aronson, Executive Director, Technology
              Evaluation Center, Blue Cross and Blue Shield
              Association
          David B. Wilson, Crime and Justice Group Cochair,
              Steering Committee, The Campbell Collaboration
          Moderator: Kay Dickersin, Professor of Epidemiology,
              Johns Hopkins Bloomberg School of Public Health

9:45   **Professional Specialty Societies Panel**
          Virginia Moyer, Section Head, Academic General
              Pediatrics, Baylor College of Medicine
          Sandra Zelman Lewis, Assistant Vice President,
              Health & Science Policy, American College of Chest
              Physicians
          Rebekah Gee, Assistant Professor of Clinical Medicine,
              Department of Obstetrics and Gynecology, Tulane
              University
          Moderator: Harold C. Sox, Editor Emeritus, *Annals of
          Internal Medicine*

10:45   Break

11:00   **The Payer Perspective Panel**
          Louis B. Jacques, Director, Coverage & Analysis Group,
              Office of Clinical Standards & Quality, Centers for
              Medicare & Medicaid Services
          Alan Rosenberg, Vice President of Technology
              Assessment, WellPoint Health Networks
          Edmund Pezalla, National Medical Director and Chief
              Clinical Officer, Aetna Pharmacy Management
          Moderator: Paul Wallace, Medical Director, The
              Permanente Federation, Kaiser Permanente

12:00   Lunch

12:30   **Consumer Panel**
          Gail Shearer, Former Director, Consumer Reports Best
              Buy Drugs, and Former Director, Health Policy
              Analysis, Consumers Union
          David Shern, President and Chief Executive Officer,
              Mental Health America
          Carol Sakala, Director of Programs, Childbirth
              Connection
          Moderator: Katie Maslow, Director, Policy Development,
              Alzheimer's Association

1:30   **Adjourn**

Questions for the Panelists

Systematic Review Experts Panel

- How do you develop your review questions?
  - o To what extent is the user involved in developing the research question?
- How do you determine the inclusion criteria for studies in your evidence synthesis?
  - o Do you incorporate observational and other nonrandomized data? If yes, what are the parameters for their use?
  - o Do you incorporate unpublished and grey literature? Please explain.
  - o How do you protect against publication and reporting (outcome) bias? What have been the challenges (if any)?
- Do you use any specific instruments or methods to ensure the quality of your SRs?
- What are the greatest challenges in producing SRs that meaningfully support users' decisions?
- How do your "customers" use your reviews?
- How are your reviews funded? Do you accept industry funding? How do you identify and address potential conflicts of interest (COIs)?
- This Institute of Medicine (IOM) committee is charged with recommending standards for SRs of comparative effectiveness research (CER). Are there steps in your SR process that could be standardized?
- What would be the implications if the IOM were to recommend a standard grading scheme for characterizing the strength of evidence?

Professional Specialty Societies Panel

- Does your organization produce its own SRs?
  - o If yes, have you developed or adopted standards or guidance for the process? Please describe.
  - o If no, who produces your SRs? To what extent does your organization participate in the review?
- What are the greatest challenges in using SRs to develop clinical practice guidelines (CPGs)?
- How are your SRs funded? Do you accept industry funding? How do you identify and address potential COIs?

- Do you use any specific instruments or methods to ensure the quality of your SRs?
- This IOM committee is charged with recommending standards for SRs of CER. Are there steps in your SR process that could be standardized?
- What would be the implications for your organization if the IOM were to recommend a standard grading scheme for characterizing the strength of evidence?

Payer Perspective Panel
- Does your organization produce its own SRs?
  - o If yes, have you developed or adopted standards or guidance for the process? Please explain.
  - o If no, who produces your SRs? Does your organization participate in the review? Please explain.
- Do you incorporate observational and other nonrandomized data in your evidence syntheses? If yes, what are the parameters for their use?
- How do use SRs to make coverage decisions?
- What are the greatest challenges in using SRs to inform coverage decisions?
- This IOM committee is charged with recommending standards for SRs of CER. Are there steps in the SR process that could be standardized?
- What would be the implications for your organization if the IOM were to recommend a standard grading scheme for characterizing the strength of evidence?

Consumer Panel
- What should be the role of the patient/consumer in the SR process?
- Who should be considered a consumer (e.g., members or representatives of organized groups; patients with personal experiences with a disease; any member of the public, caregivers, and parents)?
- What lessons can be learned from existing models of consumer involvement? Based on your personal experience, where do you think that involving consumers made a real difference to the process and to the results? What aspects of consumer involvement are working well and what aspects are not working well?
- Do consumers need training/education to participate meaningfully in the SR process?

- This IOM committee is charged with recommending standards for SRs of CER. Should the consumer role in SR be standardized?
- What would be the implications for consumers if the IOM were to recommend a standard grading scheme for characterizing the strength of evidence?

D

Expert Guidance for Chapter 2: Standards for Initiating a Systematic Review

TABLE D-1 Comparison of Chapter 2 Guidance on Conducting Systematic Reviews (SRs) of Comparative Effectiveness Research

Standards and Elements	Agency for Healthcare Research and Quality (AHRQ) Effective Health Care Program	Centre for Reviews and Dissemination (CRD)	The Cochrane Collaboration
2.1 Establish a team with appropriate expertise and experience to conduct the systematic review	Provides guidance on establishing a review team (see below).	Provides guidance on establishing a review team (see below).	Provides guidance on establishing a review team (see below).
2.1.1 Include expertise in pertinent clinical content areas	Must include an individual with relevant clinical expertise, and when indicated, access to specialists with relevant expertise.	Ideally includes an individual with knowledge of the relevant clinical/topic area.	Must include expertise in the topic area being reviewed.
2.1.2 Include expertise in systematic review methods	Must include an individual with expertise in conducting SRs.	Ideally includes an individual with expertise in SR methods, and/or qualitative research methods where appropriate.	Must include, or have access to, expertise in SR methodology.
2.1.3 Include expertise in searching for relevant evidence	Must include an individual with library expertise.	Ideally includes an individual with information retrieval skills.	Either a Trials Search Coordinator does the search, or a Trials Search Coordinator or librarian should be consulted.
2.1.4 Include expertise in quantitative methods	Must include an individual with statistical expertise.	Ideally includes an individual with expertise in statistics and health economics.	Must include, or have access to, statistical expertise.
2.1.5 Include other expertise as appropriate	Not mentioned.	Includes a range of skills.	Review authors are encouraged to seek and incorporate the views of users and stakeholders.

2.2 Manage bias and conflict of interest (COI) of the team conducting the systematic review	Provides guidance on managing bias and COI in the review team (see below).	Provides guidance on managing bias and COI in the review team (see below).	Provides guidance on managing bias and COI in the review team (see below).
2.2.1 Require each team member to disclose potential COI and professional or intellectual bias	Must disclose relevant financial, business, and professional interests.	COI should be noted early in the process and steps taken to ensure that these do not impact the review.	Financial COI should be avoided, but must be disclosed if there is any. Also, any secondary interests that might unduly influence judgments made in a review should be disclosed. All authors must sign declarations of interest.
2.2.2 Exclude individuals with a clear financial conflict	Evidence-based Practice Center (EPC) core team and any authors on the reports are barred from having any significant competing interests.	Recommends that all biases are declared. Does not specifically address the issue of whether it is appropriate to include individuals with vested financial interests in the review team.	Reviews should be free of real or perceived bias or COI. Reviews cannot be sponsored by commercial sources.
2.2.3 Exclude individuals whose professional or intellectual bias would diminish the credibility of the review in the eyes of the intended users	EPC core team and any authors on the reports are barred from having any significant competing interests.	Any COI, including professional or intellectual bias, should be declared.	Personal conflicts must be disclosed.

continued

TABLE D-1 Continued

Standards and Elements	Agency for Healthcare Research and Quality (AHRQ) Effective Health Care Program	Centre for Reviews and Dissemination (CRD)	The Cochrane Collaboration
2.3 Ensure user and stakeholder input as the review is designed and conducted	Engage a range of stakeholders across various sectors in the United States. Categories include clinicians; consumer/patients (including representative organizations); employers and business groups; federal and state partners; healthcare industry representatives; payers; health plans and policy makers; and researchers.	There may be a number of individuals or groups who are consulted at various stages, including healthcare professionals, patient representatives, service users, and experts in research methods. Some funding bodies may require the establishment of an advisory group who will comment on the protocol and final report and provide input to ensure that the review has practical relevance to likely end-users.	It may be useful to form an advisory group of people, including representation of relevant stakeholders, to ensure that authors address the questions of importance to stakeholders.
2.3.1 Protect the independence of the review team to make the final decisions about the design, analysis, and reporting of the review	The name of the EPC conducting an SR is not provided to the public until the draft report the to protect authors from external influence. Key informant and technical experts have no role in writing, analyzing, or drafting paper. Peer reviewers are selected to have no significant COI.	Not mentioned.	Sponsorship by any commercial sources with financial interests in the conclusions of Cochrane reviews is prohibited. The sponsor should not be allowed to delay or prevent publication of a review, or interfere with the independence of the authors of reviews.

continued

2.4 Manage bias and COI for individuals providing input into the systematic review	Provides guidance on managing bias and COI for individuals providing input into the SR (see below).	Not mentioned.	Not mentioned.
2.4.1 Require individuals to disclose potential COI and professional or intellectual bias	Participants, consultant, subcontracts, and other technical experts must disclose in writing any financial, business, and professional interests that are related to the subject matter of a review.	The next edition of the guidance will make explicit that all biases must be declared early in process and steps taken to ensure that these do not impact on the review.	Not mentioned.
2.4.2 Exclude input from individuals whose COI or bias would diminish the credibility of the review in the eyes of the intended user	Advisors or experts are not automatically excluded if there are conflicts, particularly for topic development and refinement. When an individual has a potential conflict and is providing input as part of a group, the conflicts must be disclosed and balanced. Experts may be excluded for conflicts depending on the stage of the review and how input is provided.	The next edition of the guidance will note that professional and intellectual bias must be declared, but should not preclude being part of an advisory group.	Not mentioned.
2.5 Formulate the topic for the systematic review	Provides guidance on topic formulation (see below).	Provides guidance on topic formulation (see below).	Provides guidance on topic formulation (see below).

TABLE D-1 Continued

Standards and Elements	Agency for Healthcare Research and Quality (AHRQ) Effective Health Care Program	Centre for Reviews and Dissemination (CRD)	The Cochrane Collaboration
2.5.1 Confirm the need for a new review	AHRQ has specific criteria to ensure the need for a new review. Topics should have strong potential for significantly improving health outcomes or for reducing unnecessary care or cost and also concern important decisions for consumers or for one or more of these groups: patients, clinicians, health system leaders, purchasers, payers, and policy makers. Should consider the available research basis for a topic and if current, high-quality research is available or underway. Try to reduce duplication of existing reviews.	Must check if there is an existing or ongoing review on topic to see if new review justified. Search Database of Abstracts of Reviews of Effects, Cochrane Database of Systematic Reviews, and others. If there is an existing review, assess for quality (using CRD critical appraisal). If high quality, see if update is justified. If completed some time ago, an update may be justified.	Many Cochrane Review Groups have developed priorities for reviews of importance. Topics suggested by review authors must be approved by the appropriate Cochrane Review Group. The background section of the protocol should clearly state the rationale for the review and should explain why the questions being asked are important. It might also mention why this review was undertaken and how it might relate to a wider review of a general problem.
2.5.2 Develop an analytic framework that clearly lays out the chain of logic that links the health intervention to the outcomes of interest and defines the key clinical questions to be addressed by the systematic review	Develop an analytic framework that portrays relevant clinical concepts and the clinical logic underlying beliefs about the mechanism by which interventions may improve health outcomes.	Communicate key contextual factors and conceptual issues relevant to review question. Explain why review is required and rationale for focus of the review.	Not mentioned.

2.5.3 Use a standard format to articulate each clinical question of interest	Topics selected for comparative effectiveness SRs are focused into research questions using the PICOTS mnemonic: population, intervention, comparator, outcome, timing, and setting.	The protocol should include the review questions framed using PICOS: population, intervention, comparator, outcome, and setting. The review question may be presented in general terms, or, more often the actual question is discussed by the review team and an objective, or series of objectives, framed by the PICOS format is agreed.	The protocol should include a well-formulated question. Questions are stated broadly as review "objectives" and specified in detail as "criteria for considering studies for this review." The clinical question should address all of the elements in PICO: population, intervention, comparator, and outcome.
2.5.4 State the rationale for each clinical question	Fully explain the rationale for formulating each clinical question.	State the objectives for undertaking the review.	The background section of the protocol should clearly state the rationale for the review and should explain why the questions being asked are important. Each review group has a title registration process. Some of their forms require statement of motivation for doing the review.
2.5.5 Refine each question based on user and stakeholder input	Topic refinement requires input from stakeholders (key informants) that represent the broad-based constituencies of the EHC (Effective Health Care Program) and for the particular topic area.	Engaging stakeholders who are likely to be involved in implementing the recommendations of the review helps to ensure that the review is relevant to their needs. The form of involvement depends on the project. Where reviews have strict time constraints, consultation may be impossible.	If present, an advisory group may be involved in making and refining decisions about the interventions of interest, the populations to be included, priorities for outcomes, and possibly subgroup analyses.

continued

TABLE D-1 Continued

Standards and Elements	Agency for Healthcare Research and Quality (AHRQ) Effective Health Care Program	Centre for Reviews and Dissemination (CRD)	The Cochrane Collaboration
2.6 Develop a systematic review protocol	Requires a protocol (see below).	Requires a protocol (see below).	Requires a protocol (see below).
2.6.1 Describe the context and rationale for the review from both a decision-making and research perspective	Fully explain the rationale for formulating each clinical question.	Explain why the review is required and provide a rationale for the inclusion criteria and focus of the review.	The background section should address the context for the review question based on an already-formed body of knowledge, the rationale for the review, and why the questions being asked are important.
2.6.2 Describe the study screening and selection criteria (inclusion/exclusion criteria)	Protocol should include detailed explanation and justification for inclusion/exclusion criteria.	Inclusion criteria should be set out in the protocol. Specify the process by which decision on the selection of studies will be made, including the number of researchers who will screen titles and abstracts and then full papers, and the method for resolving disagreements about study eligibility.	Include the criteria for selecting studies for the review, including the types of studies, types of participants, types of interventions, and types of outcome measures.
2.6.3 Describe precisely which outcome measures, time points, interventions, and comparison groups will be addressed	Define the outcome measures.	Specify the comparators and interventions that are eligible for the review, the defined set of relevant outcomes, and the timing of outcome assessment.	Review authors should consider how outcomes may be measured, both in terms of the type of scale likely to be used and the timing of measurement.

Specify the interventions of interest and the interventions against which these will be compared. When specifying drug interventions, factors such as the drug preparation, route of administration, dose, duration, and frequency should be considered.

2.6.4 Describe the search strategy for identifying relevant evidence	Describe the search strategy (including databases and search terms) in the protocol.	Include the preliminary search strategy for identifying relevant results. This should specify the databases and additional sources that will be searched, and also the likely search terms to be used.	Search methods must be described. Inclusion of the search strategy is optional.
2.6.5 Describe the procedures for study selection	Provide plans to assess evidence against inclusion/exclusion criteria.	Inclusion criteria should be set out in the protocol. Specify the process by which decision on the selection of studies will be made, including the number of researchers who will screen titles and abstracts and then full papers, and the method for resolving disagreements about study eligibility.	Include the methods used to apply the selection criteria.

continued

TABLE D-1 Continued

Standards and Elements	Agency for Healthcare Research and Quality (AHRQ) Effective Health Care Program	Centre for Reviews and Dissemination (CRD)	The Cochrane Collaboration
2.6.6 Describe the data extraction strategy	Describe how the data are extracted from each study and methods for collecting and managing the information. Identify key characteristics that might be necessary for evidence synthesis due to their role in effect modification of the intervention–treatment association and thus limit the applicability of findings.	Include the data extraction strategy. The data collected will depend on the type of question being addressed, and the types of study available. Describe the data to be extracted and provide details on the software used for recording data. Specify if authors of primary studies will be contacted to provide missing or additional data. If using foreign language papers, may need to specify translation arrangements.	Include the methods used to extract or obtain data from published reports or from original researchers.
2.6.7 Describe the process for identifying and resolving disagreement between researchers in study selection and data extraction decisions	Describe how discrepancies among researchers will be resolved in the protocol.	Describe how discrepancies between researchers will be resolved.	Include a process for identifying and resolving disagreement between researchers in study selection, data extraction, and assessment of risk of bias in included studies.
2.6.8 Describe the approach to critically appraising individual studies	Describe the approach for assessing study quality in the protocol.	Specify the method of study appraisal, including the details of how the study appraisal is to be used (e.g., will inform sensitivity analyses). Also specify the process for conducting the appraisal, the number of researchers involved, and how disagreements will be resolved.	Include the method used to assess risk of bias in individual studies.

2.6.9 Describe the method for evaluating the body of evidence, including the quantitative and qualitative synthesis strategies	Discuss how evidence will be summarized in a clinically relevant manner either as a narrative or using meta-analysis. Clearly state plans for meta-analysis and predefine clinical groups that are too heterogeneous to allow for meta-analysis or clinical groups for which the qualitative analysis will be presented separately. Identify, a priori, subgroups that will be explored to explain potential heterogeneity.	Specify the data synthesis strategy. State how hetero-geneity will be explored and quantified, under what circumstances a meta-analysis would be considered appropriate, and whether a fixed or random-effects model or both would be used. Describe any planned subgroup or sensitivity analyses or investigation of publication bias.	Address whether a meta-analysis is intended, whether to prespecify an effect measure, how to handle heterogeneity, whether to assume a fixed-effect or random-effects model, how to incorporate risk of bias, how to handle missing data, how to address reporting biases.
	Describe how the report will present findings, including the ordering of outcomes or other categorization scheme. Describe methods for prioritizing or selecting the most important outcomes to be presented in tables or summary key results (i.e., did key informants or the Technical Expert Panel help inform prioritization of outcomes?).	The approach to narrative synthesis should be outlined. Should specify the outcomes of interest and what effect measures will be used.	A qualitative synthesis strategy is not required.

continued

TABLE D-1 Continued

Standards and Elements	Agency for Healthcare Research and Quality (AHRQ) Effective Health Care Program	Centre for Reviews and Dissemination (CRD)	The Cochrane Collaboration
	Describe how criteria will be used to determine overall strength of the body of evidence for each key question and which outcomes will be graded.		
2.6.10 Describe and justify any planned analyses of differential treatment effects according to patient subgroups, how an intervention is delivered, or how an outcome is measured	Clearly state plans for meta-analysis and predefine clinical groups that are too heterogeneous to allow for meta-analysis or clinical groups for which the qualitative analysis will be presented separately. Identify, a priori, subgroups that will be explored to explain potential heterogeneity.	Any planned subgroup analyses should also be described in the data synthesis section.	Authors should, whenever possible, prespecify characteristics in the protocol that later will be subject to subgroup analyses or meta-regression.
2.6.11 Describe the proposed timetable for conducting the review	EPCs are to include time line in their workplan to AHRQ. AHRQ posts approximate final completion date.	Not mentioned.	Protocols include a date when the review is expected. Reviews must be completed within 2 years, or they may be withdrawn from the *Cochrane Database of Systematic Reviews.*

2.7 Submit the protocol for peer review	Not mentioned.	Some commissioning or funding bodies may require that they formally approve the protocol, and will provide input to the draft protocol. In addition, other stakeholders, such as clinical and methodological experts, patient groups, and service users, may be consulted in approving the protocol.	Protocols should go out for external peer review.
2.7.1 Provide a public comment period for the protocol and publicly report on disposition of comments	Public comment period is provided for key questions, but not protocol. Protocol is posted publicly, but not available for peer or public comment. The protocol is developed with input by and reviewed by a Technical Expert Panel.	Advocate where evidence base is contested: create dedicated, publicly accessible websites that provide information about all aspects of the review. These websites enable external scrutiny of the review process, and include feedback facilities for interested parties to comment, ask questions, or submit evidence for consideration.	Approved protocols are automatically published on the *Cochrane Database of Systematic Reviews*. *The Cochrane Library Feedback* tool allows users to provide comments on and feedback of Cochrane reviews and protocols in *The Cochrane Library*. If accepted, the feedback will be published.

continued

TABLE D-1 Continued

Standards and Elements	Agency for Healthcare Research and Quality (AHRQ) Effective Health Care Program	Centre for Reviews and Dissemination (CRD)	The Cochrane Collaboration
2.8 Make the final protocol publicly available, and add any amendments to the protocol in a timely fashion	Key questions are available for public review and comment prior to start of review. Protocol is made publicly available, but not for comment after start of a review. Modifications to protocol should be clearly documented and justified, then posted and available to the public.	Not mentioned. The next edition will recommend making the protocol publicly available. Modifications to the protocol should be clearly documented and justified.	Approved protocols are automatically published on the *Cochrane Database of Systematic Reviews*. Any changes to the protocol must be documented and reported in the completed review.

NOTE: Some information on methods recommended by AHRQ, CRD, and Cochrane was provided via personal communication with Stephanie Chang, EPC Program Task Order Officer, AHRQ (October 5, 2010); Lesley Stewart, Director, CRD (October 14, 2010); and Julian Higgins, Senior Statistician, MRC Biostatistics Unit, Institute of Public Health, University of Cambridge (October 4, 2010).

REFERENCES

Atkins, D., S. Chang, G. Gartlehner, D. I. Buckley, E. P. Whitlock, E. Berliner, and D. Matchar. 2010. Assessing the applicability of studies when comparing medical interventions. In *Methods guide for comparative effectiveness reviews*, edited by Agency for Healthcare Research and Quality. http://www.effectivehealthcare. ahrq.gov/index.cfm/search-for-guides-reviews-and-reports/?productid=603& pageaction=displayproduct (accessed January 19, 2011).

Chou, R., N. Aronson, D. Atkins, A. S. Ismaila, P. Santaguida, D. H. Smith, E. Whitlock, T. J. Wilt, and D. Moher. 2010. AHRQ series paper 4: Assessing harms when comparing medical interventions: AHRQ and the Effective Health Care Program. *Journal of Clinical Epidemiology* 63(5):502–512.

CRD (Centre for Reviews and Dissemination). 2009. *Systematic reviews: CRD's guidance for undertaking reviews in health care*. York, UK: York Publishing Services, Ltd.

Fu, R., G. Gartlehner, M. Grant, T. Shamliyan, A. Sedrakyan, T. J. Wilt, L. Griffith, M. Oremus, P. Raina, A. Ismaila, P. Santaguida, J. Lau, and T. A. Trikalinos. 2010. Conducting quantitative synthesis when comparing medical interventions: AHRQ and the Effective Health Care Program. In *Methods guide for comparative effectiveness reviews*, edited by Agency for Healthcare Research and Quality. http://www.effectivehealthcare.ahrq.gov/index.cfm/search-for-guides-reviews-and-reports/?pageaction=displayProduct&productID=554 (accessed January 19, 2011).

Helfand, M., and H. Balshem. 2010. AHRQ series paper 2: Principles for developing guidance: AHRQ and the Effective Health Care Program. *Journal of Clinical Epidemiology* 63(5):484–490.

Higgins, J. P. T., and S. Green, eds. 2008. *Cochrane handbook for systematic reviews of interventions*. Chichester, UK: John Wiley & Sons.

Norris, S., D. Atkins, W. Bruening, S. Fox, E. Johnson, R. Kane, S. C. Morton, M. Oremus, M. Ospina, G. Randhawa, K. Schoelles, P. Shekelle, and M. Viswanathan. 2010. Selecting observational studies for comparing medical interventions. In *Methods guide for comparative effectiveness reviews*, edited by Agency for Healthcare Research and Quality. http://www.effectivehealthcare.ahrq.gov/ index.cfm/search-for-guides-reviews-and-reports/?pageaction=displayProduct &productID=454 (accessed January 19, 2011).

Owens, D. K., K. N. Lohr, D. Atkins, J. R. Treadwell, J. T. Reston, E. B. Bass, S. Chang, and M. Helfand. 2010. AHRQ series paper 5: Grading the strength of a body of evidence when comparing medical interventions: AHRQ and the Effective Health Care Program. *Journal of Clinical Epidemiology* 63(5):513–523.

Relevo, R., and H. Balshem. 2011. Finding evidence for comparing medical interventions. In *Methods guide for comparative effectiveness reviews*, edited by Agency for Healthcare Research and Quality. http://www.effectivehealthcare.ahrq.gov/ index.cfm/search-for-guides-reviews-and-reports/?pageaction=displayProduct &productID=605 (accessed January 19, 2011).

Slutsky, J., D. Atkins, S. Chang, and B. A. Collins Sharp. 2010. AHRQ series paper 1: Comparing medical interventions: AHRQ and the Effective Health Care Program. *Journal of Clinical Epidemiology* 63(5):481–483.

White, C. M., S. Ip, M. McPheeters, T. S. Carey, R. Chou, K. N. Lohr, K. Robinson, K. McDonald, and E. Whitlock. 2009. Using existing systematic reviews to replace de novo processes in CERs. In *Methods guide for comparative effectiveness reviews*, edited by Agency for Healthcare Research and Quality. http://www.effective-healthcare.ahrq.gov/index.cfm/search-for-guides-reviews-and-reports/?page action=displayProduct&productID=329 (accessed January 19, 2011).

Whitlock, E. P., S. A. Lopez, S. Chang, M. Helfand, M. Eder, and N. Floyd. 2010. AHRQ series paper 3: Identifying, selecting, and refining topics for comparative effectiveness systematic reviews: AHRQ and the Effective Health Care Program. *Journal of Clinical Epidemiology* 63(5):491–501.

E

Expert Guidance for Chapter 3: Standards for Finding and Assessing Individual Studies

TABLE E-1 Comparison of Chapter 3 Guidance on Conducting Systematic Reviews (SR) of Comparative Effectiveness Research

Standards and Elements	Agency for Healthcare Research and Quality (AHRQ) Effective Health Care Program	Centre for Reviews and Dissemination (CRD)	The Cochrane Collaboration
3.1 Conduct a comprehensive, systematic search for evidence	Provides guidance on searching for evidence (see below).	Provides guidance on searching for evidence (see below).	Provides guidance on searching for evidence (see below).
3.1.1 Work with a librarian or other information specialist trained in performing systematic reviews to plan the search strategy	A person with library expertise is part of the review team whose responsibility is to plan the search. The person conducting the search should be involved in the development of key questions, PICOTS (population, intervention, comparator, outcome, timing, and setting), analytic frameworks, and inclusion/exclusion criteria.	An information specialist should ideally be included as part of the project team.	Review authors should work closely with the Trials Search Coordinator for assistance in searching for studies to include in their reviews.
3.1.2 Design the search strategy to address each key research question	The search strategy should be based on the concepts identified in the analytic framework, and the review question (PICOTS).	Search strategies should be highly sensitive in order to retrieve all potentially relevant studies. Use PICOS (population, intervention, comparator, outcome, and setting) to help structure the search. Consult the topic experts and the advisory team for advice.	Searches are targeted at the eligibility criteria for the review (not the review question).

3.1.3 Use an independent librarian or other information specialist to peer review the search strategy	Evidence-based Practice Centers (EPC) frequently internally peer review the electronic search strategies.	If at all possible, the final search strategy should be peer reviewed to check for errors (spelling mistakes, incorrect use of operators, or failure to include relevant MeSH) that could reduce the recall of papers.	Not mentioned.
3.1.4 Search bibliographic databases	Search at least two electronic databases. Begin with MEDLINE (including in-process and other nonindexed citations) and the Cochrane Central Register of Controlled Trials. If topic is researched primarily outside of the United States, search relevant subject-specific databases, as well as databases with stronger international coverage of languages(s) of interest, such as EMBASE.	The selection of electronic databases to search will depend upon the review topic. Importance of MEDLINE, EMBASE, and Cochrane Central Register of Controlled Trials noted. Details of scope of additional databases with narrower focus listed.	The three most important sources to search for studies are Cochrane Central Register of Controlled Trials, MEDLINE, and EMBASE.
3.1.5 Search citation indexes	Use citation indexes. If possible use Web of Science or Scopus. If you do not have access to these databases, use Google Scholar, a free citation tracking database.	Citation searching is useful for identifying a cluster of related, and therefore highly relevant, papers.	Citation searching can be conducted for additional studies.

continued

TABLE E-1 Continued

Standards and Elements	Agency for Healthcare Research and Quality (AHRQ) Effective Health Care Program	Centre for Reviews and Dissemination (CRD)	The Cochrane Collaboration
3.1.6 Search literature cited by eligible studies	Do forward citation search for any key articles. Handsearch if necessary if sources such as journals and conference abstracts are identified by key informants or technical experts.	Scanning reference lists of relevant studies may be helpful in identifying further studies of interest.	Should search reference list of included (and excluded) studies for additional studies.
3.1.7 Update the search at intervals appropriate to the pace of generation of new information for the research question being addressed	Update search at peer review draft stage.	If the initial searches were conducted some time (e.g., 6 months) before the final analysis, it may be necessary to update the literature searches.	While conducting a review, authors may be able to judge if relevant research is being published frequently, and therefore may be able to predict and suggest the need for more frequent updating of the review. (Updating is defined as including a new search.)
3.1.8 Search subject-specific databases if other databases are unlikely to provide all relevant evidence	Consult subject-specific databases that are relevant to the review topic.	Consult subject-specific databases that are relevant to the review topic. Guidance provides details of scope of additional databases with narrower focus listed.	If possible, search subject-specific databases that are relevant to the topic of the review. Access to these databases may be limited.

3.1.9 Search regional bibliographic databases if other databases are unlikely to provide all relevant evidence	If topic is researched primarily outside of the United States, search relevant subject-specific databases, as well as databases with stronger international coverage of language(s) of interest, such as EMBASE.	Using additional databases such as LILACS (Latin American and Caribbean Health Sciences Literature) that contain collections of non-English language can minimize potential language bias.	National and regional databases can be an important source of additional studies from journals not indexed in international databases.
3.2 Take action to address potentially biased reporting of research results	Provides guidance on addressing reporting bias (see below).	Provides guidance on addressing reporting bias (see below).	Provides guidance on addressing reporting bias (see below).
3.2.1 Search grey-literature databases, clinical trial registries, and other sources of unpublished information about studies	At a minimum, search grey literature for regulatory documents, clinical trial registries, and indexed conference abstracts. Search for unpublished articles, especially in areas where there is little published evidence, where the field or intervention is new or changing, where the topic is interdisciplinary, and with alternative medicine.	Searching databases of grey literature is important to minimize publication and language bias. Researchers should consult grey-literature databases and catalogues from major libraries (e.g., British Library and the U.S. National Library of Medicine). It is useful to search trials registers in order to identify unpublished or ongoing trials.	Grey literature can be an important source of studies for inclusion in reviews. Efforts should be made to identify unpublished studies. Trials registers and trials results registers are increasingly important sources of information of ongoing and unpublished trials.
3.2.2 Invite researchers to clarify information related to study eligibility, study characteristics, and risk of bias	EPC authors should prespecify if they will contact study authors for further information and describe plans in protocol.	Sometimes the amount of information reported about a study is insufficient to make a decision about inclusion, and it can be helpful to contact study authors to ask for more details.	Authors are recommended to contact the original investigators for clarification of eligibility, details of the study, and the numerical results.

continued

TABLE E-1 Continued

Standards and Elements	Agency for Healthcare Research and Quality (AHRQ) Effective Health Care Program	Centre for Reviews and Dissemination (CRD)	The Cochrane Collaboration
3.2.3 Invite all study sponsors and researchers to submit unpublished data, including unreported outcomes, for possible inclusion in the systematic review	When interventions identified in key questions involve drugs or devices, it is important to supplement the literature search with a request to the manufacturer for a scientific information packet (includes information about published and unpublished trials or studies). Public comment periods are also opportunities for industry or other study sponsors to submit other data for consideration.	Contacting experts and manufacturers may be useful for supplying information about unpublished or ongoing trials.	It may be helpful to contact colleagues, or send formal letters of request to first authors of included reports to identify unpublished data. It may be desirable to send a letter to experts and pharmaceutical companies or others with an interest in the area.
3.2.4 Handsearch selected journals and conference abstracts	Handsearch selected recent or relevant proceedings of journals if you identify journals that are highly relevant to your topic, but are not fully indexed or not indexed at all by MEDLINE, particularly as identified by key informants or technical experts. Search for information only published in abstract form.	Handsearching is an important way of identifying very recent publications that have not yet been included and indexed by electronic databases or of including articles from journals that are not indexed by electronic databases. Ideally include conference abstracts and interim results in order to avoid publication bias.	Authors are not routinely expected to handsearch journals for their reviews, but they should discuss with their Trials Search Coordinator whether in their particular case handsearching of any journals or conference proceedings might be beneficial. Conference abstracts can be an important source of studies for inclusion in reviews.

3.2.5 Conduct a web search	Use Google Scholar if you do not have access to Web of Science or Scopus.	Internet searching is useful for retrieving grey literature. Identifying and scanning specific relevant web sites is more useful than using a general search engine, such as Google.	There is little empirical evidence concerning the value of using general Internet search engines, but it might be fruitful.
3.2.6 Search for studies reported in languages other than English if appropriate	Consider when topic necessitates search of non-English studies. Discuss with expert panel whether exclusion of non-English studies would bias the report. Document decision. Consider tracking relevant non-English studies to assess the potential for bias from excluding them.	Whenever feasible, all relevant studies should be included regardless of language. This may be impossible due to time, resources, and facilities of translation. It is advisable to at least identify all non-English language papers and document their existence, but record language as the reason for exclusion in cases where they cannot be dealt with.	Whenever possible review authors should attempt to identify and assess for eligibility all possibly relevant reports of trials irrespective of language of publication.
3.3 Screen and select studies	Provides guidance on screening and selecting studies (see below).	Provides guidance on screening and selecting studies (see below).	Provides guidance on screening and selecting studies (see below).

continued

TABLE E-1 Continued

Standards and Elements	Agency for Healthcare Research and Quality (AHRQ) Effective Health Care Program	Centre for Reviews and Dissemination (CRD)	The Cochrane Collaboration
3.3.1 Include or exclude studies based on the protocol's prespecified criteria	Inclusion and exclusion criteria should be determined a priori. Determination of inclusion and exclusion criteria is made with input by technical experts. Any changes to criteria should be documented and justified.	The process by which decisions on the selection of studies will be made should be specified in the protocol.	The protocol prespecifies the criteria for including and excluding studies in the review. The eligibility criteria are a combination of relevant aspects of the clinical question (population, intervention, comparator, outcomes [PICO]) plus specification of the types of studies that have addressed these questions.
3.3.2 Use observational studies in addition to randomized controlled trials to evaluate harms of interventions	Observational studies are almost always necessary to assess harms adequately. They may provide the best (or only) evidence for evaluating harms in minority or vulnerable populations who are underrepresented in clinical trials. Observational studies should be included when there are gaps in randomized clinical trials (RCTs) evidence and when observational studies will provide valid and useful evidence.	Observational studies can provide useful information about the unintentional effects of an intervention, and in such situations it is important to assess their quality.	One of the most important roles of nonrandomized studies is to assess potential unexpected or rare harms of interventions.

3.3.3 Use two or more members of the review team, working independently, to screen and select studies	Ensure quality control mechanism; this is usually through use of independent researchers to assess studies for eligibility. Pilot testing of screening process is particularly important if there is not dual-review screening.	Good to have more than one researcher to help minimize bias and error at all stages of the review. Parallel independent assessments should be conducted to minimize the risk of errors.	At least two people, independently. Process must be transparent, and chosen to minimize biases and human error.
3.3.4 Train screeners using written documentation; test and retest screeners to improve accuracy and consistency	Pilot-testing of screening process is particularly important if there is not dual-review screening.	The selection process should be piloted by applying the inclusion criteria to a sample of papers in order to check that they can be reliably interpreted and that they classify the studies appropriately.	Pilot-testing the eligibility criteria can be used to train the people who will be applying them and ensure that the criteria can be applied consistently by more than one person.
3.3.5 Use one of two strategies to select studies: (1) read all full-text articles identified in the search, or (2) screen titles and abstracts of all articles and then read the full text of articles identified in initial screening	Screening is typically done at two stages—title/abstract and full text. Typically title/abstract-level screen may err on the side of being more inclusive.	Screening of potential studies is usually conducted in two stages: (1) initial screening of titles and abstracts against inclusion criteria to identify potentially relevant papers, and (2) screening of full papers identified in initial screening.	Typical process: (1) merge results with reference software and remove duplicates; (2) examine titles and abstracts; (3) retrieve full text of relevant reports; (4) link multiple reports of the same study; (5) examine full-text reports for compliance with eligibility criteria; (6) contact investigators, if appropriate, to clarify study eligibility; and (7) make final decisions on study inclusion.

continued

TABLE E-1 Continued

Standards and Elements	Agency for Healthcare Research and Quality (AHRQ) Effective Health Care Program	Centre for Reviews and Dissemination (CRD)	The Cochrane Collaboration
3.3.6 Taking account of the risk of bias, consider including observational studies to address gaps in the evidence from randomized clinical trials on the benefits of interventions	Observational studies should be included when there are gaps in RCT evidence and when observational studies will provide valid and useful evidence.	Because of the risk of bias, careful consideration should be given to the inclusion of quasi-experimental studies in a review to assess the effectiveness of an intervention.	Cochrane reviews focus primarily on randomized trials. Nonrandomized studies might be included (1) to provide an explicit evaluation of their weaknesses; (2) to provide evidence on interventions that cannot be randomized; or (3) to provide evidence of effects that cannot be adequately studied in randomized trials.
3.4 Document the search	Provides guidance for documenting the search (see below).	Provides guidance for documenting the search (see below).	Provides guidance for documenting the search (see below).
3.4.1 Provide a line-by-line description of the search strategy, including the date of every search for each database, web browser, etc.	While conducting the search, detailed notes about the full search strategy should be kept (e.g., database used, dates covered by search, date search was conducted, search terms used, nondatabase methods used, language restrictions).	Record the search process and results contemporaneously. Provide full detail of the searches, including the databases and interfaces searched, dates covered, full detailed search strategies (including justifications for date or language restrictions), and the number of records retrieved.	The full search strategies for each database will need to be included in an appendix. The search strategies will need to be copied and pasted exactly as run and included in full, together with the search set numbers and the number of records received. A single date should be specified to indicate when the most recent comprehensive search was started.

3.4.2 Document the disposition of each report identified including reasons for their exclusion if appropriate	Account for all citations identified from all sources. Report the list of excluded references. A flow chart accounts for all citations identified from all sources as well as accounting for all citations that were later excluded and why.	Have a record of decisions made for each article. A flow chart showing the number of studies/papers remaining at each stage is a simple and useful way of documenting the study selection process. A list of studies excluded from the review should be reported where possible, giving the reasons for exclusion. This is most useful if it is restricted to "near misses" rather than all the research evidence identified.	The review includes a characteristics of excluded studies table. This lists studies that appear to meet the eligibility criteria, but which were excluded, and the reasons for exclusion.
3.5 Manage data collection	Provides guidance on managing data collection (see below).	Provides guidance on managing data collection (see below).	Provides guidance on managing data collection (see below).
3.5.1 At a minimum, use two or more researchers, working independently, to extract quantitative or other critical data from each study. For other types of data, one individual could extract the data while the second individual checks for accuracy and completeness. Establish a fair procedure for resolving discrepancies—do not simply give final decision-making power to the senior reviewer	Quality control process for data extraction should be defined a priori. Procedure for resolving discrepancies should be defined in the protocol.	Ideally two researchers should independently perform the data extraction. At a minimum, one researcher can extract the data, with a second researcher independently checking the data extraction forms for accuracy and completeness. The process for resolving disagreements should be specified in the protocol. Disagreements should, where possible, be resolved by consensus after referring to the protocol; if necessary a third person may be consulted.	More than one person should extract data from every report. The methods section of both the protocol and the review should detail how disagreements are handled. Disagreements can generally be resolved by discussion, but may require arbitration by another person or obtain more information from the study authors.

continued

TABLE E-1 Continued

Standards and Elements	Agency for Healthcare Research and Quality (AHRQ) Effective Health Care Program	Centre for Reviews and Dissemination (CRD)	The Cochrane Collaboration
3.5.2 Link publications from the same study to avoid including data from the same study more than once	Publications from the same study are typically linked.	It is important to identify duplicate publications of research results to ensure they are not treated as separate studies in the review.	Multiple reports of the same study need to be linked together.
3.5.3 Use standard data extraction forms developed for the specific systematic review	Data abstraction forms are developed prior to data abstraction. Protocol should list elements included in data abstraction forms.	Standardized data extraction forms should be designed with both the review question and subsequent analysis in mind. Information on study characteristics should be sufficiently detailed to allow readers to assess the applicability of the findings to their area of interest.	Data collection forms are invaluable. The form should be linked directly to the review question and criteria for assessing eligibility of studies and serve as the historical record of the SR and the source of data for any analysis.
3.5.4 Pilot-test the data extraction forms and process	Data abstraction forms should be pilot tested by a sampling of studies.	Data extraction forms should be piloted to ensure that all the relevant information is captured and that resources are not wasted on extracting data not required.	All forms should be pilot-tested using a representative sample of studies to be reviewed.
3.6 Critically appraise each study	Provides guidance on appraising individual studies (see below).	Provides guidance on appraising individual studies (see below).	Provides guidance on appraising individual studies (see below).

3.6.1 Systematically assess the risk of bias, using predefined criteria	There are three steps to rating the risk of bias of individual studies (quality): (1) classify the study design (e.g., review, RCT, observational), (2) apply a predefined criteria for quality and critical appraisal (e.g., scale, checklists), and (3) arrive at a summary judgment of the study's quality (good, fair, and poor).	It is important to assess the risk of bias in included studies caused by inadequacies in study design, conduct, or analysis that may have led to the treatment effect being over- or underestimated.	A risk-of-bias table should be made for each study, including judgments of low risk of bias, high risk of bias, or unclear risk of bias for the six domains of bias. Judgments should be explicit and informed by empirical evidence, likely direction of bias, and likely magnitude of bias.
3.6.2 Assess relevance of the study's populations, interventions, and outcome measures	Must assess the relevance of the study populations in terms of severity of illness, comorbidities, and demographics (age, sex, and race). Must assess the relevance of the intervention, including drug dosing and adherence.	Assessment of risk of bias should consider whether groups were similar at outset of the study, selection bias, and attrition bias. It is important to consider the reliability or validity of the actual outcome measure being used. The outcome should also be relevant and meaningful to both the intervention and the evaluation.	Not applicable. The applicability of endpoints and outcomes can only be assessed in relation to a specific decision that needs to be made. Cochrane reviews do not have a specific implementation decision, so assessment of applicability is irrelevant.

continued

TABLE E-1 Continued

Standards and Elements	Agency for Healthcare Research and Quality (AHRQ) Effective Health Care Program	Centre for Reviews and Dissemination (CRD)	The Cochrane Collaboration
	Must assess the applicability of the study's outcomes. Outcomes should include the most important clinical benefits and harms. Surrogate outcomes are defined as important outcomes in the key questions. They may also be considered indirect outcomes of a final health outcome. Relationship between surrogate and final health outcome should be depicted by analytic framework.	It is often helpful to assess the quality of the intervention and its implementation.	
3.6.3 Assess the fidelity of the implementation of interventions	Not mentioned.	A review should assess whether the intervention was implemented as planned in the individual studies.	Not applicable. The applicability of interventions can only be assessed in relation to a specific decision that needs to be made and Cochrane reviews do not have a specific implementation decision.

NOTE: Some information on AHRQ-, CRD-, and Cochrane-recommended methods was provided via personal communication with Stephanie Chang, EPC Program Task Order Officer, AHRQ (October 5, 2010); Lesley Stewart, Director, CRD (October 14, 2010); and Julian Higgins, Senior Statistician, MRC Biostatistics Unit, Institute of Public Health, University of Cambridge (October 4, 2010).

REFERENCES

Atkins, D., S. Chang, G. Gartlehner, D. I. Buckley, E. P. Whitlock, E. Berliner, and D. Matchar. 2010. Assessing the applicability of studies when comparing medical interventions. In *Methods guide for comparative effectiveness reviews*, edited by Agency for Healthcare Research and Quality. http://www.effectivehealthcare. ahrq.gov/index.cfm/search-for-guides-reviews-and-reports/?productid=603& pageaction=displayproduct (accessed January 19, 2011).

Chou, R., N. Aronson, D. Atkins, A. S. Ismaila, P. Santaguida, D. H. Smith, E. Whitlock, T. J. Wilt, and D. Moher. 2010. AHRQ series paper 4: Assessing harms when comparing medical interventions: AHRQ and the Effective Health Care Program. *Journal of Clinical Epidemiology* 63(5):502–512.

CRD (Centre for Reviews and Dissemination). 2009. *Systematic reviews: CRD's guidance for undertaking reviews in health care.* York, UK: York Publishing Services, Ltd.

Fu, R., G. Gartlehner, M. Grant, T. Shamliyan, A. Sedrakyan, T. J. Wilt, L. Griffith, M. Oremus, P. Raina, A. Ismaila, P. Santaguida, J. Lau, and T. A. Trikalinos. 2010. Conducting quantitative synthesis when comparing medical interventions: AHRQ and the Effective Health Care Program. In *Methods guide for comparative effectiveness reviews*, edited by Agency for Healthcare Research and Quality. http://www.effectivehealthcare.ahrq.gov/index.cfm/search-for-guides-reviews-and-reports/?pageaction=displayProduct&productID=554 (accessed January 19, 2011).

Helfand, M., and H. Balshem. 2010. AHRQ series paper 2: Principles for developing guidance: AHRQ and the Effective Health Care Program. *Journal of Clinical Epidemiology* 63(5):484–490.

Higgins, J. P. T., and S. Green, eds. 2008. *Cochrane handbook for systematic reviews of interventions*. Chichester, UK: John Wiley & Sons.

Norris, S., D. Atkins, W. Bruening, S. Fox, E. Johnson, R. Kane, S. C. Morton, M. Oremus, M. Ospina, G. Randhawa, K. Schoelles, P. Shekelle, and M. Viswanathan. 2010. Selecting observational studies for comparing medical interventions. In *Methods guide for comparative effectiveness reviews*, edited by Agency for Healthcare Research and Quality. http://www.effectivehealthcare.ahrq.gov/index.cfm/search-for-guides-reviews-and-reports/?pageaction=displayProduct&productID=454 (accessed January 19, 2011).

Owens, D. K., K. N. Lohr, D. Atkins, J. R. Treadwell, J. T. Reston, E. B. Bass, S. Chang, and M. Helfand. 2010. AHRQ series paper 5: Grading the strength of a body of evidence when comparing medical interventions: AHRQ and the Effective Health Care Program. *Journal of Clinical Epidemiology* 63(5):513–523.

Relevo, R., and H. Balshem. 2011. Finding evidence for comparing medical interventions. In *Methods guide for comparative effectiveness reviews*, edited by Agency for Healthcare Research and Quality. http://www.effectivehealthcare.ahrq.gov/index.cfm/search-for-guides-reviews-and-reports/?pageaction=displayProduct&productID=605 (accessed January 19, 2011).

Slutsky, J., D. Atkins, S. Chang, and B. A. Collins Sharp. 2010. AHRQ series paper 1: Comparing medical interventions: AHRQ and the Effective Health Care Program. *Journal of Clinical Epidemiology* 63(5):481–483.

White, C. M., S. Ip, M. McPheeters, T. S. Carey, R. Chou, K. N. Lohr, K. Robinson, K. McDonald, and E. Whitlock. 2009. Using existing systematic reviews to replace de novo processes in CERs. In *Methods guide for comparative effectiveness reviews*, edited by Agency for Healthcare Research and Quality. http://www.effective-healthcare.ahrq.gov/index.cfm/search-for-guides-reviews-and-reports/?page action=displayProduct&productID=329 (accessed January 19, 2011).

Whitlock, E. P., S. A. Lopez, S. Chang, M. Helfand, M. Eder, and N. Floyd. 2010. AHRQ series paper 3: Identifying, selecting, and refining topics for comparative effectiveness systematic reviews: AHRQ and the Effective Health Care Program. *Journal of Clinical Epidemiology* 63(5):491–501.

F

Expert Guidance for Chapter 4: Standards for Synthesizing the Body of Evidence

TABLE F-1 Comparison of Chapter 4 Guidance on Conducting Systematic Reviews (SRs) of Comparative Effectiveness Research

Standards and Elements	Agency for Healthcare Research and Quality (AHRQ) Effective Health Care Program	Centre for Reviews and Dissemination (CRD)	The Cochrane Collaboration
4.1 Use a prespecified method to evaluate the body of evidence	The AHRQ method for evaluating the body of evidence is conceptually similar to the GRADE system (see below).	The planned approach to evaluating the body of evidence should be decided at the outset of the review, depending on the type of question posed and the type of studies that are likely to be available.	Adopts the GRADE system for evaluating the body of evidence.
4.1.1 For each outcome, systematically assess the following characteristics of the body of evidence: • Risk of bias • Consistency • Precision • Directness • Reporting bias	Requires the assessment of: • Risk of bias. • Consistency. • Precision. • Directness. • Applicability. • Publication bias (if there is reason to believe that relevant empirical findings have not been published). Reviewers should evaluate the applicability of a body of evidence separately from directness.	Quality assessment is likely to consider the following: • Appropriateness of study design. • Risk of bias. • Choice of outcome measure. • Statistical issues. • Quality of reporting. • Quality of the intervention. • Generalizability. The importance of each of these aspects of quality will depend on the focus and nature of the review.	Requires the assessment of: • Risk of bias. • Consistency. • Precision. • Directness. • Publication bias. Reviewers should evaluate the applicability of a body of evidence as part of the assessment of directness.

4.1.2 For bodies of evidence that include observational research, also systematically assess the following characteristics for each outcome: • Dose–response association • Plausible confounding that would change the observed effect • Strength of association	The following characteristics should be assessed if they are relevant to a particular SR. They are applied more often to evidence from observational studies than to evidence from randomized controlled trials. • Dose–response association. • Plausible confounding that would decrease an observed effect. • Strength of association.	The quality assessment should be guided by the types of study designs included in the SR.	For bodies of evidence that include observational research, assess the following characteristics for each outcome: • Dose–response association. • Plausible confounding that would decrease an observed effect. • Strength of association.
4.1.3 For each outcome specified in the protocol, use consistent language to characterize the level of confidence in the estimates of the effect of an intervention	The quality of evidence receives a single grade: high, moderate, low, or insufficient.	Not mentioned.	The quality of evidence receives a single grade: high, moderate, low, or very low.
4.2 Conduct a qualitative synthesis	All SRs should include a narrative synthesis. Provides guidance (see below).	All SRs should include a narrative synthesis. Provides guidance (see below).	A narrative synthesis should be used where meta-analysis is not feasible or not sensible. Provides guidance on some elements (see below).

continued

TABLE F-1 Continued

Standards and Elements	Agency for Healthcare Research and Quality (AHRQ) Effective Health Care Program	Centre for Reviews and Dissemination (CRD)	The Cochrane Collaboration
4.2.1 Describe the clinical and methodological characteristics of the included studies, including their size, inclusion or exclusion of important subgroups, timeliness, and other relevant factors	Summarize the available evidence using PICOTS domains in a summary table: • Characteristics of enrolled populations. Where possible, describe the proportion with important characteristics (e.g., % over age 65) rather than the range. • General characteristics of the intervention. • Comparators used. • Outcomes most frequently reported. • Range of follow-up.	Provide a clear descriptive summary of the included studies, with details about study type, interventions, number of participants, a summary of participant characteristics, outcomes, and outcome measures.	Review authors should, as a minimum, include the following in the characteristics of included studies table: methods, participants, intervention, and outcomes. Where appropriate, use an extra field to provide information about the funding of each study.
4.2.2 Describe the strengths and limitations of individual studies and patterns across studies	Assess and document decisions on "quality" and applicability of individual studies, including criteria for overall quality assessment.	Recording the strengths and weaknesses of included studies provides an indication of whether the results have been unduly influenced by aspects of study design or conduct.	Whether the synthesis is quantitative or qualitative, methodological limitations are described in detail through presentation of risk of bias tables, through written summaries of risk of bias assessments, and by footnotes in summary of findings tables.

continued

4.2.3 Describe, in plain terms, how flaws in the design or execution of the study (or groups of studies) could bias the results, explaining the reasoning behind these judgments	EPCs describe criteria for assessing risk of bias of individual studies, which, by definition, describes how the study design and execution may bias the results.	Assess the risk of bias in included studies caused by inadequacies in study design, conduct, or analysis that may have led to the treatment effect being over- or underestimated.	Assess risk of bias in all studies in a review irrespective of the anticipated variability in either the results or the validity of the included studies.
4.2.4 Describe the relationships between the characteristics of the individual studies and their reported findings and patterns across studies	EPCs should explore heterogeneity of findings. They should prespecify subanalyses or characteristics by which they analyze heterogeneity, whether for methodologic heterogeneity or clinical heterogeneity.	Provide an analysis of the relationships within and between studies.	Organizing the studies into groupings or clusters is encouraged (e.g., by intervention type, population groups, setting, etc.).
4.2.5 Discuss the relevance of individual studies to the populations, comparisons, cointerventions, settings, and outcomes or measures of interest	EPCs should describe the limitations of applicability of a body of evidence within the PICOS structure.	Not mentioned.	Not mentioned.
4.3 Decide if, in addition to a qualitative analysis, the systemic review will include a quantitative analysis (meta-analysis)	Meta-analysis is appropriate if combining studies will give a meaningful answer to a well-formulated research question.	The approach to quantitative synthesis should be decided at the outset of the review.	Describe why a meta-analysis is appropriate. The choice of meta-analysis method should be stated, including whether a fixed-effect or a random-effects model is used.

TABLE F-1 Continued

Standards and Elements	Agency for Healthcare Research and Quality (AHRQ) Effective Health Care Program	Centre for Reviews and Dissemination (CRD)	The Cochrane Collaboration
		Meta-analysis is not always possible or sensible. The type of synthesis depends on the type of question posed and the type of studies that are available. Initial descriptive phase of synthesis will be helpful in confirming that studies are similar and reliable enough to synthesize and that it is appropriate to pool results.	
4.3.1 Explain why a pooled estimate might be useful to decision makers	Authors should explain the reason a combined estimate might be useful to decision makers.	Not mentioned.	Not mentioned.
4.4 If conducting a meta-analysis, then do the following:	Provides guidance on conducting a meta-analysis (see below).	Provides guidance on conducting a meta-analysis (see below).	Provides guidance on conducting a meta-analysis (see below).
4.4.1 Use expert methodologists to develop, execute, and peer review the meta-analyses	Review team must include an individual with statistical expertise. A peer reviewer with statistical expertise should be invited as appropriate.	The review team should ideally include expertise in statistics. The team may wish to seek advice from methodological experts formally through an advisory group, or informally.	Review teams must include, or have access to, expertise in systematic review methodology (including statistical expertise).

4.4.2 Address the heterogeneity among study effects	Evaluate the amount of heterogeneity for each meta-analysis. Explore statistical heterogeneity using subgroup analysis or meta-regression or sensitivity analyses.	Variation in results across studies should be investigated informally by visual examination of the forest plot, tested using chi square test or Q statistic, quantified using the I squared statistic. If statistical heterogeneity is observed, then the possible reasons for differences should be explored. The influence of patient-level characteristics or issues related to equity can also be explored through subgroup analyses, meta-regression, or other modeling approaches.	It is important to consider to what extent the results of studies are consistent. A statistical test for heterogeneity is available, but a useful statistic for quantifying inconsistency is I^2. It is clearly of interest to determine the causes of heterogeneity among results of studies. However, most Cochrane reviews do not have enough studies to allow the reliable investigation of the reasons for heterogeneity.
4.4.3 Accompany all estimates with measures of statistical uncertainty	Appropriate measures of variance should be included with point estimates from meta-analyses.	Results should be expressed as point estimates together with associated confidence intervals and exact p-values.	Results should always be accompanied by a measure of uncertainty, such as a 95% confidence interval.
4.4.4 Assess the sensitivity of conclusions to changes in the protocol, assumptions, and study selection (sensitivity analysis)	Sensitivity analysis should be conducted to investigate the robustness of the results.	Sensitivity analyses should be used to explore the robustness of the main meta-analysis by repeating the analyses after having made some changes to the data or methods.	Sensitivity analyses should be used to examine whether overall findings are robust to potentially influential decisions.

NOTES: Some information on AHRQ-, CRD-, and Cochrane-recommended methods was provided via personal communication with Stephanie Chang, EPC Program Task Order Officer, AHRQ (October 5, 2010); Lesley Stewart, Director, CRD (October 14, 2010); and Julian Higgins, Senior Statistician, MRC Biostatistics Unit, Institute of Public Health, University of Cambridge (October 4, 2010). The order of the standards does not indicate the sequence in which they are carried out.

REFERENCES

Atkins, D., S. Chang, G. Gartlehner, D. I. Buckley, E. P. Whitlock, E. Berliner, and D. Matchar. 2010. Assessing the applicability of studies when comparing medical interventions. In *Methods guide for comparative effectiveness reviews*, edited by Agency for Healthcare Research and Quality. http://www.effectivehealthcare. ahrq.gov/index.cfm/search-for-guides-reviews-and-reports/?productid=603& pageaction=displayproduct (accessed January 19, 2011).

Chou, R., N. Aronson, D. Atkins, A. S. Ismaila, P. Santaguida, D. H. Smith, E. Whitlock, T. J. Wilt, and D. Moher. 2010. AHRQ series paper 4: Assessing harms when comparing medical interventions: AHRQ and the Effective Health Care Program. *Journal of Clinical Epidemiology* 63(5):502–512.

CRD (Centre for Reviews and Dissemination). 2009. *Systematic reviews: CRD's guidance for undertaking reviews in health care.* York, UK: York Publishing Services, Ltd.

Fu, R., G. Gartlehner, M. Grant, T. Shamliyan, A. Sedrakyan, T. J. Wilt, L. Griffith, M. Oremus, P. Raina, A. Ismaila, P. Santaguida, J. Lau, and T. A. Trikalinos. 2010. Conducting quantitative synthesis when comparing medical interventions: AHRQ and the Effective Health Care Program. In *Methods guide for comparative effectiveness reviews*, edited by Agency for Healthcare Research and Quality. http://www.effectivehealthcare.ahrq.gov/index.cfm/search-for-guides-reviews-and-reports/?pageaction=displayProduct&productID=554 (accessed January 19, 2011).

Helfand, M., and H. Balshem. 2010. AHRQ series paper 2: Principles for developing guidance: AHRQ and the Effective Health Care Program. *Journal of Clinical Epidemiology* 63(5):484–490.

Higgins, J. P. T., and S. Green, eds. 2008. *Cochrane handbook for systematic reviews of interventions.* Chichester, UK: John Wiley & Sons.

Norris, S., D. Atkins, W. Bruening, S. Fox, E. Johnson, R. Kane, S. C. Morton, M. Oremus, M. Ospina, G. Randhawa, K. Schoelles, P. Shekelle, and M. Viswanathan. 2010. Selecting observational studies for comparing medical interventions. In *Methods guide for comparative effectiveness reviews*, edited by Agency for Healthcare Research and Quality. http://www.effectivehealthcare.ahrq.gov/index.cfm/search-for-guides-reviews-and-reports/?pageaction=displayProduct&productID=454 (accessed January 19, 2011).

Owens, D. K., K. N. Lohr, D. Atkins, J. R. Treadwell, J. T. Reston, E. B. Bass, S. Chang, and M. Helfand. 2010. AHRQ series paper 5: Grading the strength of a body of evidence when comparing medical interventions: AHRQ and the Effective Health Care Program. *Journal of Clinical Epidemiology* 63(5):513–523.

Relevo, R., and H. Balshem. 2011. Finding evidence for comparing medical interventions. In *Methods guide for comparative effectiveness reviews*, edited by Agency for Healthcare Research and Quality. http://www.effectivehealthcare.ahrq.gov/index.cfm/search-for-guides-reviews-and-reports/?pageaction=displayProduct&productID=605 (accessed January 19, 2011).

Slutsky, J., D. Atkins, S. Chang, and B. A. Collins Sharp. 2010. AHRQ series paper 1: Comparing medical interventions: AHRQ and the Effective Health Care Program. *Journal of Clinical Epidemiology* 63(5):481–483.

White, C. M., S. Ip, M. McPheeters, T. S. Carey, R. Chou, K. N. Lohr, K. Robinson, K. McDonald, and E. Whitlock. 2009. Using existing systematic reviews to replace de novo processes in CERs. In *Methods guide for comparative effectiveness reviews*, edited by Agency for Healthcare Research and Quality. http://www.effectivehealthcare.ahrq.gov/index.cfm/search-for-guides-reviews-and-reports/?pageaction=displayProduct&productID=329 (accessed January 19, 2011).

Whitlock, E. P., S. A. Lopez, S. Chang, M. Helfand, M. Eder, and N. Floyd. 2010. AHRQ series paper 3: Identifying, selecting, and refining topics for comparative effectiveness systematic reviews: AHRQ and the Effective Health Care Program. *Journal of Clinical Epidemiology* 63(5):491–501.

G

Expert Guidance for Chapter 5:
Standards for Reporting
Systemic Reviews

TABLE G-1 Comparison of Chapter 5 Guidance on Conducting Systematic Reviews (SRs) of Comparative Effectiveness Research

Standards and Elements	Agency for Healthcare Research and Quality (AHRQ) Effective Health Care Program	Centre for Reviews and Dissemination (CRD)	The Cochrane Collaboration
5.1 Prepare the final report using a structured format	Use a structured format that adheres to the Evidence-based Practice Center (EPC) style guide. Report must meet Section 508 requirements for users with disabilities.	Quality of Reporting of Meta-analyses (QUORUM)/Preferred Reporting Items for Systematic Reviews and Meta-Analyses (PRISMA) are useful guides for all authors of systematic review reports. (NOTE: The next edition of the guidance will recommend adhering to PRISMA.) Commissioning bodies and journals usually have specific requirements regarding presentation and layout of the review.	Cochrane reviews all have the same format, which is facilitated by RevMan. Cochrane has endorsed PRISMA, and it will be incorporated into the next version of the Cochrane handbook.
5.1.1 Include a report title	Required.		Required.
5.1.2 Include an abstract	Required.	Include a structured abstract for reviews published as journal articles.	Required. All full reviews must include an abstract of 400 words or fewer. The abstract should primarily target healthcare decision makers.

5.1.3 Include an executive summary	Required. An executive summary is published separately as well as with the full-length report.	Include an executive summary for reviews published as full-length reports.	Not mentioned.
5.1.4 Include a summary written for the lay public	Required. Developed by the Eisenberg Center.	Not mentioned.	Required. Plain-language summaries provide findings in a straightforward style that can be understood by consumers.
5.1.5 Include an introduction (rationale and objectives)	Required in both full report as well as part of the executive summary.	Required. Include a background/introduction.	Required.
5.1.6 Include a methods section. Describe the following:			
• Research protocol	Same elements in protocol are required in methods section.	Description of the protocol is not mentioned, but the next edition will recommend that reports indicate that a protocol was written and followed, and should report the protocol registration number.	Review authors are encouraged to cite their protocol.
• Eligibility criteria (criteria for including and excluding studies in the systematic review)	Required in protocol and methods section.	Required.	Required.

continued

TABLE G-1 Continued

Standards and Elements	Agency for Healthcare Research and Quality (AHRQ) Effective Health Care Program	Centre for Reviews and Dissemination (CRD)	The Cochrane Collaboration
• Analytic framework and key questions	Required in protocol and methods section of the full report.	Not mentioned.	Not mentioned.
• Databases and other information sources used to identify relevant studies	Required in protocol and methods section.	Required. The write-up of the search should include information about the databases and interfaces searched.	Required.
• Search strategy	Required. Include a description of the search methods. Full-search strategy required in appendix. This description should be detailed enough to allow replication of search.	Required. The search process should be documented in full, including information about the databases and interfaces searched (including the dates covered), full detailed search strategies (including any justifications for date or language restrictions), and the number of records retrieved or details provided on where the strategy can be obtained. An appendix documenting the search process should be included.	Required. List all databases searched. Note the dates of the last search for each database and the period searched. Note any language or publication status restriction. List grey-literature sources. List individuals or organizations contacted. List any journals and conference proceedings specifically handsearched. List any other sources searched.

Study selection process	Required in protocol and methods section.	Required.	State the method used to apply the selection criteria.
• Data extraction process	Required in protocol and methods section.	Required.	Describe the methods for data collection.
• Methods for handling missing information	Required in protocol and methods.	Required.	Describe the strategies for dealing with missing data.
• Information to be extracted from included studies	Required in protocol and methods section.	Required.	Not mentioned.
• Methods to appraise the quality of individual studies	Required. Protocol and methods section should describe methods to assess risk of bias.	Required.	Describe the methods used to assess risk of bias.
• Summary measures (e.g., risk ratio, difference in means)	Required in protocol and methods section.	Required.	The effect measures of choice should be stated.
• Rationale for pooling (or not pooling) of included studies	Required in protocol and methods section.	Not mentioned.	Approach to determining whether a meta-analysis is considered appropriate should be included.
• Methods of synthesizing the evidence (qualitative and meta-analysis)	Required in protocol and methods section. Describing methods for grading of strength of evidence in general and of each domain is recommended.	Required.	The choice of meta-analysis method should be stated, including whether a fixed-effect or a random-effects model is used. Approaches to addressing clinical heterogeneity should be described. Method for identifying statistical heterogeneity should be stated (e.g., visually, using I^2, using a chi-squared test).

continued

TABLE G-1 Continued

Standards and Elements	Agency for Healthcare Research and Quality (AHRQ) Effective Health Care Program	Centre for Reviews and Dissemination (CRD)	The Cochrane Collaboration
• Additional analyses, if done, indicating which were prespecified	Required in protocol and methods section.	Any secondary analyses (sensitivity analyses, etc.).	All planned subgroup analyses should be listed (or independent variables for meta-regression). Any other methods for investigating heterogeneity of effects should be described.
5.1.7 Include a results section. Organize the presentation of results around key questions. Describe the following (repeat for each key question):	Organize presentation of results in logical format. This is typically done around key questions.	The results of all analyses should be considered as a whole, and overall coherence discussed.	The results section should directly address the objectives of the review.
• Study selection process	Required. Flow chart is required documenting excluded studies.	Required. Describe the details of included and excluded studies.	The results sections should start with a summary of the results of the search (e.g., how many references were retrieved by the electronic searches, and how many were considered as potentially eligible after screening?). It is essential that the number of included studies is clearly stated.

• List of excluded studies and reasons for their exclusion	Excluded studies are included in references/appendix.	Studies that may appear to meet the eligibility criteria, but which were excluded, should be listed and the reason for exclusion should be given.
• Appraisal of individual studies' quality	Required.	Required. A risk of bias table is strongly recommended.
• Qualitative synthesis	Required. Describe the findings of the review.	Not required. However, the final report should include a characteristics of included studies table and Grading of Recommendations Assessment, Development and Evaluation (GRADE) evidence tables. It should also summarize the general risk of bias in results of the included studies, its variability across studies, and any important flaws in individual studies.
	The study characteristics of eligible studies are usually included in both a text summary and a summary table, and sometimes in an evidence map as well.	
	Required. Both quantitative and narrative synthesis should begin by constructing a clear descriptive summary of the included studies. An indication of study quality or risk of bias may also be given.	
	Where possible, results of individual studies should be presented graphically, most commonly using a forest plot that illustrates the effect estimates from individual studies.	
	Highlight where evidence indicates that benefits, harms, and trade-offs are different for distinct patient groups.	
	The justification for grade and domains are required, usually provided in a grading table, sometimes in appendix.	
	Consider how the relative effects may translate into different absolute effects for people with differing underlying prognoses.	

continued

TABLE G-1 Continued

Standards and Elements	Agency for Healthcare Research and Quality (AHRQ) Effective Health Care Program	Centre for Reviews and Dissemination (CRD)	The Cochrane Collaboration
• Meta-analysis of results, if performed (explain rationale for doing one)	Required, if appropriate. Describe the findings of the review.	Required. Consistency across studies should be considered.	Required. A summary of findings table may be included to present the main findings of a review in a tabular format.
• Additional analyses, if done, indicating which were prespecified	Required as appropriate.	Required. Include any secondary analyses.	Not mentioned.
• Tables and figures	Include tables summarizing the studies and quantitative syntheses.	Where possible, results should be shown graphically. The most commonly used graphic is the forest plot. Synthesis should usually include tabulated details about study type, interventions, number of participants, a summary of participant characteristics, outcomes, and outcome measures.	Required. Tables that may be included in a review: a characteristics of included studies table, a risk of bias table, a characteristics of excluded studies table, a characteristics of studies awaiting classification table, a characteristics of ongoing studies table, and a summary of findings table. Figures that may be included in a review: forest plot, funnel plot, risk of bias graph, risk of bias summary, and other figures.
5.1.8 Include a discussion section. Include the following: • Summary of the evidence	Required, though usually in the conclusions section.	Suggests a statement of principal findings.	Required.

• Strengths and limitations of the systematic review	Recommended. Describe strengths and weaknesses of systematic review and of studies.	Required. Describe the strengths and weaknesses of the review. Appraise the methodological quality of the review, and the relation to other reviews.	Describe the quality of evidence, potential biases in the review process, and agreements / disagreements with other studies or reviews.
• Conclusions for each key question	Required. Present the benefits and harms in a manner that helps decision makers. Express benefits in absolute terms, rather than relative terms.	Should include practical implications for clinicians and policy makers.	Review authors should not make recommendations for clinical practice. May highlight different actions that might be consistent with particular patterns of values and preferences.
• Gaps in evidence	Description of gaps in evidence is required as a separate section (does not necessarily need to be in discussion section).	Gaps in evidence should be highlighted.	Describe the completeness and applicability of evidence to the review question.
• Future research needs	Required. Some reports will also require this as a more fully prioritized and fleshed-out separate paper.	The report should describe any unanswered questions and implications for further research.	Describe the implications for research.
5.1.9 Include a section describing funding sources and COI	This is done automatically in the editing process.	Required.	Required.
5.2 Peer review the draft report	Identify peer reviewers to ensure independent, unconflicted input from persons with particular clinical, methodological, and statistical expertise and submit a draft report to these individuals.	The advisory group should review the draft report for scientific quality and completeness. The commissioning body may also organize an independent peer review of the draft report.	The editorial team of the Cochrane Review Group is ultimately responsible for the decision to publish a Cochrane review on its module. The decision is made after peer review and appropriate revisions by the review authors.

continued

TABLE G-1 Continued

Standards and Elements	Agency for Healthcare Research and Quality (AHRQ) Effective Health Care Program	Centre for Reviews and Dissemination (CRD)	The Cochrane Collaboration
5.2.1 Use a third party to manage the peer review process	Use an editorial review process that provides for independent judgment of the adequacy of an EPC's response to public and peer review comments.	Not mentioned.	Peer review process is explicitly managed by the Cochrane Review Group.
5.2.2 Provide a public comment period for the report and publicly report on disposition of comments	Must post a draft report. Public report on disposition is posted 3 months after final report posted.	Public comment period not mentioned. A record of the comments and the way in which they were dealt with should be kept with the archive of the review.	Indefinite comment period: A formal feedback mechanism is in place. The review authors are required to respond to feedback on a review (usually within one month of receiving the feedback).
5.3 Publish the final report in a manner that ensures free public access	Systematic reviews are posted on the relevant AHRQ website.	The review findings need to be effectively communicated to practitioners and policy makers.	Reviews are published in the *Cochrane Database of Systematic Reviews.*

NOTE: Some information on AHRQ-, CRD-, and Cochrane-recommended methods was provided via personal communication with Stephanie Chang, EPC Program Task Order Officer, AHRQ (October 5, 2010); Lesley Stewart, Director, CRD (October 14, 2010); and Julian Higgins, Senior Statistician, MRC Biostatistics Unit, Institute of Public Health, University of Cambridge (October 4, 2010).

REFERENCES

Atkins, D., S. Chang, G. Gartlehner, D. I. Buckley, E. P. Whitlock, E. Berliner, and D. Matchar. 2010. Assessing the applicability of studies when comparing medical interventions. In *Methods guide for comparative effectiveness reviews*, edited by Agency for Healthcare Research and Quality. http://www.effectivehealthcare. ahrq.gov/index.cfm/search-for-guides-reviews-and-reports/?productid=603& pageaction=displayproduct (accessed January 19, 2011).

Chou, R., N. Aronson, D. Atkins, A. S. Ismaila, P. Santaguida, D. H. Smith, E. Whitlock, T. J. Wilt, and D. Moher. 2010. AHRQ series paper 4: Assessing harms when comparing medical interventions: AHRQ and the Effective Health Care Program. *Journal of Clinical Epidemiology* 63(5):502–512.

CRD (Centre for Reviews and Dissemination). 2009. *Systematic reviews: CRD's guidance for undertaking reviews in health care*. York, UK: York Publishing Services, Ltd.

Fu, R., G. Gartlehner, M. Grant, T. Shamliyan, A. Sedrakyan, T. J. Wilt, L. Griffith, M. Oremus, P. Raina, A. Ismaila, P. Santaguida, J. Lau, and T. A. Trikalinos. 2010. Conducting quantitative synthesis when comparing medical interventions: AHRQ and the Effective Health Care Program. In *Methods guide for comparative effectiveness reviews*, edited by Agency for Healthcare Research and Quality. http://www.effectivehealthcare.ahrq.gov/index.cfm/search-for-guides-reviews-and-reports/?pageaction=displayProduct&productID=554 (accessed January 19, 2011).

Helfand, M., and H. Balshem. 2010. AHRQ series paper 2: Principles for developing guidance: AHRQ and the Effective Health Care Program. *Journal of Clinical Epidemiology* 63(5):484–490.

Higgins, J. P. T., and S. Green, eds. 2008. *Cochrane handbook for systematic reviews of interventions*. Chichester, UK: John Wiley & Sons

Norris, S., D. Atkins, W. Bruening, S. Fox, E. Johnson, R. Kane, S. C. Morton, M. Oremus, M. Ospina, G. Randhawa, K. Schoelles, P. Shekelle, and M. Viswanathan. 2010. Selecting observational studies for comparing medical interventions. In *Methods guide for comparative effectiveness reviews*, edited by Agency for Healthcare Research and Quality. http://www.effectivehealthcare.ahrq.gov/index. cfm/search-for-guides-reviews-and-reports/?pageaction=displayProduct& productID=454 (accessed January 19, 2011).

Owens, D. K., K. N. Lohr, D. Atkins, J. R. Treadwell, J. T. Reston, E. B. Bass, S. Chang, and M. Helfand. 2010. AHRQ series paper 5: Grading the strength of a body of evidence when comparing medical interventions: AHRQ and the Effective Health Care Program. *Journal of Clinical Epidemiology* 63(5):513–523.

Relevo, R., and H. Balshem. 2011. Finding evidence for comparing medical interventions. In *Methods guide for comparative effectiveness reviews*, edited by Agency for Healthcare Research and Quality. http://www.effectivehealthcare.ahrq.gov/ index.cfm/search-for-guides-reviews-and-reports/?pageaction=displayProduct &productID=605 (accessed January 19, 2011).

Slutsky, J., D. Atkins, S. Chang, and B. A. Collins Sharp. 2010. AHRQ series paper 1: Comparing medical interventions: AHRQ and the Effective Health Care Program. *Journal of Clinical Epidemiology* 63(5):481–483.

White, C. M., S. Ip, M. McPheeters, T. S. Carey, R. Chou, K. N. Lohr, K. Robinson, K. McDonald, and E. Whitlock. 2009. Using existing systematic reviews to replace de novo processes in CERs. In *Methods guide for comparative effectiveness reviews*, edited by Agency for Healthcare Research and Quality. http://www.effective-healthcare.ahrq.gov/index.cfm/search-for-guides-reviews-and-reports/?page action=displayProduct&productID=329 (accessed January 19, 2011).

Whitlock, E. P., S. A. Lopez, S. Chang, M. Helfand, M. Eder, and N. Floyd. 2010. AHRQ series paper 3: Identifying, selecting, and refining topics for comparative effectiveness systematic reviews: AHRQ and the Effective Health Care Program. *Journal of Clinical Epidemiology* 63(5):491–501.

H

Preferred Reporting Items for Systematic Reviews and Meta-Analyses (PRISMA) Checklist

TABLE H-1 Checklist of Items to Include When Reporting a
Systematic Review or Meta-Analysis

Selection/Topic	#	Checklist Item
TITLE		
Title	1	Identify the report as a systematic review, meta-analysis, or both.
ABSTRACT		
Structured summary	2	Provide a structured summary including, as applicable: background; objectives; data sources; study eligibility criteria, participants, and interventions; study appraisal and synthesis methods; results; limitations; conclusions and implications of key findings; systematic review registration number.
INTRODUCTION		
Rationale	3	Describe the rationale for the review in the context of what is already known.
Objectives	4	Provide an explicit statement of questions being addressed with reference to participants, interventions, comparisons, outcomes, and study design (PICOS).
METHODS		
Protocol and registration	5	Indicate if a review protocol exists, if and where it can be accessed (e.g., web address), and, if available, provide registration information, including registration number.
Eligibility criteria	6	Specify study characteristics (e.g., PICOS, length of follow-up) and report characteristics (e.g., years considered, language, publication status) used as criteria for eligibility, giving rationale.
Information sources	7	Describe all information sources (e.g., databases with dates of coverage, contact with study authors to identify additional studies) in the search and date last searched.
Search	8	Present full electronic search strategy for at least one database, including any limits used, such that it could be repeated.
Study selection	9	State the process for selecting studies (i.e., screening, eligibility, included in systematic reviews, and, if applicable, included in the meta-analysis).
Data collection process	10	Describe method of data extraction from reports (e.g., piloted forms, independently, in duplicate) and any processes for obtaining and confirming data from investigators.
Data items	11	List and define all variables for which data were sought (e.g., PICOS, funding sources) and any assumptions and simplifications made.

TABLE H-1 Continued

Selection/Topic	#	Checklist Item
Risk of bias in individual studies	12	Describe methods used for assessing risk of bias of individual studies (including specification of whether this was done at the study or outcome level), and how this information is to be used in any data synthesis.
Summary measures	13	State the principal summary measures (e.g., risk ratio, difference in means).
Synthesis of results	14	Describe the methods of handling data and combining results of studies, if done, including measures of consistency (e.g., I^2) for each meta-analysis.
Risk of bias across studies	15	Specify any assessment of risk of bias that may affect the cumulative evidence (e.g., publication bias, selective reporting within studies).
Additional analyses	16	Describe methods of additional analyses (e.g., sensitivity or subgroup analyses, meta-regression), if done, indicating which were prespecified.
RESULTS		
Study selection	17	Give numbers of studies screened, assessed for eligibility, and included in the review, with reasons for exclusions at each stage, ideally with a flow diagram.
Study characteristics	18	For each study, present characteristics for which data were extracted (e.g., study size, PICOS, follow-up period) and provide the citations.
Risk of bias within studies	19	Present data on risk of bias of each study and, if available, any outcome-level assessment (see Item 12).
Results of individual studies	20	For all outcomes considered (benefits or harms), present, for each study: (a) simple summary data for each intervention group; and (b) effect estimates and confidence intervals, ideally with a forest plot.
Synthesis of results	21	Present results of each meta-analysis done, including confidence intervals and measures of consistency.
Risk of bias across studies	22	Present results of any assessment of risk of bias across studies (see Item 15).
Additional analyses	23	Give results of additional analyses, if done (e.g., sensitivity or subgroup analyses, meta-regression [see Item 16]).

continued

TABLE H-1 Continued

Selection/Topic	#	Checklist Item
DISCUSSION		
Summary of evidence	24	Summarize the main findings, including the strength of evidence for each main outcome; consider their relevance to key groups (e.g., healthcare providers, users, and policy makers).
Limitations	25	Discuss limitations at a study and outcome level (e.g., risk of bias) and at review level (e.g., incomplete retrieval of identified research, reporting bias).
Conclusions	26	Provide a general interpretation of the results in the context of other evidence and implications for future research.
FUNDING		
Funding	27	Describe sources of funding for the systematic review and other support (e.g., supply of data) and the role of funders for the systematic review.

SOURCES: Liberati et al. (2009); Moher et al. (2009).

REFERENCES

Liberati, A., D. G. Altman, J. Tetzlaff, C. Mulrow, P. Gotzsche, J. P. Ioannidis, M. Clarke, P. J. Devereaux, J. Kleijnen, and D. Moher. 2009. The PRISMA Statement for reporting systematic reviews and meta-analysis of studies that evaluate health care interventions: Explanation and elaboration. *Annals of Internal Medicine* 151(4):W11–W30.

Moher, D., A. Liberati, J. Tetzlaff, and D. G. Altman. 2009. Preferred reporting items for systematic reviews and meta-analyses: The PRISMA statement. *PLoS Medicine* 6(7):1–6.

I

Committee Biographies

Alfred O. Berg, M.D., M.P.H. (*Chair*), is a professor of family medicine at the University of Washington Department of Family Medicine in Seattle. Dr. Berg was elected to be an Institute of Medicine (IOM) member in 1996. He was a member of the IOM Immunization Safety Review Committee and chair of the Committee on the Treatment of Post-Traumatic Stress Disorder. In 2004 he received the Thomas W. Johnson Award for career contributions to family medicine education from the American Academy of Family Physicians; in 2008 he received the F. Marian Bishop Leadership Award from the Society of Teachers of Family Medicine Foundation; and in 2010 he received the Curtis Hames Research Award, family medicine's highest research honor. He has served on many national expert panels to assess evidence and provide clinical guidance, including serving as chair of the U.S. Preventive Services Task Force (USPSTF); cochair of the otitis media panel convened by the former Agency for Health Care Policy and Research; chair of the Centers for Disease Control and Prevention's (CDC's) Sexually Transmitted Disease Treatment Guidelines panel; member of the American Medical Association/ CDC panel that produced *Guidelines for Adolescent Preventive Services*; and chair of the National Institutes of Health's (NIH's) State-of-the-Science Conference on Family History and Improving Health. He currently chairs the CDC panel on Evaluation of Genomic Applications in Practice and Prevention. Dr. Berg earned his M.D. at Washington University in St. Louis and his M.P.H. at the University of

Washington. He completed residencies in Family Medicine at the University of Missouri-Columbia, and in General Preventive Medicine and Public Health at the University of Washington.

Sally C. Morton, Ph.D. (*Vice Chair*), is professor and chair of biostatistics in the Graduate School of Public Health at the University of Pittsburgh. She holds secondary appointments in the Department of Statistics and Department of Clinical and Translational Science. Previously, she was vice president for statistics and epidemiology at RTI International in Research Triangle Park, North Carolina. Prior to that position, she was head of RAND Corporation's statistics group, held the RAND-endowed chair in statistics, and was codirector of the Agency for Healthcare Research and Quality (AHRQ) Southern California Evidence-based Practice Center. She was the 2009 president of the American Statistical Association (ASA). Dr. Morton is a Fellow of the ASA and of the American Association for the Advancement of Science and an elected member of the Society for Research Synthesis Methodology. Her interests include comparative effectiveness research, the use of meta-analysis in evidence-based medicine, and the sampling of vulnerable populations. She is a founding editor of *Statistics, Politics, and Policy,* and served on the editorial boards of the *Journal of the American Statistical Association, Journal of Computational and Graphical Statistics,* and *Statistical Science.* She is a member of the National Academy of Sciences Committee on National Statistics, and has served as a member of several IOM committees concerning comparative effectiveness and systematic reviews. She has a Ph.D. in Statistics from Stanford University.

Jesse A. Berlin, Sc.D., is the vice president of epidemiology at Johnson & Johnson Pharmaceutical Research and Development. His group is involved throughout the drug development process and in the design, analysis, and interpretation of postapproval studies. At the IOM, he served on the Committee to Review the Health Effects in Vietnam Veterans of Exposure to Herbicides and, subsequently, on the committee's First Biennial Update. In 1989 he joined the faculty at the University of Pennsylvania in a unit that became the Center for Clinical Epidemiology and Biostatistics, under the direction of Dr. Brian Strom. Dr. Berlin spent several years as director of biostatistics for the University of Pennsylvania Cancer Center. He has authored or coauthored more than 220 publications in a wide variety of clinical and methodological areas. Dr. Berlin has a great deal of experience in both the application of meta-analysis and the study of meta-analytic methods as applied to both randomized trials and epidemiology. He has also served as a consultant on meta-analysis for the Australian government. Dr. Berlin received his Sc.D. in Biostatistics from the Harvard School of Public Health.

Mohit Bhandari, M.D., Ph.D., is the Canada research chair in musculoskeletal trauma at McMaster University Orthopaedic Research Unity, Clarity Research Group, at the Hamilton Health Sciences-General Site in Hamilton, Ontario, Canada. He also serves as assistant professor, Department of Surgery, and associate member, Department of Clinical Epidemiology & Biostatistics, at McMaster. Dr. Bhandari's clinical interests include the care of patients with musculoskeletal injuries. His research broadly focuses on clinical trials, meta-analyses, methodological aspects of surgery trials, and the translation of evidence into surgical practice. Specific areas of interest include identifying optimal management strategies to improve patient-important outcomes in patients with multiple injuries, lower extremity fractures, and severe soft-tissue injuries. Dr. Bhandari is currently coordinating trials of tibial fracture management and various wound irrigation techniques in open fractures. He also leads the international hip fracture research collaborative, a global consortium of surgeons focusing on the design and development of large, definitive surgical randomized trials in patients with hip fractures. In recognition of his research contributions, he has received the Edouard J. Samson Award for a Canadian orthopedic surgeon with the greatest impact on research in the past 5 years, the Founder's Medal for research, and the Royal College of Physicians and Surgeons of Canada Medal in Surgical Research. Dr. Bhandari is a graduate of the University of Toronto. He completed both his orthopedic surgery and Master's of Clinical Epidemiology and Biostatistics training at McMaster University.

Giselle Corbie-Smith, M.D., M.Sc., is a professor of social medicine and medicine at the University of North Carolina (UNC) at Chapel Hill. Dr. Corbie-Smith is the director of the Program on Health Disparities at the UNC Cecil G. Sheps Center for Health Services Research. The purpose of this program is to coordinate and enhance disparity research within the Sheps Center and throughout UNC, to build expertise in working with minority communities, and to improve collaboration and communication with minority-serving institutions in North Carolina and the nation. She served on the IOM Committee on Ethical Issues in Housing-Related Health Hazard Research Involving Children, Youth and Families. Dr. Corbie-Smith has been the Principal Investigator on grants from the NIH and the Robert Wood Johnson Foundation to examine the patient-specific and investigator-specific factors that influence participation in research. She is also director of the Community Engagement Research Core of the Carolina–Shaw Partnership for the Elimination of Health Disparities. The core's main goal is to build community–academic relationships to increase minority participation in research. Her other studies include defining the barriers and facilitators to African American elders' use of influenza vaccines; research on HIV risk among older African American women; and the impact of training in cultural competency on knowledge and skills among medical students and residents. Dr. Corbie-Smith was awarded the Jefferson-Pilot Fellowship in Academic Medicine, the highest award for assistant professors in the School of Medicine, and the National Center for Minority Health and Health Disparities Award for Leadership in Health Disparities Research. She is the deputy director of the North Carolina Translational and Clinical Sciences Institute. Her clinical work focuses on serving underserved populations in public hospitals and clinics. She earned her M.D. at Albert Einstein College of Medicine and trained as an Internal Medicine intern, resident, and chief resident at Yale University School of Medicine. She received an M.Sc. in Clinical Research from the Epidemiology Department at Emory University.

Kay Dickersin, M.A., Ph.D., is a professor of epidemiology at Johns Hopkins Bloomberg School of Public Health and director of the Center for Clinical Trials. She has served as director of the U.S. Cochrane Center (originally Baltimore Cochrane Center) since 1994 and is director of the Cochrane Eyes and Vision Group U.S. Satellite. At the IOM, she has served on numerous committees, including the Committee on Comparative Effectiveness Research Prioritization, Committee on Reviewing Evidence to Identify Highly Effective Clinical Services, and Committee on Reimbursement of Routine Patient Care Costs for Medicare Patients Enrolled in Clinical Trials. Dr. Dickersin's main research contributions have been in clinical trials, systematic reviews, publication bias, trials registers, and the development and use of methods for the evaluation of medical care and its effectiveness. Her current research is funded by the NIH, AHRQ, and Blue Shield California. Among her many honors are election as president of the Society for Clinical Trials (2008–2009) and election as a member in the American Epidemiological Society, the Society for Research Synthesis, and the IOM. Dr. Dickersin received an M.A. in Zoology, specializing in Cell Biology, from the University of California–Berkeley, and a Ph.D. in Epidemiology from Johns Hopkins University School of Hygiene and Public Health.

Jeremy M. Grimshaw, M.B.Ch.B., Ph.D., is a senior scientist in the Clinical Epidemiology Program of the Ottawa Health Research Institute and director of the Centre for Best Practice, Institute of Population Health, University of Ottawa. He holds a Tier 1 Canadian Research Chair in Health Knowledge Transfer and Uptake and is a full professor in the Department of Medicine, University of Ottawa. He served as a member of the IOM Forum on the Science of Health Care Quality Improvement and Implementation. His research focuses on the evaluation of interventions to disseminate and implement evidence-based practice. He is director of the Canadian Cochrane Network and Centre. He is coordinating editor of the Cochrane Effective Practice and Organization of Care group and he has been involved in a series of systematic reviews of guideline dissemination and implementation strategies. Dr. Grimshaw has been involved in more than 30 cluster randomized trials of different dissemination and implementation strategies conducted in a wide range of settings (including community pharmacy settings, family medicine settings, and secondary- and tertiary-care settings). Furthermore, he has evaluated a wide range of interventions (e.g., educational meetings, educational outreach, organizational interventions, computerized guidelines) relating to a wide range of behaviors. He has also undertaken research into statistical issues in the design, conduct, and analysis of cluster randomized trials. Recently his research has focused on assessing the applicability of behavioral theories to healthcare professional and organizational behaviors. He has authored more than 300 peer-reviewed publications and 60 monographs and book chapters. Dr. Grimshaw received an M.B.Ch.B. (M.D. equivalent) from the University of Edinburgh, UK. He trained as a family physician prior to undertaking a Ph.D. in Health Services Research at the University of Aberdeen.

Mark Helfand, M.D., M.S., M.P.H., is a staff physician at the Portland Veterans Affairs Medical Center and professor of medicine and medical informatics & clinical epidemiology at Oregon Health & Science University. He was a Robert Wood Johnson Generalist Faculty Scholar from 1993 to 1997 and has been director of the Oregon Evidence-based Practice Center since 1997. Dr. Helfand has been a leader in methods for comparative effectiveness research. He led a team that helped the USPSTF prioritize topics and develop evidence-based guidelines. In the area of comparative effectiveness, he was a founder of the Drug Effectiveness Review Project. His research focuses on the use of systematic reviews to inform clinical and public policy. His current projects include the Coordinating Center for the VA's Evidence-based Synthesis Program. In addition, Dr. Helfand has been editor in chief of the journal *Medical Decision Making* since 2005. He earned Bachelor of Science and Bachelor of English Literature degrees from Stanford University. He received his M.D. from the University of Illinois and completed postgraduate training in Internal Medicine at Stanford Medical School.

Vincent E. Kerr, M.D., is president of Care Solutions, UnitedHealthcare. He provides strategic leadership and a focus on customer needs in the key areas of care management, clinical operations, consumer health, and medical care advancement. He works closely with UnitedHealth Networks, United Pharmacy Management, and United Resource Networks. From this leadership position, he also represents UnitedHealthcare with a number of employer-based organizations, including the American Benefits Council, the National Business Group on Health, Bridges to Excellence, and others. The former director of healthcare management and chief medical officer for Ford Motor Co., in Dearborn, Michigan, Dr. Kerr was responsible for managing one of the largest private employer healthcare plans in the nation. During his tenure at Ford, he was responsible for managing health benefits for all Ford employees globally, for worksite health and safety, and for providing leadership to the staff at more than 100 medical centers at Ford's major manufacturing facilities around the world. Dr. Kerr also served as a lead negotiator for Ford with the United Auto Workers. Prior to joining Ford, he was the company medical director at General Electric (GE) in Fairfield, Connecticut, and focused on improving care processes using Six Sigma in GE's many medical facilities. Previously, Dr. Kerr practiced medicine as an attending physician, cofounding a multisite group practice and urgent care facility and serving as a member of the clinical teaching faculty of Yale Medical School. He has served on the boards of a number of prestigious industry groups focused on quality in health care, including the National Business Group on Health, the National Committee for Quality Assurance (NCQA), and the Voluntary Hospital Association. He also chaired the Leapfrog Group. Dr. Kerr attended Harvard University and received his M.D. from the Yale University School of Medicine. He is trained in Internal Medicine and Occupational Medicine.

Marguerite A. Koster, M.A., M.F.T., is the practice leader of the Technology Assessment & Guidelines Unit within the Southern California Permanente Medical Group, a partnership of physicians that contracts exclusively with the Kaiser Foundation Health Plan to provide medical services for more than 3 million members in Kaiser Permanente's (KP's) Southern California Region. In this position, she manages a staff of 10 evidence specialists who systematically review and critically appraise scientific evidence in support of Kaiser Permanente's clinical practice guideline, medical technology assessment, and health system implementation programs. For the past 20 years, Ms. Koster has been actively involved in the advancement of evidence-based medicine and methodology standards for guideline development and technology assessment at Kaiser Permanente's national and regional levels. She is a member of the KP Southern California Medical Technology Assessment Team, the KP Interregional New Technologies Committee, the KP National Guideline Directors, and the KP Guideline Quality Committee. Ms. Koster also has a long history of collaboration with other healthcare organizations, medical and professional societies, and accreditation groups, in the areas of evidence-based clinical guideline development, technology assessment, and performance measurement. Major interest areas include systematic review methodology, methods for synthesizing evidence, evidence grading systems, collaborative guideline development, and integration of evidence-based clinical content into electronic health systems. Prior to joining Kaiser Permanente, Ms. Koster was a research analyst at the University of Southern California's Social Science Research Institute, where she conducted survey research for grants funded by the U.S. National Institute of Justice and the Office of Juvenile Justice and Delinquency Prevention. In addition, she worked for several years as a psychotherapist specializing in long-term, residential addiction treatment and recovery programs for court-referred and homeless drug users, and is currently a licensed Marriage and Family Therapist in the State of California.

Katie Maslow, M.S.W., is a consultant on aging, dementia, and Alzheimer's care issues. She served as a member of the recent IOM Committee on Comparative Effectiveness Research Prioritization and an earlier IOM Committee to Review the Social Security Administration's Disability Decision Process Research. From 1995 to 2010, she worked for the Alzheimer's Association, focusing on practice and policy initiatives to improve the quality, coordination, and outcomes of healthcare and long-term services and support for persons with Alzheimer's and other dementias and to support their family caregivers. She directed the association's initiative on managed care, and codirected its multisite demonstration project, Chronic

Care Networks for Alzheimer's Disease. She also directed the association's demonstration project on improving hospital care for people with dementia, which included the development of training materials for hospital nurses caring for this population in partnership with the John A. Hartford Institute for Geriatric Nursing. She represented the association on the National Assisted Living Workgroup and was a primary author of the association's annual report, *Alzheimer's Disease Facts and Figures*. Before joining the Alzheimer's Association, Ms. Maslow worked for 12 years at the U.S. Office of Technology Assessment, studying policy issues in aging, Alzheimer's disease, long-term care, end-of-life issues, and case management. Ms. Maslow has served on numerous government and nongovernment advisory panels on aging, Alzheimer's disease, dementia, family caregiving, home care, assisted living, nursing home care, and care coordination. She has served on the national board of the American Society of Aging and won the Society award in 2003. She is a member of the American Geriatrics Society, Gerontological Society of America, and National Association of Social Workers. She graduated from Stanford University and received her M.S.W. from Howard University.

David A. Mrazek, M.D., F.R.C. Psych., is chair of the department of psychiatry and psychology at the Mayo Clinic. He is a child and adolescent psychiatrist with a longstanding interest in developmental psychopathology and the interaction of biological and environmental risk factors. He is currently the Principal Investigator of a large federally funded project studying the pharmacogenomics of antidepressant response. He is also director of the Samuel C. Johnson Program for the Genomics of Addiction. Before joining the Mayo Clinic, he was the Leon Yochelson Professor of Psychiatry at the George Washington University School of Medicine.

Christopher H. Schmid, Ph.D., is director of the Biostatistics Research Center in the Institute for Clinical Research and Health Policy Studies at Tufts Medical Center. He is also professor of medicine and associate director of the program in clinical and translational science at Sackler School of Graduate Biomedical Sciences at Tufts University School of Medicine. He is also adjunct professor at the Friedman School of Nutrition Science and Policy at Tufts. He is a coeditor of the *Journal of Research Synthesis Methods*; statistical editor of the *American Journal of Kidney Diseases*; a member of the editorial board for *BMC Medicine*; and a Fellow of the American Statistical Association, where he is past chair of the International Conference on Health Policy Statistics. In addition, Dr. Schmid is an elected member of the Society for Research Synthesis Methodology. He has served on study sections with several federal agencies; is a member of the Food and Drug Administration Orthopaedic and Rehabilitation Devices Panels; consults with the European Medicines Agency; and serves on the External Advisory Committee for ECRI. His major research interests include development and application of Bayesian models to clinical research, statistical methods and computational tools for meta-analysis, methods for combining and analyzing data from multiple clinical trials and clinical studies; and methods for handling missing time-dependent data in longitudinal studies. Dr. Schmid received his Ph.D. in Statistics from Harvard University.

Anna Maria Siega-Riz, Ph.D., is a professor in the Department of Epidemiology and joint appointed in the Department of Nutrition in the Gillings School of Global Public Health at the University of North Carolina–Chapel Hill. Dr. Siega-Riz is a Fellow at the Carolina Population Center and serves as associate chair of the Department of Epidemiology and director of the Nutrition Epidemiology Core for the Clinical Nutrition Research Center in the Department of Nutrition. She is also the program leader for the Reproductive, Perinatal, and Pediatric Program in the Department of Epidemiology. Dr. Siega-Riz served on the IOM Committee to Reexamine IOM Pregnancy Weight Guidelines and the IOM Committee to Review the WIC Food Packages. She has expertise in diet methodology, gestational weight gain, maternal nutritional status and its effects on birth outcomes, obesity development, and dietary trends and intakes among children and Hispanic populations. She was the lead investigator of the evidence-based review on outcomes of maternal weight gain sponsored by AHRQ. Dr. Siega-Riz uses a multidisciplinary team perspective as a way to address complex problems such as prematurity, fetal programming, and racial disparities and obesity. She received the March of Dimes Agnes Higgins Award for Maternal and Fetal Nutrition in 2007. Dr. Siega-Riz earned a B.S.P.H. in Nutrition from the School of Public Health at UNC–Chapel Hill; an M.S. in Food, Nutrition, and Food Service Management from UNC–Greensboro; and a Ph.D. in Nutrition and Epidemiology from the School of Public Health at UNC–Chapel Hill.

Harold C. Sox, M.D., recently retired after 8 years as editor of *Annals of Internal Medicine*. After serving as a medical intern and resident at Massachusetts General Hospital, he spent 2 years doing research in immunology at the NIH and 3 years at Dartmouth Medical School, where he served as chief medical resident and began his studies of medical decision making. He then spent 15 years on the faculty of Stanford University School of Medicine, where he was the chief of the Division of General Internal Medicine and director of ambulatory care at the Palo Alto VA Medical Center. In 1988 he returned to Dartmouth, where he served for 13 years as the Joseph M. Huber Professor of Medicine and chair of the Department of Medicine. He was elected to the IOM in 1993 and to a Fellowship in the American Association for the Advancement of Science in 2002. Dr. Sox has served on numerous IOM committees, including the Committee on an Evidence Framework for Obesity Prevention Decision-Making, Committee on Comparative Effectiveness Research Prioritization, Committee on Reviewing Evidence to Identify Highly Effective Clinical Services, Committee to Study HIV Transmission through Blood Products, and Committee on Health Effects Associated with Exposures Experienced in the Gulf War. Dr. Sox was president of the American College of Physicians during 1998–1999. He chaired the USPSTF from 1990 to 1995, chaired the Medicare Coverage Advisory Committee of the Center for Medicare Services from 1999 to 2003, and served on the Report Review Committee of the National Research Council from 2000 to 2005. He currently chairs the National Advisory Committee for the Robert Wood Johnson Foundation Physician Faculty Scholars Program and is a member of the Board of Directors of the Foundation for Informed Medical Decision Making. He is also a member of the Stakeholders Group for the Effective Health Care Program of the Agency for Health Research and Policy. His books include *Medical Decision Making, Common Diagnostic Tests: Selection and Interpretation*, and *HIV and the Blood Supply: An Analysis of Crisis Decisionmaking*. Dr. Sox earned a B.S. in Physics from Stanford University and an M.D. from Harvard Medical School.

Paul Wallace, M.D., is medical director of Health and Productivity Management Programs at the Permanente Federation. He is a member of the IOM Board on Population Health and Public Health Practice and served on the IOM Planning Committee for a Workshop on a Foundation for Evidence-Driven Practice: A Rapid-Learning System for Cancer Care, the IOM Planning Committee for a Workshop on Applying What We Know: Best Practices in Evidence-Based Medicine, and the IOM Subcommittee on Performance Measures. Dr. Wallace is an active participant, program leader, and perpetual student in clinical quality improvement, especially in the area of translation of evidence into care delivery using people- and technology-based innovation supported by performance measurement. At Kaiser Permanente, he leads work to extend KP's experience with population-based care to further develop and integrate wellness, health maintenance, and productivity enhancement interventions. He is also active in the design and promotion of systematic approaches to comparative effectiveness assessment and accelerated organizational learning. He was executive director of KP's Care Management Institute (CMI) from 2000 to 2005 and continues as a senior advisor to CMI and to Avivia Health, the KP disease management company established in 2005. Board certified in Internal Medicine and Hematology, he previously taught clinical and basic sciences and investigated bone marrow function as a faculty member at Oregon Health & Science University. Dr. Wallace is a Board member for AcademyHealth and for the Society of Participatory Medicine. He recently concluded terms as the Board Chair for the Center for Information Therapy, and as a Board member and Secretary for DMAA: The Care Continuum Alliance. He previously served on the National Advisory Council for AHRQ, the Medical Coverage Advisory Committee for the Centers for Medicare & Medicaid Services, the Medical Advisory Panel for the Blue Cross and Blue Shield Technology Evaluation Center, and the NCQA Committee on Performance Measurement and Standards. He received his M.D. at the University of Iowa School of Medicine and completed further training in Internal Medicine and Hematology at Strong Memorial Hospital and the University of Rochester.

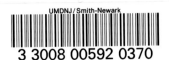